METHODS IN MOLECULAR BIOLOGY

Series Editor
John M. Walker
School of Life and Medical Sciences
University of Hertfordshire
Hatfield, Hertfordshire, AL10 9AB, UK

For further volumes:
http://www.springer.com/series/7651

Recombinant Virus Vaccines

Methods and Protocols

Edited by

Maureen C. Ferran and Gary R. Skuse

Rochester Institute of Technology, Thomas H. Gosnell School of Life Sciences, Rochester, NY, USA

Humana Press

Editors
Maureen C. Ferran
Rochester Institute of Technology
Thomas H. Gosnell School of Life Sciences
Rochester, NY, USA

Gary R. Skuse
Rochester Institute of Technology
Thomas H. Gosnell School of Life Sciences
Rochester, NY, USA

ISSN 1064-3745 ISSN 1940-6029 (electronic)
Methods in Molecular Biology
ISBN 978-1-4939-6867-1 ISBN 978-1-4939-6869-5 (eBook)
DOI 10.1007/978-1-4939-6869-5

Library of Congress Control Number: 2017934252

Printed on acid-free paper

This Humana Press imprint is published by Springer Nature
The registered company is Springer Science+Business Media LLC
The registered company address is: 233 Spring Street, New York, NY 10013, U.S.A.

Preface

Since the discovery of the prophylactic effects of the cowpox virus toward variants of the variola virus in the late eighteenth century, scientists and clinicians have fought to balance the beneficial effects of viral vaccines against the potential for undesired and potentially pathogenic side effects. In the last half century or so scientists have harnessed a variety of pathogenic viruses, from a number of species, for use and study in the laboratory and the clinic. Our increased understanding of the pathology and the molecular anatomy of those viruses has enabled us to adapt them for use as recombinant expression systems for immunogens that can be used to protect hosts from infection by a wide variety of infectious agents.

This volume is intended for scientists and clinicians who are interested in learning more about and adapting methods employed in basic and biomedical research, which are directed toward understanding the development of recombinant viruses and their use as vaccine platforms. The methods and protocols contained herein involve many of the viruses currently being used for, or under development as, vaccine platforms. Throughout this work readers will find details of the use of recombinant vaccines which are employed to either produce immunogens in vitro or elicit antibody production in vivo. Within each of the parts of this work, readers will find several chapters that are grouped according to the Baltimore Classification of viruses. Taken together, the described methods should inform individuals with interests in the current methods used to generate and develop recombinant viral vaccines.

The contributors to this volume are current or nascent leaders in the field of recombinant virus vaccine development. Taken together they have provided a large number of effective protocols that can be employed or adapted as readers see fit. While an attempt has been made to be as comprehensive as possible, inevitably there are certain platforms that are not included in this collection. We sincerely hope that you find this work informative and useful in your own laboratories and that they serve to acquaint you with the current state of the art in the use of recombinant viral vaccines.

Rochester, NY, USA

Maureen C. Ferran
Gary R. Skuse

Contents

Contributors

DAVID C. BLOOM • *Department of Molecular Genetics & Microbiology, University of Florida College of Medicine, Gainesville, FL, USA*
MATT BREWER • *Department of Microbiology and Immunology, University of Rochester, Rochester, NY, USA*
GABRIELA CALAMANTE • *Instituto de Biotecnología, CICVyAINTA, N. Repetto y de los Reseros, Hurlingham, Buenos Aires, Argentina*
YUDAN CHI • *Vaccine Research Center, Key Laboratory of Molecular Virology & Immunology, Institut Pasteur of Shanghai, University of Chinese Academy of Sciences, Shanghai, China*
JOHN H. CONNOR • *Department of Microbiology and National Emerging Infectious Disease Laboratory, Boston University School of Medicine, Boston, MA, USA*
JUAN C. CORREDOR • *Department of Pathobiology, Ontario Veterinary College, University of Guelph, Guelph, ON, Canada*
JUAN CARLOS DE LA TORRE • *Department of Immunology and Microbial Science, The Scripps Research Institute, La Jolla, CA, USA*
MARÍA PAULA DEL MÉDICO-ZAJAC • *Instituto de Biotecnología, CICVyAINTA, N. Repetto y de los Reseros, Hurlingham, Buenos Aires, Argentina; Consejo Nacional de Investigaciones Cientificas y Técnicas, Godoy Crus, Ciudad Autónoma de Buenos Aires, Argentina*
STEPHEN DEWHURST • *Department of Microbiology and Immunology, University of Rochester, Rochester, NY, USA*
REKHA DHANWANI • *Department of Veterinary and Biomedical Sciences, College of Veterinary Medicine, University of Minnesota, MN, USA; La Jolla Institute for Allergy and Immunology, La Jolla, CA, USA*
JOYCE FELLER • *Department of Molecular Genetics & Microbiology, University of Florida College of Medicine, Gainesville, FL, USA*
DÉBORA GARANZINI • *Instituto de Biotecnología, CICVyAINTA, N. Repetto y de los Reseros, Hurlinghan, Buenos Aires, Argentina; Instituto Nacional de Producción de Biológicos, ANLIS, "Dr. Carlos G. Malbrán" Ciudad Autónoma de Buenos Aires, Buenos Aires, Argentina*
SARAH C. GILBERT • *The Jenner Institute, University of Oxford, Oxford, UK*
ERIC JAMES GOWANS • *Virology Laboratory, Basil Hetzel Institute, Discipline of Surgery, University of Adelaide, Adelaide, SA, Australia*
BRANKA GRUBOR-BAUK • *Virology Laboratory, Basil Hetzel Institute, Discipline of Surgery, University of Adelaide, Adelaide, SA, Australia*
STEFAN HUTZLER • *Product Testing of IVMP, Division of Veterinary Medicine, Paul-Ehrlich-Institut, Langen, Germany*
XIANGDONG LI • *National Research Center for Veterinary Medicine, Luoyang, PR China*
QIN LI • *Department of Biology, The Catholic University of America, Washington, DC, USA*

YUYING LIANG • *Department of Veterinary and Biomedical Science, College of Veterinary Medicine, University of Minnesota, Saint Paul, MN, USA*
KENNETH LUNDSTROM • *PanTherapeutics, Lutry, Switzerland*
HINH LY • *Department of Veterinary and Biomedical Sciences, College of Veterinary Medicine, University of Minnesota, MN, USA*
LUIS MARTÍNES-SOBRIDO • *Department of Microbiology and Immunology, University of Rochester School of Medicine and Dentistry, Rochester, NY, USA*
JAKE MATTHEWS • *The Jenner Institute, University of Oxford, Oxford, UK*
JONELLE L. MATTIACIO • *Saint John Fisher College, Rochester, NY, USA*
MICHAEL D. MÜHLEBACH • *Product Testing of IVMP, Division of Veterinary Medicine, Paul-Ehrlich-Institut, Langen, Germany*
ÉVA NAGY • *Department of Pathobiology, Ontario Veterinary College, University of Guelph, Guelph, ON, Canada*
VINCENT PAVOT • *The Jenner Institute, University of Oxford, Oxford, UK*
YANLONG PEI • *Department of Pathobiology, Ontario Veterinary College, University of Guelph, Guelph, ON, Canada*
VENIGALLA B. RAO • *Department of Biology, The Catholic University of America, Washington, DC, USA*
RACHEL L. ROPER • *Department of Microbiology and Immunology, Brody School of Medicine, East Carolina University, Greenville, NC, USA*
JOHN B. RUEDAS • *Department of Microbiology and National Emerging Infectious Disease Laboratory, Boston University School of Medicine, Boston, MA, USA*
SARAH SEBASTIAN • *The Jenner Institute, University of Oxford, Oxford, UK*
SATHISH SHIVACHANDRA • *Department of Biology, The Catholic University of America, Washington, DC, USA*
FEIFEI TAN • *National Research Center for Veterinary Medicine, Luoyang, China*
PAN TAO • *Department of Biology, The Catholic University of America, Washington, DC, USA*
KEGONG TIAN • *National Research Center for Veterinary Medicine, Luoyang, Henan, PR China; College of Animal Science and Veterinary Medicine, Henan Agricultural University, Zhengzhou, China*
KHAMIS TOMUSANGE • *Virology Laboratory, Basil Hetzel Institute, Discipline of Surgery, University of Adelaide, Adelaide, SA, Australia*
ALISON V. TURNER • *The Jenner Institute, University of Oxford, Oxford, UK*
NURIA VILABOA • *Hospital Universitario La Paz-IdiPAZ, Madrid, Spain; CIBER de Bioingenieria, Biomateriales y Nanomedicine, CIBER-BBN, Madrid, Spain*
RICHARD VOELLMY • *HSF Pharmaceuticals SA, La Tour-de-Peilz, Switzerland; Department of Physiological Sciences, University of Florida College of Veterinary Sciences, Gainesville, FL, USA*
DANUSHKA WIJESUNDARA • *Virology Laboratory, Basil Hetzel Institute, Discipline of Surgery, University of Adelaide, Adelaide, SA, Australia*
CHAO ZHANG • *Vaccine Research Center, Key Laboratory of Molecular Virology & Immunology, Institut Pasteur of Shanghai, University of Chinese Academy of Sciences, Shanghai, China*
DONGMING ZHOU • *Vaccine Research Center, Key Laboratory of Molecular Virology & Immunology, Institut Pasteur of Shanghai, University of Chinese Academy of Sciences, Shanghai, China*

Part I

Double-Stranded DNA Viruses

Chapter 1

Development of Novel Vaccines Against Infectious Diseases Based on Chimpanzee Adenoviral Vector

Chao Zhang*, Yudan Chi*, and Dongming Zhou

Abstract

Vaccination is considered to be the most effective method of preventing infectious or other diseases. Adenovirus (Ad) is one the most promising vectors in vaccine research and development. It can induce not only potent humoral but also cellular immune responses, and has therefore been widely applied in basic and translational studies. Chimpanzee Ad is a rare serotype circulating in humans. This circumvents the problem of preexisting immunity to human Ad serotypes, enhancing Chimpanzee Ad prospects in vaccine development. Here we describe experimental procedures used to generate a new generation of rabies vaccine based on a chimpanzee Ad vector, which can be extended in the development of novel vaccines against other infectious diseases.

Key words Chimpanzee adenovirus, Immune response, Vaccine, Infectious disease, Rabies

1 Introduction

Adenovirus (Ad) was first discovered in 1953 by Rowe and his colleagues [1]. It is a double stranded DNA virus with icosahedral capsids. Over the past decades, Ad-based vectors have shown great potential in gene therapy and have been used to generate recombinant vaccines against cancer or infectious diseases since the first in vivo gene transfer was performed by Rosenfeld et al. in 1991 [2–4]. Nowadays, Ad vectors are widely used as gene delivery systems due to several promising features such as high biosafety levels, broad tropism, and feasibility for scale-up production [5–7]. One of the most widely used Ad vectors originates from human serotype 5(AdHu5) [8], however, the preexisting neutralizing antibodies against AdHu5 have a high seroprevalence of 74.2% in humans [9], and the preexisting antibodies dampen the vaccination effectiveness thus restricting further application in clinical

*These authors contributed equally to this work.

Maureen C. Ferran and Gary R. Skuse (eds.), *Recombinant Virus Vaccines: Methods and Protocols*, Methods in Molecular Biology, vol. 1581, DOI 10.1007/978-1-4939-6869-5_1, © Springer Science+Business Media LLC 2017

trials [10–12]. In order to circumvent the disadvantages of the AdHu5, the rare human serotype Ads and other Ads from nonhuman species have been developed [13–16].

Here, we use a chimpanzee-originated Ad, AdC68, as a model for the generation of Ad-based vaccines against infectious diseases. The construction of the AdC68 infectious clone is as previously described [17]. The E1 region is deleted, thus it is replication-deficient and can only replicate in E1-compensating cell lines such as HEK293 and PER. C6 [18]. In a previous study done in our laboratory, the AdC68 that expressed G protein of the rabies virus (rab.GP) was successfully constructed, expanded and purified. After testing, the rab.GP was found to be highly expressed in HEK 293 cells infected with the recombinant Ads, termed as AdC68-rab.GP. AdC68-rab.GP could elicit high levels of neutralizing antibodies against rabies virus in vaccinated mice. The generation of recombinant Ads in this study is based on the direct cloning method [17] which is simple and efficient and can be extended in the development of vaccines against other infectious diseases.

2 Materials

2.1 Molecular Cloning

1. Restriction enzymes: XbaI; NheI; PI-SceI; I-CeuI; BglII; SalI; XhoI.
2. T4 DNA ligase.
3. Competent cells: *Escherichia coli* strain DH5α cells; *Escherichia coli* strain Stbl2 cells.
4. Agarose G-10.
5. Low melting point agarose.
6. LB culture medium: yeast extract (5 g/L); tryptone (10 g/L); NaCl (10 g/L), amplicillin or kanamycin (0.1 g/L); agar (15 g/L., only be used for LB plate).
7. GelRed Nucleic Acid Gel Stain, 10,000× in DMSO (Biotium). (*see* **Note 1**).
8. KCM buffer (5×): 0.5 M KCl; 0.15 M $CaCl_2$; 0.25 M $MgCl_2$.
9. TAE Buffer (50×): 2 M Tris, 1 M acetic acid, 50 mM EDTA.
10. DNA size standard ladders.
11. NucleoBond Xtra Midi Plus (MACHEREY-NAGEL).
12. QIAprep® Spin Miniprep Kit (QIAGEN).
13. PUC57-rab.GP (codon-optimized for improving expression, Genscript).
14. pShuttle (as described in Ref. [17]).

2.2 Virus Production and Idetification

1. Chimpanzee Ad type 68 (AdC68, also called SAdV-25, ATCC, GenBank accession number: AF394196.1).
2. HEK 293 cell (ATCC, cat. no. CCL-243).
3. Cell culture reagents: Dulbecco's modified Eagle's medium (DMEM); fetal bovine serum; phosphate-buffered saline; penicillin–streptomycin 100× solution; trypsin (0.25%), phenol red.
4. Cell tranfection reagents: Opti-MEM; Lipofectamine 2000 transfection reagent (Invitrogen).
5. Virus purification reagents: Tris–HCl (1 M, pH 8.0); cesium chloride; Bio-Gel P-6DG (Bio-Rad); Liquid chromatography columns.
6. Pronase.
7. DNeasy® Blood & Tissue Kit (QIAGEN).

2.3 Immunoblotting

1. NuPAGE® Novex 10% Bis–Tris gel 1.0 mm, 10 Well (Thermo Fisher Scientific).
2. RIPA buffer: 25 mM Tris–HCl pH 7.6;150 mM NaCl, 1% (V/V) NP-40;1% (W/V) sodium deoxycholate; 0.1% (W/V) SDS.
3. Complete protease inhibitor cocktail tablets (Roche).
4. Running buffer (5×): 0.125 M Tris–HCl;1.25 M glycine;0.5% (W/V) SDS.
5. Transfer Buffer: 39 mM glycine;48 mM Tris;0.037% (W/V) SDS;20% (V/V) methanol.
6. PVDF membrane (0.45 μm filter).

2.4 Animals

ICR (4–6 weeks old) mice are purchased from Shanghai Laboratory Animal Center, China. The protocol for this animal experiment should be approved by the Institutional Animal Care and Use Committee.

3 Methods

3.1 In-Gel Ligation (See Fig. 1)

1. *Cloning the rab.GP gene into pShuttle.* Digest 500 ng of PUC57-rab.GP (Genscript) and 500 ng of pShuttle [17] with XbaI and NheI for 2 h at 37 °C, respectively. Conduct each digestion reaction in a total volume of 20 μl.
2. Run the digestion products on a 1% (W/V) low-melting point agarose gel in TAE buffer. Cut out the desired bands with a razor blade or scalpel to get the digested insert from PUC57-rab.GP and the digested backbone from pShuttle vector, respectively, and then place gel slices into Eppendorf microcentrifuge tubes. Incubate for 5 min at 65 °C. Cool for 1 min at room temperature

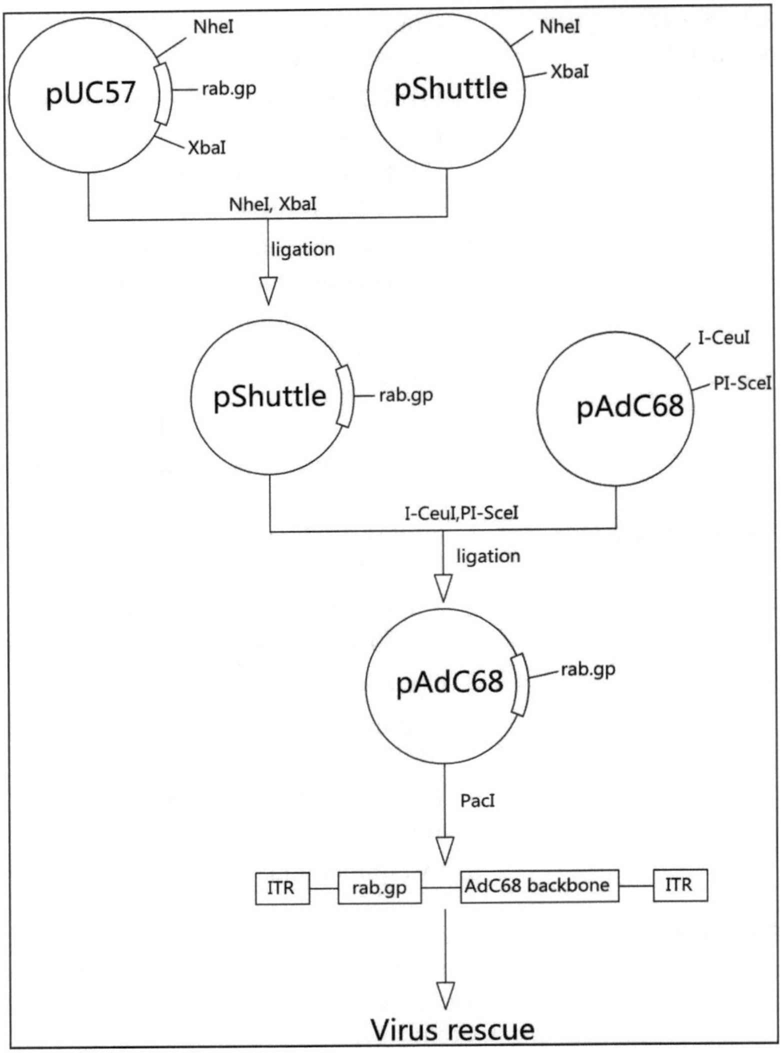

Fig. 1 Flowchart of the construction of pAdC68-rab.GP

(*see* **Note 2**). Set up the in-gel ligation with a total volume of 20 μl; use 4 μl of backbone in liquefied gel, 12 μl of insert in liquefied gel, and mix both with 1 μl T4 DNA ligase. Incubate at 16 °C overnight (*see* **Note 3**).

3. Melt the ligation products for 5 min at 65 °C, and then dilute in 180 μl of 1× KCM buffer (*see* **Note 4**), cool the system at room temperature for 1 min (*see* **Note 5**). Transform 50 μl of diluted ligation product into 100 μl of DH5α competent cells (transforming efficiency ≥10^9 CFU/μg), and then incubate on ice for 30 min. After that, perform the heat shock at 42 °C for 30 s, and spread the transformation mix onto a kanamycin-containing LB plate. Incubate plates for 14 h at 37 °C.

4. Pick up several colonies and culture each of them in 5 mL LB selective medium for 12 h in a shaker at 37 °C and 0.9 × *g* shaking speed. Extract the plasmid DNA by QIAprep® Spin Miniprep Kit based on manufacturer's instructions. Identify the plasmids by restriction enzyme digestions with Nhe1 and XbaI, respectively; choose the right clone, so the pShuttle-rab.GP was successfully generated.
5. *Clone the rab.GP gene into AdC68 vector*; digest 1 μg of the AdC68 plasmid and 1 μg of pShuttle-rab.GP with I-CeuI and PI-SceI, respectively. Conduct each reaction in a total volume of 20 μl and incubate for 4 h at 37 °C.
6. Run the digestion products on 1% (W/V) low-melting point agarose gel in TAE buffer. Cut out the desired bands with a razor blade or scalpel to get the digested insert from pShuttle-rab.GP and the digested backbone from AdC68 vector, and then place gel slices into Eppendorf microcentrifuge tubes. Incubate for 5 min at 65 °C. Cool for 1 min at room temperature. Set up the in-gel ligation with a total volume of 20 μl; use 4 μl of backbone in liquefied gel, 12 μl of insert in liquefied gel and mix both with 1 μl T4 DNA ligase. Incubate at 16 °C overnight (*see* **Note 6**).
7. Melt the ligation products for 5 min at 65 °C, and then dilute in 180 μl of 1× KCM buffer, cool the system at room temperature for 1 min. Transform 50 μl of diluted ligation product into 100 μl of Stbl2 competent cells (transforming efficiency $\geq 10^9$ CFU/μg) with heat shock as described in **step 3**, and spread the transformation mix onto an ampicillin-containing LB plate. Incubate plates for 24 h at 30 °C (*see* **Note 7**).
8. Pick up several colonies and culture each of them in 5 mL LB selective medium for 12 h in a shaker at 30 °C and 0.6 × *g* shaking speed (*see* **Note 7**). Extract each plasmid DNA by QIAprep® Spin Miniprep Kit based on manufacturer's instructions. Identify the plasmids by restriction enzyme digestions with BglII, SalI, and XhoI, respectively. Run the digested products on 1% agarose gel and verify the bands by electrophoresis (*see* Fig. 2a). Choose the right clone, so the AdC68-rab.GP vector (pAdC68-rab.GP) was successfully generated.
9. Select one correct clone and culture it in 200 mL LB medium for 20 h in a shaker at 30 °C and 0.6 × *g* shaking speed. Extract plasmid DNA using NucleoBond Xtra MidiPlus based on manufacturer's instructions.

3.2 Virus Rescue, Expansion, Purification (See Note 8)

1. *Virus rescue.* Seed HEK 293 cells on a 6-well plate 1 day before transfection, and culture cells overnight to 80–85% confluency at 37 °C and 5% CO_2 in DMEM with 10% FBS and 1× penicillin–streptomycin solution.

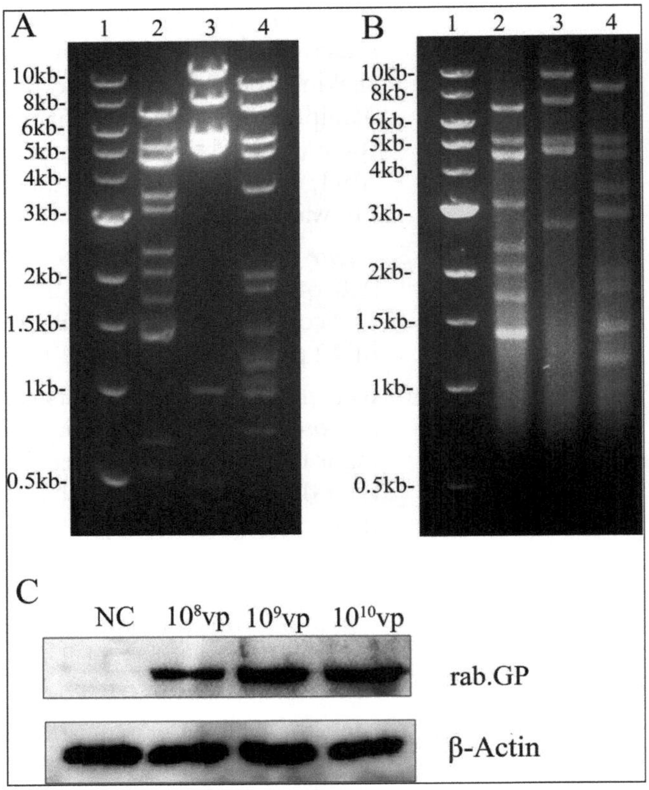

Fig. 2 Identification of the Ad. (**a**) and (**b**) illustrate the digestion of pAdC68-rab.GP and genomic DNA of AdC68-rab.GP, respectively. *Lane 1* represents a DNA ladder. *Lane 2* represents BglII digestion. *Lane 3* represents SalI digestion. *Lane 4* represents Xho1 digestion. (**c**) HEK293 cells were infected with different doses of AdC68-rab.GP. The expression of rab.GP was analyzed by western blotting and β-Actin was used as the loading control. *NC* negative control (AdC68-empty)

2. Digest 4.5 μg of pAdC68-rab.GP with 2 μl PacI to linearize the Ad plasmid. Conduct the reaction in a total volume of 300 μl. Incubate for 4 h at 37 °C. Run 20 μl digested products on 1% agarose gel by electrophoresis to check the digestion result (*see* **Note 9**).
3. Inactivate the remaining digestion mixture at 65 °C for 20 min.
4. Before transfection, replace the DMEM with 1 mL of Opti-MEM medium. Mix the inactivated linearized pAdC68-rab.GP with Lipofectamine 2000 transfection reagent according to manufacturer's instructions. Add different amounts of the transfection mixture dropwise into 3 wells (*see* **Note 10**). Gently shake plates evenly to distribute the mixture and incubate at 5% CO_2 and 37 °C. At 5 h after transfection, discard the previous cell culture medium and substitute with DMEM containing 5% FBS and 1× penicillin–streptomycin solution, incubate at 5% CO_2 and 37 °C (*see* **Note 11**).

5. Check daily for the plaque formation of the AdC68-rab.GP under a microscope. Viral plaques become visible within 8–10 days (*see* **Note 12**).
6. *Virus expansion*. Harvest transfected HEK 293 cells once cytopathogenic effect (CPE) covers 50% of the cells. Resuspend the harvested cells in 1 mL of FBS-free DMEM. Freeze and thaw cells three times (*see* **Note 13**). Centrifuge the samples at 3000 × *g* at 4 °C for 10 min, discard the pellet and harvest the supernatant.
7. Use 3/4 of the supernatant that is harvested from **step 6** to infect one T175 flask of HEK 293 cells grown to 90% confluence (*see* **Note 14**). Save the rest of the supernatant at −80 °C. After 24–48 h, once viral plaques become visible, harvest the cells by centrifugation and process the samples as described in **step 6**.
8. Use 4/5 of the supernatant that is harvested from **step 7** to infect four T175 flasks of HEK 293 cells at a confluence of 90%. After 24–48 h, harvest the infected cells, and resuspend them in 5 mL FBS-free DMEM. Repeat the above freeze-and-thaw procedure, and process the samples as described in **step 6**.
9. Use 4/5 of the supernatant that is harvested from **step 8** to infect 30–40 T175 flasks of HEK 293 cells at a confluence of 90%. After 24–48 h when the viral plaques become visible, harvest infected cells, and resuspend in 10 mL of 10 mM Tris–HCl buffer. Repeat the above freeze-and-thaw procedure, discard the pellet and save the supernatant as described in **step 6**.
10. Use the supernatant to purify the AdC68-rab.GP by CsCl gradient centrifugation (*see* **Note 15**), determine viral titer by number of vps (viral particles) by spectrophotometry (*see* **Note 16**).

3.3 Virus Identification (See Note 17)

1. *Extract genomic DNA of purified AdC68-rab.GP using modified DNeasy Blood & Tissue Kit*; aliquot 100 μl of 5 × 10^{12} vp/mL AdC68-rab.GP into an Eppendorf microcentrifuge tube, and then add 140 μl buffer ATL, 30 μl proteinase K and 30 μl of 1 μg/μl pronase. Mix thoroughly and incubate the tube in a 55 °C water bath for 3 h.
2. Vortex the tube for 20 s, add 300 μl buffer AL to the sample, and incubate the tube at 70 °C for 10 min after thorough vortexing to ensure complete mixing.
3. Add 300 μl absolute ethanol to the tube. Mix thoroughly by vortexing.
4. Pipet the mixture into a DNeasy Mini spin column, and then perform the purification per the manufacturer's instructions.
5. *Identify the genomic DNA by restriction enzyme digestions with BglII, SalI and XhoI, respectively*. Run the digested products on 1% agarose gel and verify the bands by electrophoresis (*see* Fig. 2b).

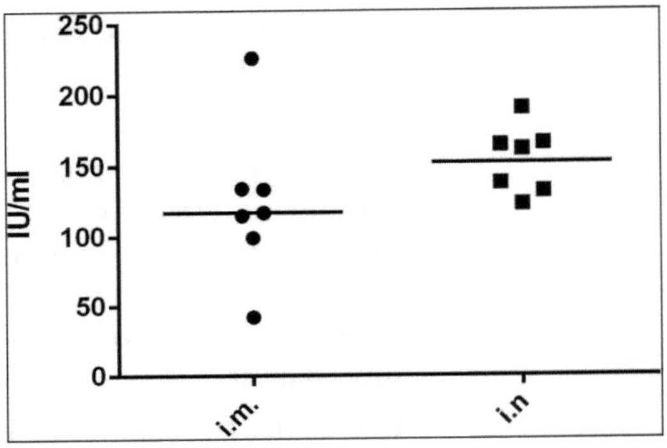

Fig. 3 Rabies virus-neutralizing antibodies in sera of vaccinated mice. 7 ICR mice in each group were immunized with AdC68-rab.GP or AdC68-empty (control group) at a dose of 2×10^{10} vp through i.m. or i.n. Antibody titers in both control groups were negative (not shown). *IU* represents international units

3.4 Antigen Expression

1. Seed HEK 293 cells in a six-well plate at a density of 5×10^5 cells/well and culture overnight.
2. When the cells growing to a confluency of 90%, infect the cells in separate wells with 10^8 vp, 10^9 vp, and 10^{10} vp of the AdC68-rab.GP, respectively, as well as 10^{10} vp of AdC68-empty as control.
3. After 24 h, harvest cells and lyze them in 100 μl of RIPA buffer with protease inhibitors cocktail.
4. Run the western blot to detect the expression of glycoprotein of rabies virus by blotting with anti-rab.GP antibody. β-Actin immunoblotting is included as a loading control (*see* Fig. 2c).

3.5 Animal Immunization and Antibody Assay.

1. Four groups of seven female ICR mice (4–6 weeks old) are to be immunized with one dose of 2×10^{10} vp AdC68-rab.GP or the same dose of AdC68-empty as control through intramuscular (i.m.) and intranasal (i.n.) administration, respectively.
2. Four weeks post vaccination, the blood of each mouse is to be harvested for antibody assays.
3. Rapid focus fluorescence inhibition test (RFFIT) will be used for the detection of the neutralizing antibodies as previously described [19]. The results should reveal that the AdC68-rab. GP administered groups had higher neutralizing antibodies while the control groups were all negative (*see* Fig. 3). Neutralizing antibody titres ≥0.5 IU/mL are considered positive according to World Health Organization (WHO) standards [19].

4 Notes

1. GelRed Nucleic Acid Stain is toxic, when handling it, please be careful and dispose of the waste according to institution-appropriate guidelines.
2. To avoid denaturing the DNA, the heating temperature for melting the gel should not exceed 70 °C. Cooling the gel at room temperature for 1 min is necessary for the ligation; otherwise, high temperatures may result in the inactivation of the ligase.
3. Incubating the ligation system at 16 °C overnight can highly increase the ligation efficiency. This can also be performed as incubation at room temperature for 2 hours, but the efficiency might be much lower.
4. The KCM stock solution remains stable at room temperature for several months.
5. High temperature will dampen the transforming efficiency of the competent cells while cooling the system at room temperature for 1 min will increase the transforming efficiency.
6. Cloning the insert from pShuttle-rab.GP into AdC68 vector is the most critical step; this ligation system should incubate at 16 °C overnight to increase the ligation efficiency, while incubation at room temperature is not recommended.
7. In order to maintain the stability of the large Ads DNA in Stbl2 competent cells, the shaking speed should not exceed 0.6 × *g* and the temperature should not be higher than 30 °C.
8. The recombinant chimpanzee Ad in this study is genetically modified; it is replication-deficient and classified as Biosafety Level 2 (BSL-2). The rescue, amplification and purification of the recombinant Ad should therefore be performed in accordance with the BSL-2 guidelines. All the related reagents, equipment and waste should also be processed according to the BSL-2 guidelines.
9. The linearization of the pAdC68-rab.GP is critical for the successful rescue of the Ad because exposure of the ITR is essential for the genomic replication.
10. To rescue the Ad virus successfully, a graded amount of pAdC68 is recommended to be transfected into HEK293 cells, usually ranging from 1 to 2 μg.
11. Lipofectamine 2000 transfection reagent is quite toxic to the HEK 293 cells. To decrease the harm to the cells, it is important to replace the tranfection medium with new medium 5 h post transfection.

12. In this period, do not change the medium because this can detach the HEK 293 cells from the culture plate. If this period lasts more than 10 days, 1 mL of fresh complete DMEM can be added to maintain the cells.
13. Freeze the samples by −80 °C freezer or liquid nitrogen is OK, but when thawing the samples, the temperature should not be higher than 37 °C as high temperature may result in the inactivation of the Ad.
14. For each round of amplification, the majority of the supernatant from the previous step is used for infecting the cells, and the rest of the supernatant should be saved in case contamination by other Ads or pathogens happens in the virus expansion
15. The CsCl gradient ultracentrifugation is performed at 4 °C at 90,000 × *g*. The CsCl gradient solution is 1.4 g/mL CsCl (53 g CsCl dissolved in 87 mL Tris–HCl (10 mM,PH8.0)) and 1.2 g/mL CsCl (26.8 g CsCl dissolved in 92 mL Tris–HCl (10 mM, PH8.0))
16. The virus titer is determined by measuring UV absorbance at 260 nm (A260) using a spectrophotometer, and determined as the following equation:

$$Viral\ titer = OD_{260} \times dilution \times 1.1 \times 10^{12}\, vp\ /\ mL(viral\ particlepermilliliter)$$

17. As a type of quality control, the genomic DNAs of the purified ads are extracted and verified by different restriction enzyme digestions.

Acknowledgment

This work was supported by grants from "Knowledge Innovation Program" (No. Y014P31503) and "100 Talent Program" (No. Y316P11503) of Chinese Academy of Sciences and Shanghai Pasteur Foundation.

References

1. Rowe WP, Huebner RJ, Gilmore LK et al (1953) Isolation of a cytopathogenic agent from human adenoids undergoing spontaneous degeneration in tissue culture. Proc Soc Exp Biol Med 84(3):570–573
2. Breyer B, Jiang W, Cheng H et al (2001) Adenoviral vector-mediated gene transfer for human gene therapy. Curr Gene Ther 1(2):149–162
3. Uusi-Kerttula H, Hulin-Curtis S, Davies J et al (2015) Oncolytic adenovirus: strategies and insights for vector design and immuno-oncolytic applications. Viruses 7(11):6009–6042. doi:10.3390/v7112923
4. Rosenfeld MA, Siegfried W, Yoshimura K et al (1991) Adenovirus-mediated transfer of a recombinant alpha 1-antitrypsin gene to the lung epithelium in vivo. Science 252(5004):431–434
5. Legrand V, Leissner P, Winter A et al (2002) Transductional targeting with recombinant adenovirus vectors. Curr Gene Ther 2(3):323–339
6. Xu ZL, Mizuguchi H, Sakurai F et al (2005) Approaches to improving the kinetics of

adenovirus-delivered genes and gene products. Adv Drug Deliv Rev 57(5):781–802. doi:10.1016/j.addr.2004.12.010
7. Heilbronn R, Weger S (2010) Viral vectors for gene transfer: current status of gene therapeutics. Handb Exp Pharmacol 197:143–170. doi:10.1007/978-3-642-00477-3_5
8. Xiang Z, Gao G, Reyes-Sandoval A et al (2002) Novel, chimpanzee serotype 68-based adenoviral vaccine carrier for induction of antibodies to a transgene product. J Virol 76(6):2667–2675
9. Wang X, Xing M, Zhang C et al (2014) Neutralizing antibody responses to enterovirus and adenovirus in healthy adults in China. Emerg Microbes Infect 3(5):e30. doi:10.1038/emi.2014.30
10. Perreau M, Pantaleo G, Kremer EJ (2008) Activation of a dendritic cell-T cell axis by Ad5 immune complexes creates an improved environment for replication of HIV in T cells. J Exp Med 205(12):2717–2725. doi:10.1084/jem.20081786
11. Zaiss AK, Machado HB, Herschman HR (2009) The influence of innate and pre-existing immunity on adenovirus therapy. J Cell Biochem 108(4):778–790. doi:10.1002/jcb.22328
12. Lasaro MO, Ertl HCJ (2009) New insights on adenovirus as vaccine vectors. Mol Ther 17(8):1333–1339. doi:10.1038/mt.2009.130
13. Peruzzi D, Dharmapuri S, Cirillo A et al (2009) A novel Chimpanzee serotype-based adenoviral vector as delivery tool for cancer vaccines. Vaccine 27(9):1293–1300. doi:10.1016/j.vaccine.2008.12.051
14. Reddy PS, Ganesh S, Limbach MP et al (2003) Development of adenovirus serotype 35 as a gene transfer vector. Virology 311(2):384–393. doi:10.1016/S0042-6822(03)00161-2
15. Cheng C, Wang LS, Ko SY et al (2015) Combination recombinant simian or chimpanzee adenoviral vectors for vaccine development. Vaccine 33(51):7344–7351. doi:10.1016/j.vaccine.2015.10.023
16. Stone D, Ni SH, Li ZY et al (2005) Development and assessment of human adenovirus type 11 as a gene transfer vector. J Virol 79(8):5090–5104. doi:10.1128/Jvi.79.8.5090-5104.2005
17. Zhou DM, Zhou XY, Bian A et al (2010) An efficient method of directly cloning chimpanzee adenovirus as a vaccine vector. Nat Protoc 5(11):1775–1785. doi:10.1038/nprot.2010.134
18. Havenga MJE, Holterman L, Melis I et al (2008) Serum-free transient protein production system based on adenoviral vector and PER.C6 technology: high yield and preserved bioactivity. Biotechnol Bioeng 100(2):273–283. doi:10.1002/bit.21757
19. Nguyen KA, Nguyen TT, Nguyen DV et al (2015) Evaluation of rapid neutralizing antibody detection test against rabies virus in human sera. Trop Med Health 43(2):111–116. doi:10.2149/tmh.2014-35

Chapter 2

Development of Recombinant Canarypox Viruses Expressing Immunogens

Débora Garanzini, María Paula Del Médico-Zajac, and Gabriela Calamante

Abstract

Canarypox viruses (CNPV) are excellent candidates to develop recombinant vector vaccines due to both their capability to induce protective immune responses and their incompetence to replicate in mammalian cells (safety profile). In addition, CNPV and the derived recombinants can be manipulated under biosafety level 1 conditions. There is no commercially available system to obtain recombinant CNPV; however, the methodology and tools required to develop recombinant vaccinia virus (VV), prototype of the *Poxviridae* family, can be easily adapted. This chapter provides protocols for the generation, plaque isolation, molecular characterization, amplification and purification of recombinant CNPV.

Key words Canarypox, Transfer vector, Nonessential region, Transfection, Homologous recombination, Visual screening

1 Introduction

Canarypox viruses (CNPV) have been widely used as vectors for vaccine development due to their safety profile and for the protection they induce against infectious diseases [1–3]. Recombinant viruses are based on an attenuated (vaccine) strain of CNPV which can be amplified in the laboratory in avian cell culture such as primary chicken embryo fibroblasts (CEFs) or in several cell lines.

Poxviruses, such as the canarypox virus, have large DNA genomes (175–375 kbp) making it impossible to directly manipulate them genetically to obtain recombinant viruses for expressing foreign antigens. Instead, recombinant viruses are produced inside the cell by homologous recombination between the poxvirus genome and a plasmid vector (named here as "transfer vector," TV) carrying the desired gene flanked by viral sequences. Afterwards, the viral progeny are a mixed population of recombinant and nonrecombinant poxviruses, however only a small percentage

Maureen C. Ferran and Gary R. Skuse (eds.), *Recombinant Virus Vaccines: Methods and Protocols*, Methods in Molecular Biology, vol. 1581, DOI 10.1007/978-1-4939-6869-5_2, © Springer Science+Business Media LLC 2017

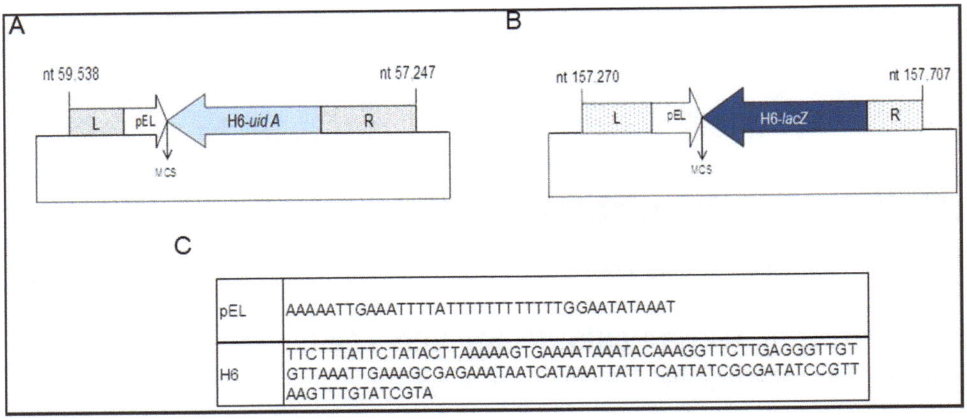

Fig. 1 Scheme of transfer vectors TV-048GUS and TV-134lacZ. TVs have been designed to obtain recombinant CNPV that express a maker enzyme that (**a**) interrupts the CNPV048 gene or (**b**) into the intergenic region between the CNPV134 and CNPV135 genes. *pEL* synthetic vaccinia early/late promoter, MCS: multiple cloning site (containing 1 to 5 unique restriction enzyme recognition sites), H6-lacZ: *lac Z* gene (codes for β-galactosidase enzyme) under regulation of vaccinia virus H6 gene promoter, H6-uidA: *uid A* gene (codes for β-glucuronidase) under regulation of vaccinia virus H6 gene promoter, R and L.: viral regions which serve as points of recombination with CNPV genome. Genomic nucleotide positions are indicated according to Tulman et al. [14]. (**c**) DNA sequence of pEL and H6 promoters

(10^{-4}–10^{-3}) correspond to recombinant virus. Therefore the selection of recombinant viruses, which represent low frequency virus in that mixed progeny, is a vital step for isolation of recombinant CNPVs. The methodology described for the isolation of recombinant canarypox viruses is based on visual screening (through colored lysis plaques) for expression of a marker enzyme (such as β-galactosidase or β-glucuronidase) from the transfected DNA (Fig. 1a, b). This method is not as efficient as those based on direct selection but it is required because no antibiotic/drug resistance gene should be included in the recombinant viral genome that will be used as a vaccine.

2 Materials

2.1 Reagents and Equipment

1. Ultrapure water to prepare solutions.
2. Plasmid purification kits: QIAGEN® Midi, Maxi Kits or Zyppy™ Plasmid Midiprep Kit (Hilden, Germany).
3. Lipofectamine 2000® Reagent (Thermo Fisher Scientific, MA, USA).
4. Phosphate-buffered saline (PBS).
5. 2× Extraction Buffer: 200 mM Tris–HCl pH 8; 20 mM EDTA pH 8; 200 mM NaCl; 2% SDS; 20 mM 2-mercaptoethanol.
6. 5 M potassium acetate.

7. Isopropyl alcohol (99.9%).
8. Ethyl alcohol (70% w/w in distilled water).
9. Cell Scrapers, sterile.
10. NP-40 lysis buffer: 50 mM Tris–HCl pH 8, 150 mM NaCl, 1% Nonidet P-40.
11. 6× SDS-Sample Buffer: 375 mM Tris–HCl pH 6.8, 6% SDS, 48% glycerol, 9% 2-mercaptoethanol, 0.03% bromophenol blue.
12. Neutral red (1 mg/mL in water), filter-sterilized.
13. TMN buffer: 0.01 M Tris–HCl pH 7.5, 1.5 mM $MgCl_2$, 10 mM NaCl.
14. Humidified incubator at 37 °C, 5% CO_2.
15. Water baths (37 and 42 °C).
16. Laminar flow cabinet BSL 2.
17. Inverted microscope.
18. Ultrasonic bath sonicator (e.g., Elmasonic S 30).
19. Ultracentrifuge (e.g., Beckman Coulter), rotor (SW41), and tubes.

2.2 Cells and Virus

1. Cell monolayers of Chicken Embryo Fibroblasts (CEFs) prepared from 11-day-old specific pathogen-free (SPF) embryos [4] or cell lines (e.g., ATCC DF-1, ATCC QM-7, ProBioGen AGE1.CR.pIX®).
2. Canarypox virus: live attenuated vaccine strain (*see* **Note 1**)

2.3 Cell Culture Media (See Note 2)

1. DMEM: Dulbecco's Modified Eagle Medium, high glucose (4.5 g/mL D-glucose; Gibco®, Thermo Fisher Scientific) supplemented with 3.7 mg/mL sodium bicarbonate, 0.3 mg/mL L-glutamine, 50 μg/mL gentamicin, 66 μg/mL streptomycin, 100 U/mL penicillin.
2. Growth medium: DMEM containing 10% fetal calf serum (FCS).
3. Maintenance medium: DMEM containing 2% FCS.
4. Semisolid overlay medium (first overlay): DMEM containing 2% FCS and 0.7% Low Gelling Temperature (LGT) agarose (SeaPlaque™ Agarose, Lonza, Basel, Switzerland).
5. Semisolid overlay medium with substrate (second overlay): semisolid overlay medium containing enzyme substrate 0.2 mg/mL X-Gluc (5-bromo-4-chloro-3-indolyl-β-D-glucuronic acid, Inalco S.p. A, Italy) or 0.35 mg/mL Bluo-gal (halogenated indolyl-β-galactoside, Inalco) for β-glucuronidase or β-galactoside, respectively.

2.4 Cell Culture Flasks

1. 25 cm^2 Tissue Culture Flask (T25).
2. 60 mm cell culture-dish plates (P60).
3. 175 cm^2 Tissue Culture Flask (T175).

3 Methods

The desired sequence is cloned into the transfer vector (*see* **Note 3**), under regulation of an early (or early/late) poxvirus promoter (*see* **Note 4**). The transfer vector is then transfected into CNPV infected CEFs, where the recombination between the viral genome and the TV occurs. Due to the fact that non-recombinant (receptor) CNPV replicate normally, an effective selection/screening method as to be performed to obtain the recombinant CNPV. One strategy involves the screening of the recombinant viruses based on their capability to produced colored (blue) lysis plaques by the expression of a marker enzyme such as β-galactosidase or β-glucuronidase in the presences of a specific chromogenic enzyme substrate. The blue plaques (recombinant virus) are picked and the screening by plaque purification is repeated until a homogenous stock (100% blue plaques) is obtained. Then, the recombinant CNPV is amplified in CEFs to evaluate the presence and expression of the antigen coding sequence. Finally, the recombinant virus is amplified in CEFs and purified through a sucrose cushion.

3.1 Construction and Purification of Transfer Vector

Transfer vectors (TV) carry foreign genes flanked by viral regions which are target sites for recombination with the CNPV genome. In our laboratory two TV have been designed to obtain recombinant CNPV interrupting the CNPV048 gene or the intergenic region between CNPV134 and CNPV135 genes (Fig. 1; [5]). The construction of TV was performed by standard genetic engineering techniques (PCR amplification and cloning). It is also possible to acquire the desired sequences through a service of gene synthesis

1. Subclone the coding sequence of the desired antigen into the CNPV transfer vector downstream of a poxviral promoter. The gene of interest must include its authentic start (ATG) and stop (TAA/TAG/TGA) codons.
2. The correct orientation and identity of the cloned DNA fragment is confirmed by DNA sequencing (*see* **Note 5**).
3. Prepare a stock of TV plasmid DNA using plasmid purification kits to obtain supercoiled and clean DNA (ultrapure transfection-grade; *see* **Note 6**)

3.2 Transfection of CNPV-Infected CEFs

Use the following procedure to transfect CEFs monolayer grown on 25 cm^2 Tissue Culture Flask (T25).

1. One day before transfection seed 3.5–4.5 × 10^6 cells in a T25 to obtain 70–80% confluent the next day (*see* **Note 7**).

2. Discard the medium, wash the monolayer and add 1 mL of CNPV viral stock to get a multiplicity of infection (moi) of 0.5 (*see* **Note 8**).
3. Incubate 2 h at 37 °C (with agitation every 20 min) in a humidified CO_2 incubator.
4. Add 5 ml of maintenance medium and incubate 2 h at 37 °C. During this incubation step, prepare complexes for transfection.
5. For each transfection reaction, prepare 5–8 μg DNA (transfer vector) in 20 μl of H_2O and mix with 100 μl DMEM without serum. Mix gently.
6. Mix Lipofectamine 2000® gently before use, then dilute 6.25 μl in 93.75 μl of DMEM (or other medium) without serum. Incubate for 20–30 min at room temperature (without mixing) to stabilize the cationic lipid into cell culture medium.
7. Combine DNA solution with diluted Lipofectamine 2000®. Mix 4–6 times by pipetting and incubate for 15 min at room temperature (complexes are stable for 6 h at room temperature).
8. Remove medium from flask and wash cells two times with DMEM (without serum).
9. For each transfection, add 2 mL of DMEM to the tube containing the complexes DNA/Lipofectamine 2000® and add to each T25 (total volume = 2.24 mL). Mix gently by rocking.
10. Incubate at 37 °C for at least 2 h.
11. To each T25 add 3 mL of growth medium and 40 μl of FCS without removing the transfection mixture. Incubate overnight.
12. Replace medium with fresh maintenance medium.
13. Incubate until cytopathic effect (CPE) is observed (normally between 4 and 5 days).
14. Harvest cells and supernatant, release virus by three freeze–thaw cycles and store at −80 °C before starting the screening of recombinant virus.

3.3 Visual Screening and Plaque Isolation of Recombinant CNPV

Plaque purification of recombinant CNPV will ensure complete removal of the parental virus. Several consecutive rounds (between 8 and 12) of plaque purification have to be performed.

One day before transfection seed 5 × 10^6 cells in a 60 mm cell culture-dish plates (P60) to obtain 80–90% confluent the next day.

1. Dilute the virus (infection/transfection cell lysate) 1/5 and 1/10 in DMEM (serum free).
2. Add 0.5–1 mL of each dilution to CEFs from which the growth medium has been previously discarded. Infect at least three dish plates per dilution.

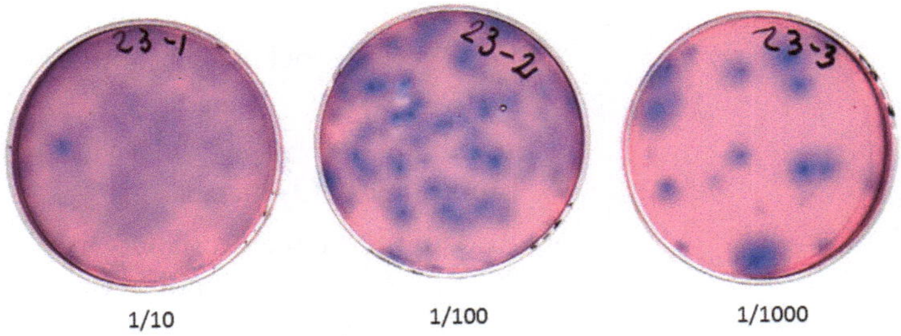

Fig. 2 Screening of recombinant CNPV based on visualization of blue plaques. CEFs grown on 60 mm cell culture-dish plates were infected with recombinant CNPV (diluted 10^{-1}, 10^{-2}, and 10^{-3}) and a second overlay containing X-gluc was added at 4–5 days post-infection

3. Leave the virus on the cells to adsorb for 1 h at 37 °C (tilt dishes every 15–20 min).
4. Remove the inoculum by aspiration or pipetting.
5. Add 3 mL of semisolid overlay medium (first overlay) and incubate for 4–5 days.

   Semisolid overlay: prepare DMEM 2× concentrated and add 4% FCS, keep solution at 37 °C. Prepare 1.4% LGT in water, melt using microwave oven (2–3 min at maximum) and keep at 42 °C. Mix equal volume of DMEM/FCS and molten LGT agarose (maintaining the solution at 37 °C), gently add to cell monolayer and leave at room temperature for allowing medium to solidify before introducing into the humidified incubator.
6. CNPV plaques can easily be seen by holding the dish up to the light or using optical microscopy. Add 2.5 mL of semisolid overlay medium with substrate (second overlay).
7. Hopefully the next day it should be possible to see individual blue plaques.
8. Blue plaques are picked with a filtered pipette tip into 500 μl aliquots of DMEM (serum free) in 1.5 mL microfuge tubes.
9. Freeze-thaw × 3 and store at −80 °C.
10. Prepare dilutions (1/5, 1/10 and 1/50 in DMEM) for each picked blue plaque.
11. Repeat **steps 2–6**.
12. The next day blue plaques have to be seen, picked, freeze-thawed × 3 and stored at −80 °C. This is the first plaque purification step.
13. Prepare dilutions (1/10, 1/100 and 1/1000 in DMEM) for each picked blue plaque.
14. Repeat **steps 2–6** until 100% blue plaques are visualized in the greatest dilution (1/1000) (Fig. 2).

15. Amplify recombinant CNPV viral stock by infection with 1 mL of virus (1/10 dilution in DMEM serum free) into a T25 flask of CEFs. Specifically, discard the growth medium, add virus, incubate 45 min, add 4 mL maintenance medium without discarding the inoculum and harvest cells and supernatant when generalized CPE is observed.

3.4 Characterization of Recombinant CNPV Genomes by PCR

Since the screening of recombinant CNPV is based on marker enzyme expression it is important to analyze the presence of the desired gene by PCR. Detection of the foreign gene can be evaluated after four rounds of screening, even though total DNA is obtained from a mixed (wild type, wt) and recombinant) viral population.

Additionally, once the viral progeny produces blue-plaques, it is necessary to confirm the purity of recombinant CNPV stock (absence of wt virus). Thus, a PCR analysis using a combination of three primers in the reaction should be performed. According to the design of those primers, fragments of different length are amplified from wt and recombinant CNPV genomes (*see* **Note 9** for details of this PCR screen, also *see* Fig. 3).

It is important to keep sterile conditions while performing **steps 1–5** (CEFs infection and harvest).

1. Infect CEFs grown in a P60 (80% confluent) with 500 μl of a 1/10 dilution of recombinant virus (different clones producing blue-plaques), wt CNPV or DMEM (labeled as non-infected cells).
2. Four to five days post infection (dpi) discard medium and wash the monolayer twice with 2–3 mL of sterile PBS (*see* **Note 10**).
3. Add 1 mL of PBS resuspend the cells by pipetting, and transfer to a microcentrifuge tube.
   Remove the cells by pipetting or scrap the cells off in 1 mL of PBS. Transfer the cells to a microcentrifuge tube, spin down by centrifugation (5 min at 200 × g), remove the supernatant, carefully resuspend cells in 1 mL of PBS, centrifuge as before, discard supernatant and resuspend cells in 1 mL of PBS
4. Freeze-thaw three times and store at −80 °C.
5. Transfer 350 μl of each cell lysate to a new microcentrifuge tube. Store the remaining sample at −80 °C as a viral stock.
6. Add one volume of 2× Extraction Buffer.
7. Mix by vortexing and incubate at 65 °C for 10 min.
8. Add 250 μl of 5 M potassium acetate, mix thoroughly by inverting the tube (and incubate on ice for 20 min).
9. Centrifuge at 10,000 × *g*, 30 min, 4 °C.
10. Transfer 700 μl the supernatant into a clear microcentrifuge tube.

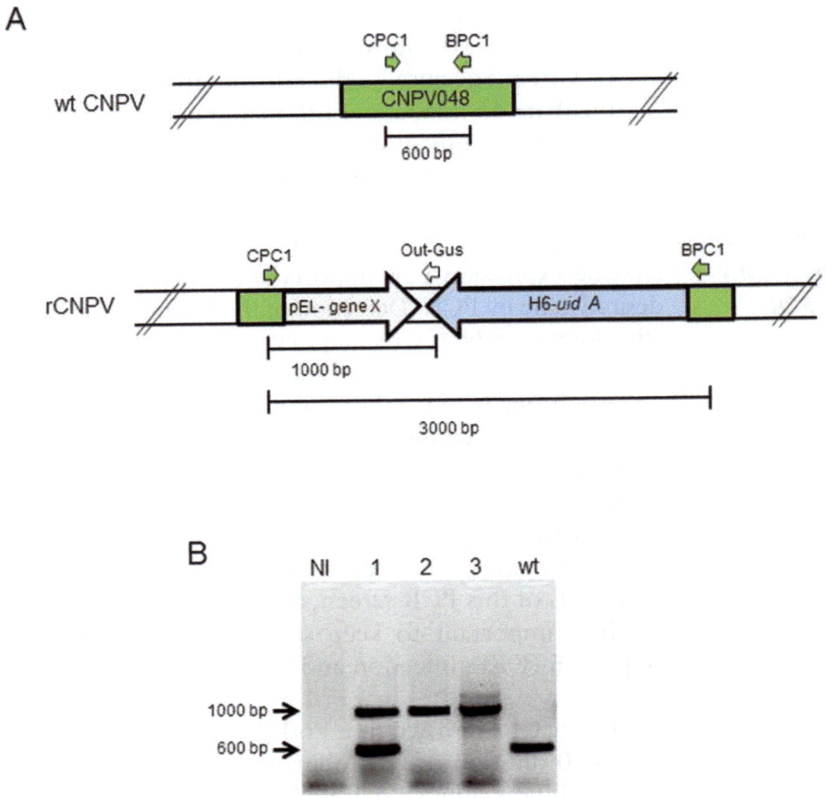

Fig. 3 Determining the purity of recombinant viral stocks by PCR amplification. (**a**) Schematic representation of wild type (wt) and recombinant (r) CNPV genome. Position of the primers used for PCR and expected sizes of amplified products are shown. (**b**) PCR amplification using CPC1 (2× concentrated), BPC1 and Out-Gus primers to analyze rCNPV purity. Total DNA was purified from non-infected cells (NI), non-recombinant CNPV (wt) and different clones (1, 3, to) of recombinant CNPV–infected CEFs. The length of the elongation step in the PCR was not long enough to allow amplification of the 3000 bp fragment on rCNPV genome. Recombinant CNPV clones 2 and 3 are pure (absence of wt CNPV)

11. Add 700 μl of absolute isopropanol and mix by inverting. Incubate at least 1 h on ice or keep overnight at −20 °C.
12. Centrifuge at 10,000 × *g*, 20 min at room temperature.
13. Discard supernatant and wash the pellet twice with 500 μl of 70% ethanol and centrifuge as before. Discard supernatant by pipetting.
14. Dry the pellet to allow ethanol evaporation.
15. Dissolve the pellet in 50 μl sterile distilled deionized water and store at −20 °C.
16. Use 1.5 μl of DNA for each PCR reaction to ensure that the desired gene was properly inserted in CNPV genome.

3.5 Total Protein Sample Preparation for Western Blot Analysis

Once the recombinant CNPV (rCNPV) is obtained and the presence of the foreign gene was confirmed by PCR analysis, the expression of the desired antigen must be evaluated by Western blot.

1. Infect CEFs grown in a P60 (80% confluent) with rCNPV (different clones), wt CNPV or DMEM (labeled as non-infected cells). Use a viral dilution to obtain a moi of 1–5.
2. Allow the virus to adsorb for 45 min (mix by rocking every 15 min).
3. Add 3 mL of maintenance medium and incubate 24 h at 37 °C.
4. Discard supernatant, wash the cell monolayer twice with PBS, scrape the cells off in 1 mL of PBS and transfer to a microcentrifuge tube.
5. Centrifuge 5 min at 200 × *g*, 4 °C. Discard the supernatant.
6. Resuspend each pellet in 50 μl NP-40 lysis buffer by vortexing.
7. Incubate on ice during 45 min and mix by vortexing every 10 min.
8. Centrifuge 5 min at 10,000 × *g*.
9. Recover each supernatant to a new microcentrifuge tube (approximately 40 μl) and add 8 μl of 6× SDS-Sample Buffer.
10. Boil on hot plate for 10 min and spin samples briefly to bring condensation to bottom.
11. Load 15–20 μl of each sample into 0.75 mm wells of a polyacrylamide gel.
12. Perform electrophoresis and Western blot as described elsewhere [6].

3.6 Evaluation of Recombinant CNPV Replication by Multiple-Step Growth Curves

The recombinant CNPV is usually obtained by insertion of the foreign gene into a target site identified as nonessential by genomic sequence homology or bioinformatics prediction. However it is important to confirm that this site is nonessential for in vitro replication. This is done by performing multiple-step growth curves in permissive cells.

1. Infect CEF monolayers (grown in P60) with wt CNPV or rCNPV at a moi of 0.01.
2. Allow the virus to adsorb for 45 min (mix by rocking each 15 min), remove the inoculum, and wash the cell monolayers twice with DMEM.
3. Add 3 mL of maintenance medium and incubate al 37 °C.
4. At different times (e.g., 0, 6, 12, 16, 20, 24, 36, 48, and 72 h) post-infection collect separately the cells (which contain the intracellular virus), and the supernatant (which contains the

extracellular virus). Freeze at −80 °C and thaw these fractions three times and store at −80 °C.

5. Determine the virus titer by performing plaque assays (*see* Subheading 3.7) at each time point. This should be done in duplicate.

3.7 Titration of CNPV: Determining Pfu/ mL

Titration of viral stocks is a critical step before any experimental use of the virus. The plaque assay is one of the most used methods to determine the infective titer of a virus stock. Briefly, cell monolayers are infected with different dilutions of virus suspension and a semisolid agarose overlay is added over the infected cells. As dilution is increasing, sporadic cells become infected. The agarose overlay keeps the cells stable and limits the spread of virus. When the virus lyses the cells, only the immediately adjacent cells become infected. After a few days the viral cytopathic effect can be distinguished as plaques (clear areas) in the cell monolayer. Then, these plaques can be easily visualized by staining with a vital dye (e.g., neutral red) for wt virus or with a second overlay containing the substrate for the expressed marker-enzyme for recombinant CNPV.

1. Thaw virus suspension at room temperature and homogenize by vortexing.
2. Make 10-fold serial dilution (from 10^{-1} to 10^{-8}) of virus in DMEM.
3. Infect cell monolayers (grown in P60, 80% confluent) with 0.5 mL of viral dilution in duplicate (*see* **Note 11**).
4. Allow the virus to adsorb for 1 h (mix by rocking each 20 min), remove the inoculum and wash cell monolayers twice with DMEM.
5. Add 3 mL of semisolid overlay medium (first overlay) and incubate for 4–5 days until plaques can be seen by holding the dish up to the light.
6. To stain wt virus plaques add 2.5 mL of the first overlay containing 50 μg/mL neutral red: for rCNPV add 2.5 mL of the second overlay containing the appropriate enzyme substrate.
7. Let solidify at room temperature and incubate overnight at 37 °C.
8. Count plaques visually (*see* **Note 12**). For wt virus is critical to confirm that the dots are viral lysis plaques by inspection under a microscope.
9. Calculate the titer of the initial viral suspension in pfu/mL using the following formula:

$$pfu\ /\ mL = No.\text{of plaques} / (D \times V)$$

D = dilution factor.

V = Volume of diluted virus/P60.

3.8 Amplification and Purification of CNPV

This protocol is useful for amplification and purification of recombinant and non-recombinant CNPV. It is recommended to prepare a "master seed" viral stock (e.g., from approximately 15 infected T175) that is used to amplify "working" virus stocks of wt and recombinant CNPV.

1. Infect CEFs monolayers grown on 15–20 T175 by adding 2–4 mL of diluted viral suspension to obtain a moi of 0.1–0.3.
2. Allow virus to adsorb for 1 h at 37 °C, mix by rocking every 15–20 min.
3. Add 30 mL of maintenance medium per flask.
4. Incubate 4–5 days until generalized CPE is observed.
5. Collect cells and supernatants, release virus by three cycles of freeze −80 °C–thaw and store at −80 °C as "primary" viral stock or carry on with following steps for viral purification.
6. Homogenize virus material using an ultrasonic bath sonicator. Fill sonicator with ice-water, place tubes containing viral suspension (25 mL of virus in a 50 mL polypropylene conical tube) and sonicate using sweep frequency mode for 3 min. Repeat three times with 1 min interval between each sonication step.
7. Centrifuge 20 min at 500 × *g*, 4 °C to discard cell debris.
8. Recover supernatant to another tube filtering through sterile gauze.
9. Resuspend the pellet in 10 mL DMEM and repeat **steps 6–8** (*see* **Note 13**).
10. Collect supernatant. *This is a possible stop point, keeping the supernatant at 4 °C overnight.*
11. Centrifuge 1.5 h at 48,000 × *g*, 4 °C to concentrate viral suspension.
12. Discard supernatant and resuspend pellets in 10–15 mL of TMN buffer by vortexing and pipetting.

    Resuspend each pellet in 1–1.5 mL of TMN buffer by vortexing and pipetting (use a filtered tip) to ensure complete resuspension. Then, pool viral suspensions, wash each ultracentrifuge tube with 0.5–1 mL of TMN buffer and pool. Complete with TMN buffer until a final volume of 10–15 mL.
13. Sonicate the viral suspension as before and centrifuge 5 min at 500 × *g*, 4 °C.
14. Prepare sucrose cushions by filling an ultracentrifuge tube (for SW41 rotor) with 4 mL of 25% (w/v) sucrose in TMN buffer.
15. Overlay the viral suspension (supernatant of **step 13**) onto the sucrose cushion (*see* **Note 14**).
16. Centrifuge 2 h at 160,000 × *g*, 4 °C.

17. Discard supernatant (cell debris and sucrose) and resuspend pelleted viral suspension in TMN buffer using approximately 1 mL/10 T175 (*see* **Note 15**). Separate a 10–20 μl aliquot for viral titration.
18. Store purified viral stock at −80 °C, in aliquots of 0.5–1 mL.

4 Notes

1. Recombinant CNPV vaccines are based on strain ALVAC (Aventis Pasteur) or Abbatista95 (Instituto de Biotecnología, INTA). To our knowledge is quite difficult to find a supplier for a canarypox vaccine. Poximune C (Ceva) or Diftervac (LaDiPreVet, Argentina) are not producing these vaccines anymore. A critical start point is the obtainment of an attenuated strain of canarypox.
2. All media used on cells has to be warmed at 37 °C before use.
3. Unfortunately, there are not commercially available systems to obtain recombinant canarypox virus. So, the platform has to be set up in each laboratory interested in develop it. For example the transfer vectors (TV) have to be designed and constructed and an attenuated strain of CNPV has to be available. Otherwise, collaborative agreements are signed between research groups where one provides the platform and the other evaluates the recombinant CNPV as a vaccine.
4. The first step in designing a transfer vector is the selection of a nonessential target gene. Briefly, selection of a target gene can be done through searching bibliographic databases or by bioinformatics analysis on genome sequences of (avi)poxvirus available on GenBank. The foreign sequences have to be under regulation of poxviral early promoters, which are highly conserved between different members of the *Poxviridae* family [7]. It has been shown that vaccinia virus promoters can efficiently direct the expression of foreign genes in recombinant CNPV [8–10]. Among those are the synthetic vaccinia early/late promoter (pE/L.; [11]), the promoter of 7.5 kDa protein (p7.5; [12]) and vaccinia virus H6 gene promoter (pH 6; [13]). The TV also provides a poxviral transcription stop sequence (TAAATAAATAATTTTTAT) downstream of the polylinker where the desired gene is cloned.
5. This is an important check-point to guarantee both that there are no nucleotide mutations (mainly if the desired gene was amplified by PCR) and the initiation of translation occurs from the proper start (ATG) codon.
6. Plasmid DNA for transfection into eukaryotic cells must be clean and free from phenol and sodium chloride as these con-

taminants may kill cells. In addition, salt will interference with formation of lipid complexes, decreasing transfection efficiency.

7. Seed at least 2 T25 flasks with different amount of cells to guarantee that one will be 80% confluence the next day. Viability of primary cell culture can vary a little each time they are prepared.

8. Multiplicity of infection (moi) is the average number of virus particles infecting each cell.

   moi = Plaque form ing units (pfu) of virus used for infection/ number of cells.

9. In the example of Fig. 3 the primers used were BPC1 (5′ TCCGCTTGTACAGATGGT), CPC1 (5′ GATTGAAGATACAGGATTCT) and OutGus (5′ CAGCCTCGGGAATTGCTAC). The protocol for a routine Taq PCR of 25 μl reaction contains Taq Reaction Buffer (1×), MgCl2 (2 mM), dNTPs (200 μM), BPC1 and OutGus primers (50 ng of each), CPC1 primer (100 ng), template DNA from Subheading 3.4 (1.5 μl) and Taq DNA polymerase (0.6 U). For these primers the cycling conditions are:

1 cycle	**Initial denaturation**	**94 °C, 5 min**
30 cycles	*Denaturation*	*94 °C, 1 min*
	Annealing	*50 °C, 1 min*
	Extension	*72 °C, 1 min*
1 cycle	*Final extension*	*72 °C, 10 min*

10. CNPV infected CEFs at 4–5 dpi normally show generalized CPE but the monolayer is still fixed to the dish plate. Alternatively, the monolayer can be easily washed by gently adding 1–2 mL of PBS directly to the cell monolayer grown on P60, washing by rocking and discarding the buffer by pipetting. Then, 1 mL of PBS is added to recover cells by pipetting and transferring to a new microcentrifuge tube.

11. Use an appropriate dilution series based on the expected titer. The following expected titers can be used as a guideline: 10^{-4} to 10^{-8} for sucrose-cushion purified virus, 10^{-1} to 10^{-4} for picked viral plaques, 10^{-3} to 10^{-6} for tittering virus in a multiple-step growth curve.

12. Select the virus dilution that produces 20–100 lysis plaques/ P60 to calculate the titer. Neutral red stains healthy cells and the plaques will appear as clear areas. In the case of rCNPV, the

blue lysis plaques are visualized after addition of the second overlay containing X-Gluc or Bluo-gal.

13. During the purification protocol, the greatest loss of virus occurs in the first low speed centrifugation. Repeat **steps 6** to **8** two or three times in order to increase recovery.
14. Complete each tube with TMN buffer until 2 mm from the top to prevent the tube from collapsing.
15. CNPV stocks purified by sucrose cushion are fine for animal work (veterinary vaccines).

References

1. Poulet H, Minke J, Pardo MC et al (2007) Development and registration of recombinant veterinary vaccine. The example of the canarypox vector platform. Vaccine 25(30):5606–5612
2. Draper SJ, Heeney JL (2010) Viruses as vaccine vectors for infectious diseases and cancer. Nat Rev Microbiol 8(1):62–73
3. Weli SC, Tryland M (2011) Avipoxviruses: infection biology and their use as vaccine vectors. Virol J 8:49
4. Staib C, Drexler I, Sutter G (2004) Construction and Isolation of Recombinant MVA. In: Isaacs SN (ed) Vaccinia virus and poxvirology methods and protocols, 1st edn. Humana, Totowa, NJ
5. Calamante G, Conte Grand MD, Carrillo EC (2010) Argentinian Patent AR052743B1
6. Green MR, Sambrook J (2012) Molecular cloning: a laboratory manual, 4th edition. In: Inglis J, Boyle A, Gann A (eds) Expressing cloned genes for protein production, purification and analysis, chapter 19, vol 3. Cold Spring Harbor Laboratory Press, New York, pp 1602–1630
7. Boyle DB (1992) Quantitative assessment of poxvirus promoters in fowlpox and vaccinia virus recombinants. Virus Genes 6:281–290
8. Taylor J, Meignier B, Tartaglia J et al (1995) Biological and immunogenic properties of a canarypox-rabies recombinant, ALVAC-RG (vCP65) in non-avian species. Vaccine 13:539–549
9. Amano H, Morikawa S, Shimizu H et al (1999) Identification of the canarypoxvirus thymidine kinase gene and insertion of foreign genes. Virology 256:280–290
10. Zanetti FA, Conte Grand MD, Mitarotonda RC et al (2014) Canarypox virus expressing infectious bursal disease VP2 protein as immunogen for chickens. Braz J Microbiol 45:231–234
11. Blasco R, Moss B (1995) Selection of recombinant vaccinia viruses on the basis of plaque formation. Gene 158:157–162
12. Coupar BE, Andrew ME, Both GW, Boyle DB (1986) Temporal regulation of influenza hemagglutinin expression in vaccinia virus recombinants and effects on the immune response. Eur J Immunol 16:1479–1487
13. Rosel J, Earl P, Weir J, Moss B (1986) Conserved TAAATG sequence at the transcriptional and translational initiation sites of vaccinia virus late genes deduced by structural and functional analysis of the HindIII H genome fragment. J Virol 60:436–449
14. Tulman ER, Afonso CL, Lu Z et al (2004) The genome of canarypox virus. J Virol 78:353–366

Chapter 3

Fowl Adenovirus-Based Vaccine Platform

Juan C. Corredor, Yanlong Pei, and Éva Nagy

Abstract

Nonpathogenic fowl adenoviruses (FAdVs) are amenable for engineering multivalent vaccine platforms due to large stretches of nonessential DNA sequences in their genomes. We describe the generation of FAdV-9-based vaccine platforms by targeted homologous recombination in an infectious clone (pPacFAdV-9 or wild type FAdmid) containing the entire viral genome in a cosmid vector. The viral DNA is subsequently released from the cosmid by restriction enzyme digestion followed by transfection in a chicken hepatoma cell line (CH-SAH). Virus is harvested, propagated, and verified for foreign gene expression.

Key words Homologous recombination, FAdV-9, Fowl adenovirus-9, FAdmid, Virus vector, Recombinant virus vaccine, Lambda red recombinase

1 Introduction

Mammalian adenoviruses, including those of humans, are best characterized and used as vectors for various purposes such as gene delivery, vaccination, and oncolytic therapeutics [1]. Fowl adenoviruses are less characterized, though their potential as gene delivery and vaccine vectors have been demonstrated [2–9].

Fowl adenovirus 9 (FAdV-9), strain A-2A, is nonpathogenic for poultry and has a large dsDNA genome (45 kb) with dispensable regions for virus replication in vitro. Large and simultaneous deletions of such regions can be tolerated while in vitro replication is maintained at wild-type levels [2, 10, 11]. In general, homologous recombination in *Escherichia coli* BJ5183 has been used for cloning entire genomes of mammalian and fowl adenoviruses into plasmid vectors to facilitate manipulation [12–14]. We have previously generated an infectious clone (pPacFAdV-9 or parental wild type, wt, FAdmid) consisting of the entire FAdV-9 genome in a cosmid vector [10]. Next, we engineered new viable parental FAdmid versions (FAdmids Δ1, Δ4, ΔTR2, ΔORF11, etc.) as platforms for recombinant viruses [2, 10, 11]. Importantly, FAdV-9-based recombinant viruses stimulate antibody response to foreign protein in chickens [3], suggesting their potential as vaccine candidates.

Maureen C. Ferran and Gary R. Skuse (eds.), *Recombinant Virus Vaccines: Methods and Protocols*, Methods in Molecular Biology, vol. 1581, DOI 10.1007/978-1-4939-6869-5_3, © Springer Science+Business Media LLC 2017

We describe two methods for the generation of FAdV-9-based vaccine platforms: intermediate construct- and lambda Red recombinase-mediated deletion/foreign gene replacement. The first method consists of cloning foreign gene expression cassettes into viral DNA sequences in intermediate constructs such as pFAP-2 and pleftΔ491–2782 [10, 11]. The protocol described for this method is applicable to any intermediate construct. For simplicity, our protocol describes the use of pleftΔ491–2782 for cloning foreign genes at the left end region of the viral genome. This construct contains the first 7.5 kb of the left end region with a deletion at nts 491–2782 that includes ORFs 1, 1A, 1B, 1C, and 2. SwaI restriction sequence was incorporated at the deletion site [11]. First, the foreign gene is directionally cloned into an expression plasmid vector containing a strong promoter (CMV, CAG, etc.) and downstream sequences consisting of a poly-A signal and transcription termination sites. Subsequently, the entire expression cassette (promoter, foreign gene and downstream sequences) is PCR-amplified and blunt-end cloned into the SwaI site of pleftΔ491–2782. The orientation of foreign gene cassette is then verified through different approaches such as restriction mapping, PCR or direct sequencing. Subsequently, the gene expression cassette along with flanking viral DNA arms is PCR-amplified, purified, and co-transformed with SgfI-digested parental FAdmids (either wt or FAdmidΔ1 with a deletion at nts 1194–2342) or SwaI-digested parental FAdmidΔ4 (deletion at nts 491–2782) into *E. coli* BJ5183. Recombinant FAdmids are generated through homologous recombination [11].

The lambda Red recombinase-mediated foreign gene cloning allows the exquisite targeting of nonessential regions for deletion anywhere in the FAdmid DNA through the insertion of an antibiotic resistance gene (chloramphenicol acetyl transferase, kanamycin resistance gene, etc.). So far, targetable viral DNA sequences for deletion/foreign gene replacement without compromising virus replication in vitro include ORFs 0, 1, 1A, 1B, 1C, and 2 at the left and TR-2 and ORF11 at the right end regions [2, 4, 10]. Our protocol describes the use of chloramphenicol acetyl transferase (CAT) gene as a selection marker for targeted deletions. CAT amplicon is generated from pKD3 (or any other plasmid containing CAT gene) with high-fidelity KOD DNA polymerase using 78–81 nt primers containing around 50 nt viral DNA homologous arms, a SwaI restriction site and at least the first 20 nt sequence of the CAT expression cassette. *E. coli* H10B harboring the parental wt FAdmid and pJW103 (carrying lambda Red recombinase gene) is transformed with the CAT amplicon. Lambda Red recombinase enhances homologous recombination [15], and bacterial clones carrying the "CAT-marked parental FAdmids" are selected with chloramphenicol. CAT expression cassette is subsequently removed by SwaI and replaced with the foreign gene cassette of interest, either by conventional blunt-end ligation with T4 DNA ligase or homologous recombination in *E. coli* BJ5183 [2].

Recombinant (r) FAdmids generated by either method are verified with NotI or any other restriction enzyme digestion. Subsequently, rFAdmids are digested with PacI to release the viral genome from the cosmid vector and transfected into chicken hepatoma cells (CH-SAH line). After cytopathic effect (CPE) is evident, recombinant virus is harvested, titrated, propagated and verified by sequence and restriction analyses. Foreign gene expression is then detected by either fluorescence microscopy (for fluorescent proteins such as GFP) or Western blotting [4]. The recombinant FAdVs as potential vaccines are assessed in vivo (in chickens) using different routes (e.g., oral, intramuscular, or subcutaneous), doses and boosting inoculations [3, 16, 17].

2 Materials

2.1 Plasmid Vectors and Constructs, and Plasmid Preparation Kits

1. Plasmids: pKD3 (or any other plasmid vector carrying the CAT gene expression cassette), pJW103 (carrying lambda Red recombinase and kanamycin resistance genes) and eukaryotic expression vector containing a strong promoter, poly-A signal, and transcription termination site (pEGFP-N1, pCI-neo, etc.).
2. Constructs: pleftΔ491–2782 [11], parental wild-type (wt) FAdmid [10], FAdmidΔ1 and FAdmidΔ4 [4, 11].
3. Plasmid preparation kits are available from different sources (e.g., PureLink® HiPure Plasmid Midiprep Kit, Invitrogen, *see* **Note 1**).

2.2 Primers

1. Primers located at the left end terminus [11]: FAdE1F (5′ TACATGAATGACGCTGCTG 3′), FAdE1R (5′ CCCCCGCAGAGAATTAAAA 3′) and FAD-1 primer (5′ TGCAGCACTTACTTCCTTAT 3′) (*see* **Note 2**).
2. CAT primers [2]: CAT forward primer (5′ $[N]_{50}$-ATTTAAAT gtgtaggctggagctgcttc3′) and CAT reverse primer (5′ $[N]_{50}$-AT TTAAATcatatgaatatcctccttagttc). N, viral DNA homologous arms (around 50 bases). Capital letters represent SwaI site; small letters represent CAT cassette-specific sequence (*see* **Note 3**).
3. Foreign gene specific primers for directional cloning (*see* **Note 4**).
4. Verification primers: design primers that anneal viral DNA sequences upstream and downstream of the CAT insertion site.

2.3 Equipment

1. Microcentrifuge.
2. NanoDrop 2000 spectrophotometer.
3. Vortex.
4. Electronic pipettor.

5. Water baths (37 and 42 °C).
6. Mini autoclave sterilizer.
7. Analytical scale.
8. Horizontal gel electrophoresis apparatus.
9. PCR thermocycler.
10. Orbital shaker incubator.
11. Electroporation system (Bio-Rad) along with electroporation cuvettes 0.2 cm-gap (Fisher Scientific).
12. Incubators (30 and 37 °C).
13. CO_2 incubator.
14. Laminar flow hood biosafety level 2.
15. Centrifuge (Beckman Coulter AllegraTM X-22, SX4250 rotor).
16. Manual cell counter.
17. Inverted brightfield and fluorescence microscopes.
18. Rocking shaker and electronic pipettor (pipette aid).
19. Sonicator.
20. Heating block.
21. SDS-PAGE gel and transfer apparatuses.
22. Micropipettes (10, 20, 200, and 1000 μL).

2.4 Enzymes

1. SgfI.
2. SwaI.
3. NotI.
4. PacI.
5. T4 polynucleotide kinase (PNK).
6. Antarctic phosphatase.
7. T4 DNA ligase (1 U/μL and 5 U/μL, Invitrogen).
8. KOD DNA polymerase (Novagen®).

2.5 Cell Line and *Escherichia coli* Strains

1. Chicken hepatoma cell line (CH-SAH).
2. *E. coli* DH5-α, BJ5183, and DH10B.

2.6 Antibiotics

1. Ampicillin: 100 mg/mL in dH_2O.
2. Chloramphenicol: 34 mg/mL in ethanol.
3. Kanamycin: 50 mg/mL in dH_2O.
4. Tetracycline: 10 mg/mL in dH_2O.
5. Streptomycin: 30 mg/mL in dH_2O.

2.7 Bacterial and Cell Culture

1. LB medium (1 L): Dissolve 10 g tryptone, 5 g yeast extract, and 10 g NaCl in 950 mL MQ water. Adjust the pH to 7.0 with 1 N

NaOH and complete volume to 1 L. Autoclave on liquid cycle for 20 min at 15 psi. After cooling, add antibiotic as required.

2. LB agar-plates: Prepare LB medium as above plus 15 g agar before autoclaving. Autoclave as above. If antibiotic is required, allow medium to cool to approximately 55 °C, add antibiotic and pour onto petri dishes. Let the medium harden, wrap them in plastic sleeves and store at 4 °C.
3. Concentrations of antibiotics in LB medium (liquid or agar): ampicillin (Amp), 100 μg/mL; chloramphenicol (Cam), 34 μg/mL; kanamycin (Kan), 50 μg/mL; streptomycin (Str), 30 μg/mL and tetracycline (Tet), 10 μg/mL.
4. Arabinose (10% w/v in MQ water). Sterilize through a 0.2 μm filter.
5. SOC medium (Invitrogen).
6. Dulbecco modified Eagle's medium/F12 (DMEM-F12, Sigma).
7. Fetal bovine serum (FBS, Sigma).
8. 0.5% trypsin–EDTA.
9. 200 mM L-glutamine (100×).
10. Cell culture antibiotics (100×): 10,000 IU/mL penicillin, 10,000 μg/mL streptomycin.
11. DMEM-F12 growth medium: add 50 mL FBS, 5 mL 100× L-glutamine and 5 mL 100× penicillin/streptomycin to the bottle containing 500 mL medium. Mix well and store at 4 °C.
12. Serum-free medium: add L.-glutamine and antibiotics as described above, but no FBS.
13. 2× DMEM: pour all DMEM powder bottle (10 g/L., Sigma) into 470 mL MQ water while steering. Once dissolved, add 3.7 g sodium bicarbonate, steer to dissolve and adjust pH to 7.4 with either 1 N NaOH or 1 N HCl. Complete to 500 mL with MQ water and mix well. Sterilize with 0.2 μm filters and store in aliquots (e.g., in 100 mL bottles) at 4 °C.
14. Low-melting point agarose (Seakem).
15. DMEM-agarose: For one 6-well plate, weigh 0.14 g low-melting point agarose and pour it into a 100 mL Erlenmeyer flask containing 10 mL distilled water. Cover flask with cotton plugs wrapped in gauze and sterilize in a mini autoclave for 30 min at 121 °C (15 psi, liquid cycle). Carefully, place flask with molten agarose in a waterbath at 42 °C for at least 10 min. In a sterile 100 mL bottle, mix 8.6 mL 2× DMEM, 1 mL FBS, 0.2 mL L-glutamine, and 0.2 mL penicillin/streptomycin. Mix contents well and place bottle at 42 °C for at least 10 min. Mix agarose and 2X DMEM preparations in a laminar flow hood and place it back to the waterbath at 42 °C. DMEM-agar should be immediately used after completion of virus adsorption time (1 h).

16. 0.015% neutral red-containing medium: add 0.2 mL 0.3% neutral red in 4 mL DMEM-F12, 5% FBS.
17. Phosphate buffer saline (PBS).
18. Transfection reagents: Opti-MEM (serum-reduced medium, GIBCO), Lipofectamine 2000 (1 mg/mL, Invitrogen) and antibiotic-free DMEM-F12, 10% FBS.
19. Cell culture plasticware: T75 and T25 flasks, 6 and 15 cm diameter dishes, 6-well plates, sterile disposable pipettes (5, 10, and 25 mL) and 15 mL centrifuge tubes.

2.8 Bacteria Transformation

1. Glassware and plasticware: Ultra cleaned Erlenmeyer flasks (for competent bacteria only), 1.5 mL microcentrifuge tubes, 15 mL centrifuge tubes, 200 and 1000 μL micropipette tips.
2. RF1 buffer for competent bacteria preparation: For 100 mL solution, add 4 mL 2.5 M KCl, 5 mL 1 M $MnCl_2$, 3 mL 1 M potassium acetate, pH 6.0, 1 mL 1 M $CaCl_2$, and 18.8 mL 80% glycerol. Add MQ water to just below 100 mL volume and stir. Adjust pH to 5.8 with 0.5 M acetic acid (usually less than 500 μL). If pH drops below 5.8, discard solution and prepare a fresh one. Adjust volume to 100 mL with MQ water and filter-sterilize with a 0.2 μm filter. Store at 4 °C (*see* **Notes 5, 6** and **8**).
3. RF2 buffer competent bacteria preparation. For 100 mL solution, add 1 mL 1 M MOPS, 0.4 mL 2.5 M KCl, 7.5 mL 1 M $CaCl_2$, 18.8 mL 80% glycerol and MQ water. Adjust pH to 6.8 with around 50 μL 1 N NaOH. Complete to 100 mL final volume with MQ water and filter-sterilize with a 0.2 μm filter. Store at 4 °C (*see* **Notes 5,** 7 and **8**).
4. Sterile 10% glycerol in MQ water.

2.9 Viral DNA Preparation

1. 10× TNE buffer (100 mM Tris pH 7.5, 1 M NaCl, 10 mM EDTA pH 8.0): for 100 mL, add 10 mL 1 M Tris–HCl pH 7.5, 20 mL 5 M NaCl, 2 mL 0.5 M EDTA and 68 mL MQ water. Sterilize by autoclaving.
2. 1× TNE buffer (10 mM Tris–HCl pH 7.5, 100 mM NaCl, 1 mM EDTA pH 8.0): dilute 10× TNE buffer ten times in sterile MQ water according to volume required.
3. 30% sucrose in TNE buffer: for 100 mL, pour 30 g sucrose into a beaker containing around 70 mL MQ water while stirring. Allow the sucrose to dissolve and add 10 mL 10× TNE buffer. Adjust the volume to 100 mL with MQ water. Mix well and filter sterilize through a 0.2 μm filter.
4. Proteinase K (Promega): 100 mg/mL.
5. 2× lysis buffer (10 mM Tris–HCl pH 8.0, 10 mM EDTA, 1% SDS, 100 μg/mL proteinase K). Add proteinase K only when samples are ready for the lysis step.

6. Plasticware: 6-well plates, sterile and disposable plastic pipettes (5, 10, and 25 mL), 200 μL- and 1 mL-filtered tips, 200 μL and 1 mL micropipettes, sterile 1.5 mL tubes, 1.5 mL-tube racks, desktop autoclavable biohazard bag and stand, and ultracentrifuge tubes (Beckman centrifuge tubes, 1 × $3^{1/2}$ in or 25 × 89 mm).

2.10 Detection of Foreign Protein Expression

1. Plasticware: 1.5 mL tubes, 200 μL and 1 mL tips and 1.5 mL-tube lid locks.
2. RIPA buffer: 150 mM NaCl, 1.0% NP-40, or Triton X-100, 0.5% sodium deoxycholate, 0.1% and 50 mM Tris–HCl, pH 8.0.
3. 6× Laemmli buffer: 375 mM Tris–HCl, 9% SDS, 50% glycerol, 0.03% bromophenol blue. Add ß-mercaptoethanol (9% v/v) before use.

2.11 In Vivo Testing of Candidate Recombinant Vaccines

1. Housing conditions: chickens are grouped for each recombinant virus in separate isolators. Housing conditions must be followed according to the local and institutional animal care guidelines. Such conditions include temperature, feed, drinking water, and humidity. Animals must be monitored daily by trained personnel.
2. Wing tagging: wing tags and pliers.
3. Blood collection: 70% ethanol, 1.5 mL tubes, 1.5 mL tube racks, 25 G needles (5/8 inch) and sterile gauze pads.
4. Virus inoculation: virus preparation on ice, tuberculin syringes with 25 G needles, gloves and Sharpie markers.

3 Methods

3.1 Passage of CH-SAH Cells

1. When cells reach high density, remove supernatant and rinse cells with PBS (10 mL in T75 or 5 mL in T25 flasks).
2. Add 0.5% trypsin–EDTA (2 mL for T75 or 0.5 mL for T25 flasks) and incubate at room temperature for 5 min.
3. Tap cells to detach and add 5 mL DMEM-F12 containing 10% FBS.
4. Mix gently by pipetting up and down and centrifuge at 100 × *g* (Beckman Coulter AllegraTM X-22, SX4250 rotor) for 5 min.
5. Discard medium and resuspend the cells in 3 mL fresh growth medium.
6. Subculture 1 mL cells in 10 mL or 0.5 mL cells in 5 mL DMEM-F12, 10% FBS, in T75 or T25 flasks, respectively. Incubate at 37 °C, 5% CO_2 incubator and monitor cells daily (*see* **Note 9**).

3.2 Intermediate Construct-Mediated Deletion/Foreign Gene Replacement (Traditional Method): Foreign Gene Amplification and Purification

1. Extract nucleic acids from which the foreign gene originates using conventional methods [18] or extraction kits (e.g., ChargeSwitch® gDNA Mini Bacteria Kit, DNAzol® or PureLink® Viral RNA/DNA Mini kit).
2. If foreign gene originates from viral RNA, reverse transcription must be performed by preparing the RNA mix reaction that comes with the SuperScript® III First-Strand Synthesis System for RT-PCR (Invitrogen) in a 0.2 or 0.5 mL tube as follows: 1 μL random hexamers (50 ng/μL, *see* **Note 10**), 1 μL dNTP mix (10 mM), and 1 pg-5 μg RNA. If necessary, complete reaction volume to 10 μL with sterile RNase-free water.
3. Incubate reaction at 65 °C for 5 min, then chill on ice for at least 1 min.
4. In a separate tube, prepare reverse transcription mix as follows: 2 μL 10× reverse transcription buffer, 4 μL 25 mM $MgCl_2$, 2 μL 0.1 M DTT, 1 μL RNaseOUT™ (40 U/μL), and SuperScript® III RT (200 U/μL).
5. Combine RNA and reverse transcription mix.
6. Perform reverse transcription in a thermocycler as follows: 25 °C for 10 min, 50 °C for 50 min, 85 °C for 5 min and 4 °C for indefinitive time.
7. Optional: Add 1 μL *E. coli* RNase H (2 U/μL) and incubate at 37 °C for 20 min.
8. Prepare PCR reaction with high-fidelity KOD Hot Start DNA polymerase (Novagen®) as follows: 5 μL 10× buffer for KOD Hot Start, 3 μL 25 mM $MgSO_4$, 5 μL 2 mM dNTPs, 1.5 μL 10 μM forward primer, 1.5 μL 10 μM reverse primer, template DNA (50–100 ng genomic DNA or 2–5 μL reverse transcription reaction prepared in **step 2**), and 1 μL KOD Hot Start DNA Polymerase (1 U/μL). Complete to 50 μL with sterile deionized water.
9. Program thermocycler as follows: 95 °C for 2 min for polymerase activation followed by 20–40 cycles. Each cycle is performed as follows: 95 °C for 20 s, lowest primer Tm°C for 10 s and 70 °C for 10 s/kb (<500 bp), 15 s/kb (500–1000 bp) or 25 s/kb (3000 bp) (*see* **Note 11**).
10. Run 5 μL PCR reaction in agarose gel with appropriate concentration for amplicon size and 0.2–0.5 μg/mL ethidium bromide. Alternative DNA dyes can be used.
11. Verify amplicon size with appropriate DNA ladders.
12. Purify the PCR product using QIAquick II® Gel Extraction Kit (Qiagen) according to manufacturer's instructions (*see* **Notes 11–15**).

13. Run 1 μL in an agarose gel to verify PCR product and size.
14. Quantitate PCR product in a NanoDrop spectrophotometer.

3.3 Intermediate Construct-Mediated Deletion/Foreign Gene Replacement (Traditional Method): Foreign Gene Cloning Into Expression Vector

1. If plasmid vector (*see* **Note 16**) is in bacteria, perform plasmid mini or midi-prep with plasmid preparation kits (e.g., Qiagen Plasmid mini or midi kits) according to manufacturer's instructions. Alternatively, prepare plasmid using classical methods [18].
2. Quantitate plasmid DNA concentration and verify a small aliquot in an agarose gel.
3. Cut plasmid vector and amplicon (0.5–1 μg) with the appropriate restriction enzymes and conditions (temperature and buffer). In general, 1–2 μg DNA is digested in 50 μL. It is not necessary to digest amplicon for blunt-end cloning.
4. Run 5 μL of digested vector in 1% agarose gel along with DNA ladder. Verify that linearized vector corresponds to the expected size.
5. Purify the digested plasmid and amplicon with QIAquick II® Gel Extraction Kit (Qiagen) following the manufacturer's instructions.
6. Determine DNA concentration in a NanoDrop spectrophotometer.
7. Perform ligation (1:3 vector–insert) in a final volume of 20 μL using Invitrogen reagents as follows: 4 μL 5× T4 DNA ligase buffer, vector (3–30 fmol for sticky- or 15–60 fmol for blunt-end ligation), insert (9–90 fmol for sticky- or 45–180 fmol for blunt-end ligation) and 1 μL T4 DNA ligase (1 U/μL for sticky end and 5 U/μL for blunt-end ligation). Complete to 20 μL with sterile distilled water. Incubate for 1 h at room temperature for sticky end ligation or 16–24 h at 14 °C for blunt end ligation.
8. Transform competent *E. coli* DH5-α by either electroporation or chemical methods reported elsewhere [19]. Plate transformed bacteria onto LB plates containing an appropriate antibiotic for selection. Incubate overnight at 37 °C.
9. Grow single colonies in 2 mL LB (with the appropriate antibiotic) at 37 °C overnight with vigorous agitation.
10. Perform plasmid miniprep using classical methods [19] or kits (e.g., Qiagen plasmid mini kit).
11. Run plasmids in a 0.8% agarose gel. Use empty vector as reference (*see* **Note 17**). It is not necessary to load DNA ladder. Select plasmids that migrate slower than the reference.
12. Digest selected plasmids with an appropriate restriction enzyme and conditions.

13. Run digested plasmids in an agarose gel along with a DNA ladder. Confirm the size of insert.
14. Confirm insert orientation by restriction mapping, PCR or direct sequencing if foreign gene is not directionally cloned (e.g., blunt- or sticky-end cloning with the same restriction sites).

3.4 Intermediate Construct-Mediated Deletion/Foreign Gene Replacement (Traditional Method): Foreign Gene Cloning Into pleftΔ491–2782

1. Phosphorylate foreign gene cassette specific primers with PNK according to manufacturer's instructions. The final concentration of primers in the phosphorylation reaction should be 10 μM. Use 1.5 μL of PNK reaction for PCR.
2. Perform PCR to amplify foreign gene expression cassette DNA from expression vector using KOD DNA polymerase and conditions described in **steps 9** and **10**, Subheading 3.2 (*see* **Note 11**).
3. Purify amplicons with QIAquick II® Gel Extraction Kit (Qiagen). Quantitate amplicon and run agarose gels with DNA ladder to verify amplicon size.
4. Digest pleftΔ491–2782 with SwaI (New England Biolabs) as follows: 5 μL 10× NEB3.1 buffer, 0.5–1 μg pleftΔ491–2782 and 1 μL SwaI (2 U/μL, *see* **Note 18**). Complete to 50 μL with sterile distillated water. Incubate for 1 h at 25 °C.
5. Dephosphorylate SwaI-digested pleftΔ491–2782 with 1 μL Antarctic phosphatase (5 U/μL) at 37 °C for 30 min. Inactivate phosphatase at 70 °C for 5 min.
6. Purify digested pleftΔ491–2782 with QIAquick II® Gel Extraction Kit (Qiagen).
7. Ligate SwaI-digested pleftΔ491–2782 and foreign gene expression cassette using ligation conditions for blunt-end cloning as mentioned in **step** 7, Subheading 3.3.
8. Transform *E. coli* DH5-α by chemical or electroporation methods [19] and grow bacteria in LB-Amp plates. Incubate overnight at 37 °C.
9. Grow single colonies in 2 ml LB-Amp. Incubate overnight at 37 °C with agitation in an orbital shaker.
10. Perform plasmid miniprep using classical methods [19] or kits (e.g., Qiagen plasmid mini kit).
11. Run plasmid DNA in a 0.8% agarose gel. Use empty pleftΔ491–2782 as reference. Select plasmids that migrate slower than the reference (*see* **Note 17**).
12. Confirm the presence of the foreign gene by restriction analysis or PCR with foreign gene specific primers. Determine the orientation of foreign gene by PCR with FAD1 forward primer (nts 281–300 in the viral genome) and foreign gene specific

reverse primer. Rightward orientation generates discrete PCR products while leftward orientation does not. Select clones with both orientations (*see* **Note 19**).

3.5 Intermediate Construct-Mediated Deletion/Foreign Gene Replacement (Traditional Method): Amplification of Foreign Gene Expression Cassette from pleftΔ491–2782

1. PCR amplify foreign gene expression cassette with primers FAdE1F and FAdE1R as described in **step 8**, Subheading 3.2.
2. Program thermocycler as follows: 95 °C for 2 min for polymerase activation followed by 20–40 cycles. Each cycle is performed as follows: 95 °C for 20 s, 50 °C for 10 s, and 70 °C for 25 s (or over, *see* **Note 11**).
3. Verify amplicon size in a 1% agarose gel and purify amplicons with QIAquick II® Gel Extraction Kit (Qiagen).
4. Quantitate DNA with a NanoDrop spectrophotometer.
5. Proceed to Subheading 3.11.

3.6 FAdmid Preparation

1. When DNA of parental FAdmid clones (wt FAdmid, FAdmidΔ1 or FAdmidΔ4) is in low quantities, transform *E. coli* DH5-α using either electroporation or chemical methods [19]. Place bacteria onto LB-Amp plates and incubate overnight at 37 °C.
2. Perform plasmid midi prep with PureLink® HiPure Plasmid Midiprep Kit (Invitrogen) and quantitate FAdmid DNA.
3. When FAdmidΔ4 is used as platform, digest with SwaI as described in **step 4**, Subheading 3.4. When either wt FAdmid or FAdmidΔ1 is used as platform, digest with SgfI (Promega) in a 50 μL reaction as follows: sterile distilled water (to 50 μL final volume), 1–2 μL FAdmid DNA, 5 μL 10X buffer C, 1 μL SgfI (8 U/μL) (*see* **Note 20**). Mix well and gently, and briefly centrifuge to bring all contents to the bottom. Incubate at 37 °C for 1 h.
4. Load around 10 μL reaction in a 0.8% agarose gel to verify complete digestion. Two bands should be clearly visible for wt FAdmid when digested with SgfI: 48 and 1.1 kb. One 48 kb-band should appear for FAdmidΔ1 when digested with SgfI. Digestion of FAdmidΔ4 with SwaI gives one fragment of around 47 kb (Fig. 1a).
5. Purify digested FAdmid(s) with QIAquick II® Gel Extraction Kit (Qiagen). Alternatively, extract with phenol–chloroform followed by ethanol precipitation as follows: (1) Complete total volume to 300 μL with sterile distilled water. (2) Add 1 volume of phenol–chloroform (300 μL), mix well and centrifuge at 16,000 × *g* for 5 min. (3) Take the upper aqueous phase and transfer it to a fresh 1.5 mL tube. (4) Add 1 volume of chloroform (300 μL), mix well and centrifuge for 5 min. (5) Transfer upper aqueous phase to a fresh tube and add 30 μL 3 M sodium

acetate (pH 5.2). Mix well. (6) Add 750 μL cold ethanol (100%), mix well and incubate at −20 °C for at least 20 min. (7). Centrifuge at 16,000 × *g* for 15 min at 4 °C. (8) Discard supernatant and wash the pellet with 300 μL cold 70% ethanol. (9) Centrifuge at 16,000 × *g* for 5 min, discard ethanol and let it evaporate (do not let the pellet overdry, as it would be difficult to resuspend). (10) Resuspend DNA in 30 μL 10 mM Tris–HCl, pH 8.0 and quantify DNA with a NanoDrop.

6. Proceed to Subheading 3.11.

3.7 Lambda Red Recombinase-Mediated Deletion/Foreign Gene Replacement: Generation of CAT Gene Expression Cassette Amplicon from pKD3

1. Perform PCR reaction with CAT forward and reverse primers (Subheading 2.2) as described in **step 8**, Subheading 3.2. In cycling conditions, use 55 °C for annealing temperature.
2. Purify CAT gene expression cassette amplicon (1.1 kb) with QIAquick II® Gel Extraction Kit (Qiagen).

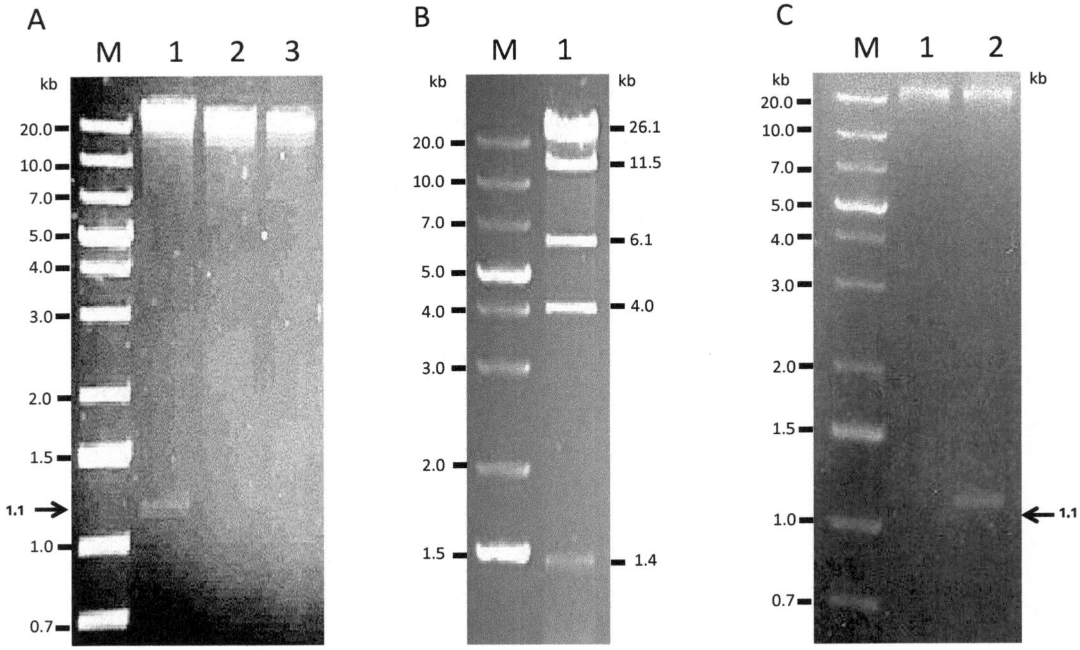

Fig. 1 *Lanes M* correspond to GeneRulerTM 1 kb Plus DNA Ladder (Biogen). Panel (**a**) Banding patterns of wtFAdmid and FAdmidΔ1 digested with SgfI (*lanes 1* and *2*, respectively), and FAdmidΔ4 digested with SwaI(*lane 3*); Panel (**b**) DNA banding pattern of wtFAdmid digested with NotI (*lane 1*); Panel (**c**) SwaI digestion of wtFAdmid (*lane 1*) and CAT-marked FAdmid (*lane 2*). SwaI sites are absent in wtFAdmid while insertion of CAT through homologous recombination incorporates these restriction sites

3.8 Lambda Red Recombinase-Mediated Deletion/Foreign Gene Replacement: Generation of *E. coli* DH10B-Wt FAdmid Stock

1. Pick one colony of *E. coli* DH10B and place it in 25 mL LB-edium. Incubate overnight at 37 °C with vigorous shaking.
2. Add 1 mL overnight culture into 100 mL LB. Incubate at 37 °C with vigorous shaking for around 3 h. Verify that OD_{600} is 0.5. If not, incubate bacteria longer until OD_{600} is 0.5.
3. Chill on ice for 15 min and centrifuge at 3,300 ×*g* (Beckman Coulter, JA-25.50 rotor) for 15 min.
4. Discard supernatant and wash bacterial pellet 2–3 times with 100 mL ice-cold 10% glycerol.
5. Resuspend pellet in 2 mL of ice-cold 10% glycerol.
6. Optional: Make competent bacteria aliquots (200 μL) and store at −80 °C. Stocks are optimal for around 6 months.
7. Transfer 200 μL of bacteria to 0.2 gap electroporation cuvettes and add 2 μg wt FAdmid (*see* **Note 21**).
8. Electroporate at 2500 V for 5 ms. Immediately, add 800 μL of SOC medium onto bacteria, mix and transfer them into culture tubes (*see* **Note 22**). Incubate at 37 °C for 1 h with shaking.
9. Spin down bacteria, discard supernatant, and resuspend pellet in 200 μL LB.
10. Plate bacteria onto LB-Amp agar plates and incubate overnight at 37 °C.
11. Pick individual colonies and grow them in 5 mL LB-Amp. Next day, perform plasmid mini prep and verify wt FAdmid with NotI (Fig. 1b).
12. Grow bacteria with verified wt FAdmid in LB-Amp plates and incubate overnight at 37 °C.
13. Pick one colony and grow bacteria in 5 mL LB-Amp overnight at 37 °C.
14. Centrifuge bacteria at 800 ×*g* (Beckman Coulter, JA-25.50 rotor) for 10 min.
15. Resuspend bacterial pellet in 5 mL of fresh LB-Amp containing 30% glycerol.
16. Aliquot bacteria stock and store at −80 °C.

3.9 Lambda Red Recombinase-Mediated Deletion/Foreign Gene Replacement: Generation of *E. coli* DH10B-Wt FAdmid-pJW103 Stock

1. Pick one colony of *E. coli* DH10B-wt FAdmid and place it in 25 ml LB-Amp, and incubate overnight at 37 °C with vigorous shaking.
2. Prepare competent *E. coli* DH10B-wt FAdmid for electroporation as described in **steps 2–6** of Subheading 3.8, except that bacteria have to be cultured in LB-Amp.
3. Electroporate 2 μg pJW103 (carrying the kanamycin resistance gene and lambda Red recombinase) into *E. coli* DH10B-FAdmid as described in **steps 8** and **9** of Subheading 3.8, except that the incubation temperature is 30 °C.

4. Plate culture onto LB-Amp-Kan agar plates at 30 °C.
5. Pick one colony and prepare *E. coli* DH10B-wt FAdmid-pJW103 stock as described in **steps 12–16**, Subheading 3.8, except that the incubation temperature is 30 °C.

3.10 Lambda Red Recombinase-Mediated Deletion/Foreign Gene Replacement: Generation of CAT-Marked FAdmids

1. Scratch a frozen stock of *E. coli* DH10B-FAdmid-pJW103 (prepared in Subheading 3.9) with a sterile inoculating loop and seed bacteria onto a LB-Amp-Kan plate. Incubate overnight at 30 °C. Bacterial colonies are usually visible at 16–20 h.
2. Prepare competent *E. coli* DH10B-FAdmid-pJW103 as described in **steps 2–5**, Subheading 3.8.
3. Add 1 μg (in 50 μL maximum volume) of purified CAT amplicon (generated in Subheading 3.7) into 350 μL of freshly prepared *E. coli* DH10B-wt FAdmid-pJW103.
4. Electroporate as described in **step 8**, Subheading 3.8.
5. While bacteria are in the cuvette, immediately add 600 μL SOC plus 10 μL 10% arabinose (0.1% final concentration). Mix well and transfer bacteria into sterile tubes and incubate overnight at 30 °C with vigorous shaking (*see* **Note 22**).
6. The following day, plate bacteria onto LB-Amp-Cam agar plates. Incubate at 37 °C for 16–24 h.
7. Pick individual colonies (*see* **Note 23**) and grow them in 5 ml LB-Amp-Cam at 37 °C overnight with vigorous shaking.
8. Perform plasmid mini prep using classical methods or kits. Analyze "CAT-marked FAdmids" by SwaI digestion (49 and 1.1 kb fragments, Fig. 1c). Alternatively, perform PCR using primers located upstream and downstream the deletion/CAT insertion sites. PCR products can increase or decrease in size with respect to parental wt FAdmid depending on size of deleted ORFs.
9. Remove CAT gene expression cassette by SwaI digestion as mentioned in **step 4**, Subheading 3.4. Purify FAdmid DNA as described in **step 5**, Subheading 3.6.
10. When cloning by homologous recombination (Subheading 3.11), PCR amplify foreign gene expression cassette from expression vector (prepared in Subheading 3.3) with primers containing 50 bp viral DNA homologous arms, a restriction site (optional) and the first 20 bp of foreign gene expression cassette. Use the same PCR reaction and cycling conditions as described in Subheading 3.2.
11. When cloning by classical ligation, PCR amplify foreign gene expression cassette from expression vector as described in **steps 9** and **10**, Subheading 3.2 followed by purification with QIAquick II® Gel Extraction Kit (Qiagen) and quantitation.
12. Perform blunt-end ligation (1:3 vector–insert) as described in **step 7**, Subheading 3.3.

3.11 Generation of Recombinant FAdmid Clones by homologous Recombination in *E. coli* BJ5183

1. Scratch a frozen bacterial stock of *E. coli* BJ5183 with a sterile inoculation loop and transfer bacteria to an LB-agar-Str plate. Do not let the bacterial stock thaw (*see* **Note 24**).
2. Incubate overnight at 37 °C, and the following day move the plate to room temperature. Do not place it at 4 °C.
3. Pick one colony and place it into 10 mL LB-Str. Incubate overnight at 37 °C with vigorous shaking.
4. Take 0.5 mL overnight culture and transfer into 50 mL LB-Str medium containing 10 mM $MgSO_4$.
5. Incubate at 37 °C with vigorous shaking for about 2–4 h until OD_{600} is 0.5.
6. Chill on ice for 10 min. Transfer bacterial culture into a pre-chilled 50 mL tube and centrifuge at 800×*g* (Beckman Coulter JA-25.50 rotor) for 10 min at 4 °C. Downstream procedures should be done on ice.
7. Discard supernatant and resuspend bacterial pellet with 10 mL of cold RF1 buffer.
8. Incubate on ice for 1 h.
9. Centrifuge at 400×*g* (Beckman Coulter, JA-25.50 rotor) for 15 min. Discard supernatant and resuspend pellet with 2 mL RF2 buffer. Incubate on ice for 15 min.
10. Take 100 μL bacterial aliquot per transformation. Discard the rest of competent bacteria.
11. Co-transform bacteria with 100–200 ng of gene expression cassette amplicon (prepared in Subheadings 3.5 or 3.7) with 10–20 ng restriction enzyme digested FAdmids (prepared in Subheadings 3.6 or 3.10).
12. Mix gently and incubate on ice for 30 min.
13. Heat-shock bacteria by rapidly placing them at 42 °C (in waterbath) for 1.5 min.
14. Chill bacteria on ice for 5 min.
15. Add 800 μL SOC or LB medium (without antibiotics) and incubate for 1 h at 37 °C in a water bath.
16. Centrifuge bacteria at 500 × *g* for 10 min. Discard medium leaving 200 μL medium.
17. Resuspend bacteria gently by pipetting up and down and plate them onto LB-Amp plates using a sterile glass rod.
18. Incubate overnight at 37 °C.
19. Using sterile toothpicks, pick several colonies and place them in tubes containing 2 mL LB-ampicillin medium.
20. Perform plasmid mini preps using classical method [18].

21. Run FAdmids in a 0.8% agarose gel. Use empty parental FAdmid as a reference. Choose plasmids that migrate differently from empty FAdmids.
22. Digest selected recombinant (r) FAdmids with NotI or any other restriction enzyme that allows the identification of foreign gene. If foreign gene cannot be clearly verified by restriction analysis, perform PCR with foreign gene specific primers (*see* **Note 25**).
23. Transform verified rFAdmids in *E. coli* DH5-α (*see* **Note 26**).
24. Perform plasmid midi preps and quantitate rFAdmid DNA.
25. Digest rFAdmids with PacI (New England Biolabs) and purify as follows: (1) Add distilled water (up to 300 μL), 30 μL 10× CutSmart® Buffer (or 10× NEBuffer 1.1), 10 μg rFAdmid DNA, and 2 μL PacI (10 U/μL). (2) Mix gently and briefly centrifuge to bring down all reaction to the bottom of the tube. (3) Incubate for 1–2 h at 37 °C. (4) Purify DNA with QIAquick II® Gel Extraction Kit (Qiagen) or with phenol–chloroform extraction and ethanol precipitation as described in **step 5**, Subheading 3.6). Quantitate digested DNA.
26. For transfection, subculture 2 × 10^6 CH-SAH cells in 35 mm dishes as described in Subheading 3.1 using antibiotic-free DMEM-F12 medium (Sigma-Aldrich), 10% FBS. The total volume for 35 mm diameter dishes should be 2 mL. Incubate the cells overnight at 37 °C in 5% CO_2 (*see* **Note 27**).
27. Proceed to Subheading 3.12.

3.12 Transfection to Generate Recombinant Viruses

1. Transfection control (no DNA, *see* **Note 28**). For one dish, dilute 10 μL Lipofectamine 2000 in 300 μL Opti-MEM.
2. DNA transfection: For one dish, prepare 2 tubes (tubes A and B) containing 150 μL Opti-MEM each. Add 10 μL Lipofectamine 2000 in tube A and 2–4 μg PacI-digested rFAdmids (generated in Subheading 3.11, **step 25**) in tube B. Mix gently and incubate for 5 min. Combine tubes A and B and mix gently. Incubate for another 20–30 min.
3. Add the whole mixture of either transfection control or DNA transfection reaction (300 μL) onto dishes containing cells and medium. Incubate overnight at 37 °C, 5% CO_2. Check for toxicity the following day. If toxicity is evident, withdraw the lipofectamine–DNA complexes and replace with growth medium. CPE should appear at 3–5 days post-transfection (Fig. 2b).
4. After CPE is complete (Fig. 2c), place dishes at −80 °C and perform three cycles of freezing and thawing.
5. Harvest cells and virus and split them into 1.5 mL tubes. Centrifuge at 16,000 × *g* for 30 s and transfer supernatant (virus) to fresh 1.5 mL tubes.

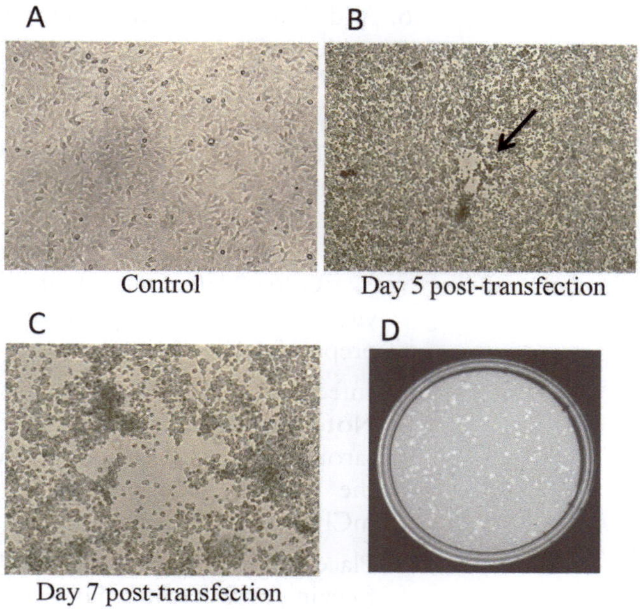

Fig. 2 Cytopathic effect (CPE) at different days post-transfection of CH-SAH cells with PacI-digested wtFAdmid. Panel (**a**) Uninfected cells. First, CPE is localized to one region of the monolayer (panel (**b**); *arrow*) and continues to expand throughout the cell culture (panel (**c**)). Panel (**d**) Wild-type FAdV-9 plaques in CH-SAH cells

3.13 Plaque Assay to Titrate Recombinant Virus

1. Subculture CH-SAH cells as described in cell culture passage (**steps 1–5**, Subheading 3.1). Count cells with hemocytometer or cell counter and adjust concentration of CH-SAH cells to seed 2.2×10^6 cells/well in 6-well plates.
2. Make tenfold serial dilutions of the virus in six 1.5 mL tubes from 10^{-1} to 10^{-6}. Using 1 mL-filter tips, add 900 μL serum-free DMEM-F12 in each tube. Transfer 100 μL of virus to the first tube (10^{-1}) with a 200 μL-filter tip. Discard tip and mix by vortexing. Transfer 100 μL virus to the next tube with a fresh 200 μL-tip. Repeat this step up to 10^{-6} dilution. Change tips for each dilution. Discard 100 μL from last dilution.
3. Remove cell culture medium from cells and add 0.5 mL of serum-free DMEM-F12. Add 100 μL/well from each virus dilution (vortex prior) to infection).
4. Incubate cells at room temperature with gentle rocking for 1 h.
5. In a laminar flow hood, remove virus from cells, rinse the cells twice with PBS and quickly (but gently) add DMEM-agarose (Subheading 2.7, and *see* **Note 29**). Let medium harden for 10 min with the lid partially open to remove excess of moisture. Close the lids and incubate cells at 37 °C, 5% CO_2, for 3 days.

6. Add 0.5 mL 0.015% neutral red-containing DMEM-F12 medium, 5% FBS, for each well (see Subheading 2.7). Incubate at 37 °C, 5% CO_2, for another 2–3 days.
7. Count plaques (Fig. 2d) and calculate the virus titer as follows: number of plaques × 10× dilution factor; express titer as plaque forming unit/mL (pfu/mL).

3.14 Preparation of Recombinant Virus Stock

1. Seed 6 × 10^7 cells in 15 cm diameter dishes. Incubate cells at 37 °C for 24 h. One set of dishes is used for preparation of virus stocks and at least one dish is used for viral DNA preparation.
2. Infect cells at multiplicity of infection (MOI) of 0.1 (*see* **Note 30**). Incubate cells at 37 °C until CPE is complete (around 5 days). Use an inverted fluorescent microscope when the foreign gene product is a fluorescent protein (GFP, mCherry, YFP, RFP, etc.).
3. Place dishes with cells at −80 °C and perform three cycles of freezing and thawing. Harvest virus and cells (after mixing by pipetting up and down) and transfer them into sterile centrifuge tubes.
4. Centrifuge cells at 3,300 × *g* (Beckman Coulter, rotor JA-25.50) at 4 °C, for 15 min. Collect supernatants and centrifuge again.
5. Collect supernatants to fresh tubes. For storage of virus stocks, aliquot virus in cryovials and store at −80 °C. Thaw one cryovial and titrate virus stock as described in Subheading 3.13. For viral DNA preparation, proceed to Subheading 3.15.

3.15 Viral DNA Preparation and Restriction Enzyme Analysis

1. For virus concentration slowly and gently add cleared supernatant onto ultracentrifuge tubes containing prechilled 30% sucrose in TNE buffer (Subheading 2.9). Tubes must be filled 2–3 mm from the top (*see* **Note 31**). This procedure is performed on ice.
2. Balance the tubes and centrifuge them at 100,000 × *g* using an SW-28 (or SW-32Ti) rotor in a Beckman Coulter (e.g., OptimaTM L.-80 XP) ultracentrifuge at 4 °C for 2 h.
3. Carefully remove all liquid from the viral pellet (whitish color).
4. Add 200 μL TNE buffer to viral pellet. Do not resuspend pellet by pipetting up and down. Cover tubes with Parafilm and incubate at 4 °C overnight. Next day, resuspend the pellet by gentle pipetting and transfer the virus to a sterile 1.5 mL tube.
5. Determine the final volume of the concentrated virus. Take one volume of 2× lysis buffer and add 1 μL 100 mg/mL proteinase K for 1 mL 2× lysis buffer (Subheading 2.9). Mix virus preparation with 2× lysis buffer (1:1) and incubate at 37 °C overnight.

6. Extract DNA with one volume of phenol–chloroform. Mix well and centrifuge at 16,000 × *g* for 5 min. Transfer the upper aqueous phase to a fresh tube and add one volume of chloroform. Centrifuge at 16,000 × *g* for 5 min.
7. Transfer aqueous phase into a fresh 1.5 mL tube and add 2.5 volumes of cold absolute ethanol (around 1 mL). Incubate at −20 °C for 1 h, and centrifuge at 16,000 × *g* for 15 min.
8. Wash pellet with 70% ethanol, discard ethanol and allow the reminder to evaporate. Do not overdry the pellet; otherwise, it will be difficult to resuspend.
9. Resuspend viral DNA in 50–100 μL 10 mM Tris–HCl, pH 8.0 and quantitate it.
10. Digest 1–2 μg DNA with NotI or any other restriction enzyme that can help confirm the presence of foreign gene (*see* **Note 25**). The presence of the foreign gene can be also detected by PCR using specific primers.

3.16 Detection of Foreign Gene Expression

1. Seed 5 × 10^6 cells in 6 cm diameter dish and incubate at 37 °C for 24 h.
2. Remove medium and infect the cells with a recombinant virus at an MOI of 5–10.
3. Incubate the cells at room temperature for 1 h in a rocking platform.
4. Remove virus and add 4–5 mL of DMEM-F12 medium containing 5% FBS. Incubate cells at 37 °C for various time points (*see* **Note 32**).
5. Discard medium (unless foreign protein is secreted) and immediately place dishes on ice. Wash cells with ice-cold PBS.
6. Aspirate PBS and add 0.5 mL ice-cold lysis buffer (RIPA, *see* Subheading 2.10 and **Note 33**).
7. Scrape cells off the dish using a cold plastic cell scraper, then gently transfer the cell suspension into a precooled 1.5 mL-microcentrifuge tube.
8. Incubate on ice for 20 min.
9. Sonicate three times (10 min pulse, 10% amplitude) (*see* **Note 33**).
10. Centrifuge in a refrigerated microcentrifuge at 16,000 × *g* for 20 min.
11. Transfer supernatant to a fresh ice-cold 1.5 mL-tube. Quantitate protein (e.g., Bradford assay).
12. Calculate the volume required to take 10–20 μg protein. Add Laemmli buffer to have a final concentration of 1×.

13. Heat-treat the samples at 95–100 °C for 5 min.
14. Quickly chill samples on ice for at least 5 min.
15. Prepare SDS-PAGE gels and running buffers as described elsewhere [20] taking into account the size of the foreign protein for appropriate gel concentration. Load protein in SDS-PAGE gel and run it according to manufacturer's instructions: For example, Mini-PROTEAN® vertical electrophoresis chamber can be run at 100 V for approximately 1.5 h.
16. Perform Western blot analysis as described [20].

3.17 *In Vivo* Testing of Recombinant Viruses: Housing, Grouping and Wing Tagging

1. Plan the number of chickens needed for animal experiment according to the number of recombinant viruses to be tested. One-day-old chicks are housed according to federal, provincial and/or institutional animal care and use policies.
2. Group chicks in separate isolators for each treatment. Normally, each group consists of 15–20 chicks. One group is the mock-infected control (usually PBS) while other groups are inoculated with recombinant viruses. A group of chickens inoculated with wtFAdV-9 (or the parental deleted virus) should be also included (*see* **Note 34**).
3. At 1 week of age the chicks are wing tagged (*see* **Note 35**).

3.18 *In Vivo* Testing of Recombinant Viruses: Blood Collection

1. Restrain by holding the bird with the nondominant hand and ensure that its head is between the base of the index and middle fingers. Tuck the legs under the body and against the palm. Extend the left wing and hold it between the tip of the index and middle fingers.
2. Locate the brachial vein and disinfect the area with 70% ethanol using a gauze pad.
3. With a 25-G needle, quickly puncture the brachial vein and collect blood by placing a 1.5 mL tube at the puncture site. Place a gauze pad for around 1 min to stop the bleeding. Collected blood before virus inoculation corresponds to day 0. Collect blood samples at days 7, 14, 21, 35, and 42 (or according to the experimental design) after virus inoculation (Subheading 3.19).

3.19 *In Vivo* Testing of Recombinant Viruses: Virus Inoculation

1. Prepare the required amount of virus in PBS so that 2×10^6 to 5×10^6 pfu/chicken can be delivered in 0.2 mL.
2. Use 12.5 mm (1/2″), 19 gauge needles and 200 μL tips for intramuscular and oral inoculations, respectively (*see* **Notes 19** and **36**).
3. Boost-inoculate 2 weeks after the first inoculation.

3.20 In Vivo Testing of Recombinant Viruses: Serum Preparation, Animal Euthanization and Detection of Antibody to Foreign Protein

1. Incubate blood at 4 °C overnight. Centrifuge at 100 × *g* for 10 minutes and transfer sera to fresh 1.5 mL tubes. Store at −20 °C.
2. Euthanize chickens according to animal care and use policies.
3. Perform ELISA assays using specific conditions for detection of antibodies to foreign protein.

4 Notes

1. In our experience, PureLink® HiPure Plasmid Midiprep Kit renders high FAdmid yields relative to other commercial midi prep kits. Classical methods for FAdmid preparation can also produce high yields.
2. FAdE1F and FAdE1R primers generate a PCR product size of 2078 bp without foreign expression cassette. Insertion of foreign gene will increase the PCR product size. PCR extension times should be 25 s or over depending on the whole amplicon size.
3. Design CAT primers with 49–50 bp homologous flanking arms (N). SwaI is a rare-cutter restriction enzyme that is not present in the FAdmid DNA and has been used for cloning foreign genes [4]. Other rare-cutter restriction sites can be incorporated into FAdmid in place of SwaI. PCR conditions using 78–81 nt long oligonucleotides may require optimization such as annealing and extension times and temperatures.
4. Primers with different restriction sites should be designed for directional cloning of foreign gene into expression vectors. We recommend performing nucleotide sequence analysis prior to primer design to avoid the incorporation of restriction sites present inside the foreign gene. Online programs are available for restriction enzyme analysis such as Nebcutter [21]. Restriction sites in primers should be located at certain distance downstream the 5′ end. For example, BamHI requires at least three nucleotides from the end for efficient cutting. For further information about restriction digestion close to the end of DNA fragments, go to https://www.neb.com/tools-and-resources/usage-guidelines/cleavage-close-to-the-end-of-dna-fragments.
5. Use ultraclean plasticware or glassware for preparation of reagents RF1 and RF2. Also, use designated glassware for preparation of competent bacteria only. Glassware should be cleaned thoroughly and rinsed with MQ water several times. To ensure glassware cleanness, fill with MQ water and autoclave for 30 min. Discard autoclaved water and let glassware dry. Traces of detergent can significantly decrease the efficiency of competent bacteria.

6. If the pH of RF1 buffer drops below 5.8, discard and prepare a fresh buffer. Raising the pH with a base will cause $MnCl_2$ to precipitate. $MnCl_2$ also precipitates if autoclaved.
7. Autoclaving RF2 buffer is not recommended due to MOPS. Though its buffer capacity is not compromised after autoclaving, MOPS turns to yellow. The yellow breakdown identity is unknown and the effects on bacterial competency have not been determined.
8. RF1 and RF2 buffers should be freshly prepared at least 1 day before preparation of competent bacteria.
9. Subculture CH-SAH cells to achieve 70–80% confluency within 18–24 h. Lower cell densities can cause cell death or significant delays in cell division. When cells reach full confluency, split cells 1/3–1/4 to fresh flasks. Alternatively, count cells and subculture between 5×10^6 and 1×10^7 cells in T75 flasks to achieve 70–80% [22]. Passage number should be recorded in each passage. For optimal virus yields, use low passage cells (below 70). Cells beyond passage 70 usually undergo morphological changes, significant decrease in proliferation and death.
10. In our experience, random primers (hexamers) render higher yields of target cDNA for PCR amplification.
11. PCR reaction and cycling conditions for each foreign gene have to be optimized to generate high amplicon yields. Normally, around 5% of DNA is lost after purification with QIAquick II® Gel Extraction Kit (Qiagen).
12. QIAquick II® Gel Extraction Kit (Qiagen) is suitable for fragments from 40 bp to 50 kb. Use QIAquick Nucleotide Removal Kit for purification of smaller fragments.
13. Thin agarose gels usually leads to better DNA recovery when using the QIAquick II® Gel Extraction Kit (Qiagen). It is extremely important that agarose gels be completely melted for optimal recovery. During DNA elution from gel, do not vortex when fragments are larger than 10 kb (e.g., FAdmid DNA).
14. Agarose gels beyond 2% requires 6 volumes of QX1 buffer and longer incubation times at 50 °C to ensure complete melting. DNA recovery decreases as the concentration of regular agarose increases. We recommend low melting point agarose gels when high concentrations (>2%) are required. Low melting point agarose gels require less QX1 buffer and incubation times.
15. We recommend 10 mM Tris–HCl buffer instead of water for elution of DNA.

16. Strong promoters such as CMV and CAG can be used for foreign gene expression. In addition to promoters, expression vectors should also contain foreign gene downstream elements (promoter, poly-A signal, and transcription termination site).
17. Uncut plasmids appear as three bands in an agarose gel. The supercoiled DNA, the fastest migrating form, is predominant in optimal plasmid preparations.
18. SwaI comes at 10,000 U/μL. The enzyme can be diluted to the desired concentration in storage buffer (10 mM Tris–HCl, 400 mM NaCl, 1 mM DTT, 0.1 mM EDTA, 200 μg/mL BSA, 50% glycerol, pH 7.4 at 25 °C).
19. Plasmid with both orientations should be selected for generation of recombinant viruses. Recombinant viruses with foreign gene at both orientations are tested in vitro (in cells) to determine differences in foreign protein levels. Subsequently, these viruses are tested in vivo (chickens). Regardless of orientation and protein levels in in vitro, recombinant virus that best elicits seroconversion to foreign protein is regarded as the best candidate vaccine.
20. AsiSI restriction enzyme (New England Biolabs) can be used in place of SgfI (isoschizomer of AsiSI).
21. Volumes up to 400 μL of competent bacteria can fit into 0.2 mm Gap electroporation cuvette. We recommend using between 10 and 50 μL amplicon DNA for transformation.
22. Transformation efficiency dramatically decreases when SOC medium is not added immediately onto bacteria after electroporation.
23. Few colonies are generally visible after overnight incubation. However, over 90% of colonies carry CAT-marked FAdmids.
24. *E. coli* BJ5183 competent bacteria for homologous recombination purposes should be freshly prepared. Homologous recombination efficiency drops when competent bacteria is stored at −80 °C. Preparation of competent bacteria from colonies in plates stored at 4 °C has significant decreases in homologous recombination and transformation efficiencies.
25. Nucleotide sequence analysis is strongly recommended before generation of recombinant FAdmid. Complete nucleotide sequence of FAdV-9 is available in the Genebank database (accession NC_000899). Online software programs (NEBcutter, New England Biolabs) are available for prediction of restriction patterns. In some situations, the size of foreign gene cassette does not clearly show differences with NotI with respect to parental FAdmid. In other situations, NotI banding patterns change depending on location of deletion/replacement, size and presence of internal NotI sites in the foreign

gene. Alternatively, PCR using foreign gene specific primers or primers flanking the deletion/insertion regions can be used. If primers flanking the deletion/insertion regions are used, expected PCR product sizes can vary depending on size of deleted viral DNA fragments and foreign gene.

26. Phenol–chloroform extraction is very important when classical methods are used [18] to prepare FAdmids from *E. coli* BJ5183. Transformation efficiency in *E. coli* DH5-α is very low with FAdmids that are not phenol–chloroform extracted. Furthermore, very low FAdmid yields are recovered from *E. coli* BJ5183. For screening of recombinant FAdmids from *E. coli* BJ5183 by restriction analysis, use at least half the FAdmid preparation.
27. CH-SAH cells at low passage (50–65) should be used for transfection. Transfection efficiency significantly decreases in cells over passage 70. Cells should be subcultured at densities not less than 90% to compensate toxicity by lipofectamine. If chicken hepatoma cell lines (CH-SAH, LMH) are not available, primary chicken embryo liver (CELi) cells can be used instead.
28. Lipofectamine 2000 alone has moderate toxicity in CH-SAH cells after incubation overnight. Always include a lipofectamine control (no DNA) to monitor toxicity.
29. DMEM-agarose should be kept warm to prevent agarose from hardening. When several 6-well plates are used, it is recommended to pour between 2 and 4 plates at a time to avoid cells to dry out (after virus removal) and DMEM-agarose to cool down quickly and harden. Place DMEM-agarose back to the 42 °C waterbath, allow it to warm up for a few minutes and mix to ensure even warming. Then, repeat this procedure with the next 2–4 plates. Though this procedure should be quickly performed to avoid agarose from hardening, DMEM-agarose should be gently poured onto cells to prevent detachment.
30. Low MOI is recommended for preparation of virus stocks and viral DNA. Infections at higher MOIs may generate defective interfering particles (DIPs) [23].
31. Virus-containing supernatant has to be added onto the sucrose cushion slowly and gently. It is important to perform this step on ice. Tubes will collapse if not completely filled. If amount of supernatant is not sufficient to reach the recommended volume, complete with medium up to 2–3 mm from the top.
32. We recommend harvesting cells before complete CPE develops. Extensive CPE can cause foreign protein degradation. Incubation times may require optimization according to foreign protein stability and cellular location.

33. RIPA buffer is generally recommended for protein extraction. Cell surface proteins are known to solubilize well in RIPA buffer. Alternatively, use NP-40 lysis buffer (150 mM NaCl, 1.0% NP-40, 50 mM Tris–HCl, pH 8.0) to solubilize cell surface proteins. Treatment of cells with trypsin is not recommended for analysis of cell surface proteins. Sonication is recommended for optimal lysis, although optional. Samples should become nearly transparent after sonication. Sonication should be performed on ice.
34. Animal work requires careful planning. Materials should be ready in advance and restricted to the given isolator. To avoid cross contamination among animal groups, the workflow should be as follows: (1) mock-infected controls, (2) recombinant virus groups, (3) parental viruses with deletions (e.g., FAdV-9Δ1, Δ4, ΔORF11), and/or (4) wtFAdV-9 group.
35. For convenience, list wing tag numbers for each group. Personnel must be trained for animal handling. Animals should be monitored daily.
36. Virus dose may require optimization depending on the antigenicity of foreign protein.

Acknowledgments

This work was supported by grants from the Natural Sciences and Engineering Research Council of Canada (NSERC), the Canadian Poultry Research Council (CPRC), and the Ontario Ministry of Agriculture, Food and Rural Affairs (OMAFRA) to É.N.

References

1. Wold WS, Toth K (2013) Adenovirus vectors for gene therapy, vaccination and cancer gene therapy. Curr Gene Ther 13:421–433
2. Pei Y, Griffin B, de Jong J et al (2015) Rapid generation of fowl adenovirus 9 vectors. J Virol Methods 223:75–81
3. Corredor JC, Nagy E (2011) Antibody response and virus shedding of chickens inoculated with left end deleted fowl adenovirus 9-based recombinant viruses. Avian Dis 55:443–446
4. Corredor JC, Nagy E (2010) The non-essential left end region of the fowl adenovirus 9 genome is suitable for foreign gene insertion/replacement. Virus Res 149:167–174
5. Cherenova LV, Logunov DY, Shashkova EV et al (2004) Recombinant avian adenovirus CELO expressing the human interleukin-2: characterization in vitro, in ovo and in vivo. Virus Res 100:257–261
6. Francois A, Chevalier C, Delmas B et al (2004) Avian adenovirus CELO recombinants expressing VP2 of infectious bursal disease virus induce protection against bursal disease in chickens. Vaccine 22:2351–2360
7. Johnson MA, Pooley C, Ignjatovic J et al (2003) A recombinant fowl adenovirus expressing the S1 gene of infectious bronchitis virus protects against challenge with infectious bronchitis virus. Vaccine 21:2730–2736
8. Sheppard M, Werner W, Tsatas E et al (1998) Fowl adenovirus recombinant expressing VP2 of infectious bursal disease virus induces protective immunity against bursal disease. Arch Virol 143:915–930
9. Shashkova EV, Cherenova LV, Kazansky DB et al (2005) Avian adenovirus vector CELO-TK displays anticancer activity in human cancer cells and suppresses established murine melanoma tumors. Cancer Gene Ther 12:617–626

10. Ojkic D, Nagy E (2001) The long repeat region is dispensable for fowl adenovirus replication in vitro. Virology 283:197–206
11. Corredor JC, Nagy E (2010) A region at the left end of the fowl adenovirus 9 genome that is non-essential in vitro has consequences in vivo. J Gen Virol 91:51–58
12. Chartier C, Degryse E, Gantzer M et al (1996) Efficient generation of recombinant adenovirus vectors by homologous recombination in *Escherichia coli*. J Virol 70:4805–4810
13. Michou AI, Lehrmann H, Saltik M et al (1999) Mutational analysis of the avian adenovirus CELO, which provides a basis for gene delivery vectors. J Virol 73:1399–1410
14. Ojkic D, Nagy E (2000) The complete nucleotide sequence of fowl adenovirus type 8. J Gen Virol 81:1833–1837
15. McVey D, Zuber M, Ettyreddy D et al (2002) Rapid construction of adenoviral vectors by lambda phage genetics. J Virol 76: 3670–3677
16. Deng L, Sharif S, Nagy E (2013) Oral inoculation of chickens with a candidate fowl adenovirus 9 vector. Clin Vaccine Immunol 20: 1189–1196
17. Gay M, Castro F, Paz G et al. (2015) Development of a vectorized fowl adenovirus vaccine expressing the hemagglutinin gene of influenza virus subtype H5. 9th International Symposium on avian influenza. Athens, Georgia, USA. April 12–15, 2015
18. Green MR, Sambrook J (2012) Isolation and quantification of DNA. In: Inglis J, Boyle A, Gann A (eds) Molecular cloning: a laboratory manual, Fourth edn, vol 1. Cold Spring Harbor laboratory Press, Cold Spring Harbor, NY, pp 11–71
19. Green MR, Sambrook J (2012) Cloning and transformation with plasmid vectors. In: Inglis J, Boyle A, Gann A (eds) Molecular cloning: a laboratory manual, Fourth edn, vol 1. Cold Spring Harbor laboratory Press, Cold Spring Harbor, NY, pp 157–258
20. Green MR, Sambrook J (2012) Expressing cloned genes for protein production, purification, and analysis. In: Inglis J, Boyle A, Gann A (eds) Molecular cloning: a laboratory manual, Fourth edn, vol 1. Cold Spring Harbor laboratory Press, Cold Spring Harbor, NY, pp 1483–1634
21. Vincze T, Posfai J, Roberts RJ (2003) NEBcutter: a program to cleave DNA with restriction enzymes. Nucleic Acids Res 31:3688–3691
22. Alexander HS, Huber P, Cao J et al (1998) Growth characteristics of fowl adenovirus type 8 in a chicken hepatoma cell line. J Virol Methods 74:9–14
23. Wickham TJ, Davis T, Granados RR et al (1991) Baculovirus defective interfering particles are responsible for variations in recombinant protein production as a function of multiplicity of infection. Biotechnol Lett 13:483–488

Chapter 4

Development of Recombinant HSV-Based Vaccine Vectors

Richard Voellmy, David C. Bloom, Nuria Vilaboa, and Joyce Feller

Abstract

Herpes simplex virus (HSV) causes significant morbidity on the human population through such clinical syndromes as cold sores, genital herpes, herpes stromal keratitis, and encephalitis. Attempts to generate efficacious vaccines to date have failed. We have recently described the use of a conditionally replication-competent HSV-1 vector to immunize mice against a lethal challenge of HSV-1. The unique feature of this vaccine vector is that its replication is tightly controlled and can only occur in the presence of local heat and the presence of a small molecule inducer (an antiprogestin). This gives it the safety advantage of a replication-defective vaccine vector as well as the advantage of a replication-competent vector in that it is able to stimulate innate and adaptive aspects of the immune response in a natural context that a replication-defective vector cannot. In this chapter we provide a brief overview of HSV vaccines followed by the methodology used to propagate and utilize replication-conditional HSV vectors as vaccines.

Key words Herpesvirus, Vaccine, Vector, Heat-inducible, Heat shock promoter, Antiprogestin

1 Introduction

Human herpes simplex virus (HSV-1, HSV-2) belongs to the subfamily of alpha-herpesviruses (*see* Ref. 1 for a review). They are enveloped, double-stranded DNA viruses that infect epithelial cells as well as other types of cells. HSV has a linear DNA genome of >150 kbp that contains >90 ORFs and encodes about 80 proteins. Gene expression occurs sequentially, immediate-early genes being activated before early genes, and early genes before late genes. Generally, immediate-early genes express regulatory proteins, early genes express enzymes and late genes encode structural proteins. The viruses cause efficient cell lysis but are also capable of latently infecting sensory nerve cells from which they may be induced to reactivate, causing virus shedding and symptomatic disease in a fraction of infected individuals.

HSV-1 is primarily transmitted by oral–oral contact which results in orolabial herpes (cold sores). In developed countries, HSV-1 is also the most common cause of sporadic encephalitis in children and adults. HSV-1 is highly prevalent, and the infection is

Maureen C. Ferran and Gary R. Skuse (eds.), *Recombinant Virus Vaccines: Methods and Protocols*, Methods in Molecular Biology, vol. 1581, DOI 10.1007/978-1-4939-6869-5_4,

life-long, i.e., it is never cleared. The most recent estimate has the worldwide prevalence at 67% (3709 million people aged 0–49 years) [2, 3]. Genital infections by HSV-1 have been on the rise, in particular in developed countries in which an estimated 140 million people are infected. HSV-2 is almost entirely sexually transmitted and is, therefore, most closely associated with genital herpes which involves symptomatic or asymptomatic virus shedding and, in a fraction of those affected, the periodic appearance of often painful genital lesions. The 2012 global prevalence of HSV-2 infection has been estimated at 11.3% or approximately 417 million people aged 15–49 years.

Although not for lack of effort, there is presently no effective vaccine available for HSV-1 or HSV-2. Nevertheless, in a large study on HSV-1/HSV-2 seronegative women, a HSV-2 glycoprotein D (gD2 or, generically, gD) subunit vaccine was 35% effective in preventing HSV-1 infection and 58% effective against HSV-1 genital disease [4]. Herpes zoster virus (VZV) is an alphaherpesvirus that causes varicella in the young and that can reactivate to cause herpes zoster in aged persons. That a highly effective live attenuated vaccine (delivered in two doses) against varicella as well as a reasonably efficacious vaccine against herpes zoster disease has been developed suggests that it should also be possible to create effective vaccines against HSV, although it has been pointed out that HSV and VZV display significantly different pathophysiologies [5, 6].

Most HSV vaccine strains have been derived from HSV-2 isolates. This choice appears rational given that most efforts have been directed at genital herpes, and genital herpes is specifically caused by HSV-2. Furthermore, as mentioned above, HSV-2 antigens were found to cross-protect against HSV-1. It is noted, however, that the converse is also true: certain HSV-1 vaccine strains were shown to protect against HSV-2-mediated genital disease in animal models [7–9]. Proposed vaccine strains are either replication-defective, replication-competent attenuated or replication-competent controlled.

1.1 Recombinant HSV-Based Vaccine Vectors Currently Under Preclinical and Clinical Development

1.1.1 Replication-Defective Viral Vectors

HSV529 (dl5–29) is a replication-defective HSV-2 that has its UL5 (a subunit of tripartite helicase) and UL29 (major single strand DNA-binding protein ICP8) genes deleted [10]. In mice and guinea pigs, the mutant strain (administered subcutaneously (SC)) is effective in attenuating acute and recurrent disease and in reducing latent virus as well as is capable of inducing more potent humoral and cell-mediated immune responses than recombinant gD2 [11]. HSV529 is currently undergoing phase I clinical testing as a prophylactic or therapeutic vaccine.

Another strategy employed an HSV-2 mutant deleted for the US6 gene ($\Delta gD^{-/+gD-1}$) [12]. As gD, the product of the US6 gene, is essential for virus entry and cell-to-cell spread, $\Delta gD^{-/+gD-1}$ is replication-defective. In a mouse model of lethal intravaginal challenge, $\Delta gD^{-/+gD-1}$ protected against HSV-2 disease as well as prevented establishment of latent virus in dorsal root ganglia. Note that the term "protection" as used herein encompasses both full and partial protective effects. Corresponding results were obtained in a mouse skin scarification model in which animals were challenged with either HSV-1 or HSV-2. The observed protection appeared to be due to induction of high levels of antibodies against multiple viral proteins, which antibodies exhibited antibody-dependent cell-mediated cytotoxicity.

Protection against HSV-2-mediated genital disease and induction of neutralizing antibodies and T cell responses to HSV-1 and HSV-2 were observed in mice vaccinated (SC) with replication-defective recombinant HSV-1 strain CJ9-gD in which the genes for ICP0 (immediate-early regulatory protein) were replaced with a tetracycline repressor-controlled gene cassette for UL9-C535C and the gene for UL9 was substituted with an extra gene for gD [8, 13]. UL9-C535C is a dominant-negative form of the replication-essential UL9 origin of replication-binding protein. Immunization with CJ9-gD also reduced HSV-2 challenge virus replication in the vagina and shortened the period of virus shedding. Furthermore, CJ9-gD also protected against HSV-1 skin disease in guinea pigs as well as reduced the amount of HSV-1 present in dorsal root ganglia [13]. An analogous vaccine vector, CJ2-gD2, was derived from an HSV-2 strain [14]. Immunization (SC) with this strain protected well against HSV-2-induced genital herpes disease and mortality. Reduced vaginal replication of challenge virus could also be demonstrated. It is noted that infection of dorsal root ganglia by challenge virus was not prevented. Neutralizing antibodies as well as robust $CD4^+$ and $CD8^+$ T cell responses were detected.

Expression from a replication-defective (UL29-deleted) HSV-2 strain of co-stimulation molecule B7-2 enhanced the T cell response elicited in wild type mice [15]. Immunization with B7-2-expressing virus (SC; no boost) decreased replication of a vaginally introduced HSV-2 challenge virus as well as reduced disease severity and mortality more effectively than a comparison virus that did not express the co-stimulatory molecule.

1.1.2 Attenuated Replication-Competent Viral Vectors

Attenuated replication-competent HSV-2 strain ImmunoVEX^{HSV2} that is functionally mutated in the US5 (glycoprotein J), US12 (ICP47, a TAP-binding protein), UL41 (virion-host shut off (VHS)), UL43 (membrane protein), and $\gamma_1 34.5$ (neurovirulence factor) genes was entered into a phase I clinical study in 2010 [16]. No additional information about the results of that study appears to be available at this time.

HSV-2 strain ICP10ΔPK has a deletion of the protein kinase domain of the ICP10 gene encoding the large subunit of ribonucleotide reductase [17]. The virus is growth-compromised both in vitro and in vivo and has at most a low propensity for latent infection. Using a mouse footpad immunization and challenge model, immunization with ICP10ΔPK rendered mice resistant to a lethal challenge with HSV-2. Three sequential administrations of high doses of virus completely prevented replication of the challenge virus in the footpad. HSV-2-directed humoral and cellular immune responses which included induction of $CD8^+$ CTL (that inhibited HSV-2 replication in adoptive transfer experiments) were detected in the immunized animals [18]. A clinical trial tested the efficacy of ICP10ΔPK as a therapeutic vaccine [19]. Patients with documented occurrences of herpetic disease received three successive doses of the vaccine. During the observation period, 37.5% of vaccinated patients were lesion-free, and the remainder exhibited a statistically significant reduction in the number of recurrences compared to patients in the placebo group. Apparently, the development of the ICP10ΔPK vaccine has not been continued.

HF10 is a naturally occurring attenuated HSV-1 strain that lacks functional expression of UL43, UL49.5 (membrane-associated protein, TAP inhibitor), UL55 (nuclear matrix protein), UL56 (membrane protein), and latency-associated transcripts [7]. Immunization (SC) of mice with this strain protected (80%) against lethal vaginal challenge with a wild type HSV-2 strain. Clearance of challenge virus was substantially accelerated in the immunized animals. It appears that the latter protective effects were due to T cells resident in the vaginal mucosa responding to multiple viral antigens.

AD472 was derived from HSV-2 (G) and is deleted for $\gamma_1 34.5$ genes, UL55-56, UL43.5 (transcript mapping antisense to UL43 encoding a membrane protein) and the US10-12 region (US10 being a tegument protein and US11 an RNA-binding protein) [20]. The mutant strain is severely replication-impaired and is devoid of neurovirulence. Intramuscular (IM) immunization of guinea pigs induced detectable neutralizing antibody titers. However, challenge virus replication in vaginal tissue was not significantly reduced. Nevertheless, AD472-immunized guinea pigs were protected against HSV-2-induced vaginal disease as well as showed reduced reactivation of challenge virus from dorsal lumbosacral ganglia. It is noted that, unlike most other studies discussed, the latter study involved only a single administration of immunizing vector.

The immediate-early protein ICP0 enhances viral gene transcription by counteracting chromatinization of the viral genome and it antagonizes interferon-mediated antiviral responses. HSV-2 virus 0ΔNLS contains a deletion in the nuclear localization signal (NLS) of the ICP0 gene resulting in a mutant protein that cannot access the nucleus [21]. The virus is replication-competent but avirulent. Immunization of mice (SC in the footpad) with 0ΔNLS protected nearly all animals against subsequent lethal ocular or vaginal challenge with HSV-2 wild type virus. Vaginal shedding of challenge virus was strongly reduced. A strong antibody response was elicited as also evidenced by an elevated titer of neutralizing antibodies. A subsequent study demonstrated that this humoral response was an essential aspect of the efficacy of this vaccine [22].

gE-del virus was derived by deleting a portion of the glycoprotein E-coding region of a highly virulent HSV-2 isolate [23]. The mutant virus was demonstrated to be replication-competent but defective in neural spread. LD_{50} doses were 10^2 to 10^5 times higher than those of the wild type virus, depending on the route of administration. Intramuscular, and to a lesser degree subcutaneous, immunization effectively prevented HSV-2-induced vaginal disease and mortality as well as reduced vaginal titers of challenge virus in mouse and guinea pig models. Protection was vaccine dose-dependent and enhanced by booster immunization. Nevertheless, dorsal root ganglia were not completely protected against infection, and recurrent lesions and vaginal shedding occurred in some of the vaccinated and challenged animals. gE-del virus was also tested in a therapeutic setting. A significant reduction of the cumulative number of genital lesions over the observation period was reported.

Generally, live vaccines are thought to be more effective than subunit vaccines, in part because of their ability to induce substantial cellular immune responses. The effectiveness of such vaccines may be limited by the restricted migration of effector T cells to peripheral tissues such as the vaginal mucosa, particularly in the absence of an inflammation. A "prime and pull" strategy was designed to facilitate the establishment of a resident pool of effector T cells [24]. To facilitate tracking HSV-2-specific T cells, mice were transplanted with congenically marked $CD8^+$ T cells that recognized an epitope within HSV glycoprotein B and then immunized/"primed" (SC) with an attenuated HSV-2 strain defective for thymidine kinase [25]. An effective "pull" consisted of an intravaginal administration of CXCL9/CXCL10 during the effector phase of the T cell response. This non-inflammatory regimen resulted in a recruitment of an antigen-specific $CD8^+$ T cell population to vaginal tissue, which population was retained in this tissue for an extended period of time. The "prime and pull" regimen substantially enhanced the survival and reduced the disease severity in animals subjected to a lethal vaginal challenge with HSV-2. Vaginal shedding of challenge virus was not significantly reduced. In contrast, an effective pull resulted in a substantial further reduction of virus titers in the dorsal root ganglia of immunized animals.

Recently, HSV-1-derived strain VC2 carrying small deletions in the glycoprotein K and UL20 (membrane protein mediating cell fusion in a complex with glycoprotein K) genes was tested as a potential vaccine against genital herpes disease [9]. The virus replicated well in Vero cells but did not cause clinical disease after intranasal or intramuscular administration to mice. Intramuscular administration of a high dose (10^7 pfu) of this virus induced significant humoral and cellular immune responses, protected fully against lethal vaginal challenge with either HSV-1 or HSV-2 and significantly reduced vaginal shedding of challenge virus. Viral DNA was not detected in dorsal root ganglia.

1.1.3 Replication-Competent Controlled Viral Vectors: HSV-GS

We recently developed the concept of subjecting the replication of a vaccine strain to deliberate spatiotemporal control rather than disabling or attenuating the virus ((*26*); *see* **Note 1**). Hence, the vaccine virus would be administered to a body region in which it cannot cause disease and be specifically activated in this region to undergo one or more rounds of unimpeded replication. While this concept may be elaborated in different ways, our first solution was to subject two replication-essential genes (ICP4, ICP8) of wild type HSV-1 strain $17syn^+$ to the control of a two-component gene switch that is activated in a cell by transient heat in the presence of an antiprogestin [27]. In vitro, the latter controlled virus, HSV-GS3, could be induced to replicate as efficiently as $17syn^+$. Both in vitro and in vivo, the virus was essentially incapable of replication in the absence of activation. Cutaneous administration of HSV-GS3 to wild type mice followed by activation by heat directed to the site of administration in the systemic presence of antiprogestin induced localized virus replication and resulted in strong protective effects upon lethal challenge [26, 27].

1.2 Basis for Using HSV as Platform for the Delivery of Heterologous Antigens

The concept of using replication-defective or attenuated viruses as vectors for the delivery of heterologous antigens has been explored extensively. There are several reasons that render HSV attractive as a vector [1, 26]: (1) it is able to infect a broad range of host cells and cause efficient lysis; (2) its genome is not integrated into the host genome, avoiding issues of effects on host gene expression or even transformation; (3) replication of its genome is by a high-fidelity DNA polymerase, (4) its genome is relatively large and tolerant of insertion of sizeable DNA segments; (5) inserted heterologous genes are, typically, expressed in a stable fashion. Regions of the viral genomes are known that tolerate gene insertions without negative effects on virus growth or virulence. In HSV-1, the UL43/44 and UL37/38 intergenic regions are such desirable recipient regions; (6) HSV is lethal only under exceptional circumstances, and HSV thymidine kinase renders the virus susceptible to drugs such as acyclovir; (7) it is endemic in the human population (in particular HSV-1), but preexisting immunity does not appear to substantially interfere with its use as vaccine vector; (8) robust methods have been developed that allow for the manipulation of the viral genome; and (9) the virus can typically be grown to high titers in cell lines. A complication is that HSV latently infects sensory nerve cells and that reactivation can occur.

Reactivation could be avoided by employing replication-defective or replication-competent controlled but not replication-competent attenuated HSV vectors. One may wonder whether partial reactivation could be beneficial for the maintenance of resident immunity. If this were the case, ideal vectors would be HSV strains in which one or more late genes are disabled or subjected to deliberate control and that are, therefore, capable of expressing most viral proteins.

Immune responses to heterologous antigens have been examined in multiple studies. In one proof-of-principle study, a CMV promoter–ovalbumin gene cassette was inserted into the UL41 locus of a mutant HSV-1 strain defective in the immediate-early proteins ICP4, ICP22 and ICP27 to create T0H-OVA [28]. Immunization (IM) of DO11.10 mice (expressing transgenic T cell receptor specific for $OVA_{323-339}$/MHC class II I-A^d) with T0H-OVA but not with control vector induced a strong CD8+ effector T cell response that protected against a lethal infection with high doses of *L. monocytogenes* bacteria expressing OVA. T0H-OVA induced a far superior effector T cell response and protected significantly better against the intracellular pathogen than a DNA vaccine delivered by gene gun. Several studies were aimed at developing an HIV/AIDS vaccine. A CMV promoter-driven SIV ENV-NEF expression cassette was inserted into the thymidine kinase gene of attenuated HSV-1 strain KOS1.1 or strain d27 defective for ICP27 [29]. Seven rhesus macaques were vaccinated (SC/IM with two boosts) with one or the other strain. HSV- and SIV envelope protein-specific antibody and CTL responses were detected. Two of the animals were solidly protected against a lethal rectal challenge with SIV239. In a more recent study, expression cassettes for SIV ENV, GAG and a REV-TAT-NEV fusion protein were inserted into HSV-1 mutant strain d106 (defective for ICP4, 22, 27, and 47) [30]. Six rhesus macaques were either administered (IM/SC) a combination of the d106-derived vaccine strains (at weeks 0, 4, 12 and 20) or a DNA vaccine (at weeks 0 and 4) prior to boosting with the d106-derived vaccine strains (at weeks 12 and 20). Humoral and cellular immune responses could be documented. When challenged with SIV239 (i.v.), all animals became infected. However, when compared to pre-challenge sera, plasma SIV RNA levels in the surviving vaccinated animals [5] were significantly reduced at weeks 2 and 12 after challenge.

2 Materials

1. MEM: Modified Eagle's Medium (Life Sciences, Bethesda, MD) supplemented with 5% calf serum, 250 U penicillin, 250 μg/mL streptomycin, and 292 μg/mL L-glutamine/mL.

2. Rabbit skin or Vero cells (American Type Culture Collection).
3. Trypsin: 1.25 g trypsin dissolved in 50 mL dH2O at 37 °C. Add 0.5 g EDTA, 20 g NaCl, 1 g KCl, 2.5 g dextrose, 0.5 g penicillin, and 0.25 g streptomycin. Bring volume up to 200 mL with dH_2O. Filter-sterilize and store at 4 °C. Dilute 1:10 for working stock.
4. T75 flasks and 60-mm dishes.
5. Sterile 5 mL falcon tubes.
6. Water bath with adjustable heating.
7. Solution A: 0.1 M NaOH, 1.5 M NaCl.
8. Solution B: 0.2 M Tris–HCl, pH 7.6.
9. Solution C: 2 × SSPE. 20 × SSPE: 3.6 M NaCl, 0.2 M NaH_2PO_4. H_2O, 0.02 M EDTA; adjust pH to 7.0 to 7.5 with NaOH. Autoclave.
10. 2.5 M $CaCl_2$: filter-sterilize and store at room temperature.
11. 1× TE: 10 mM Tris–HCl, pH 8.0, 1 mM EDTA in dH_2O. Autoclave.
12. 10% SDS: 100 g in 900 mL dH_2O dissolved by heating to 68 °C. pH to 7.2 and q.s. to 1 l.
13. 2× HEPES (for 100 mL): 1.6 g NaCl, 74 mg KCl, 37 mg $Na_2HPO_4{:}7H_2O$, 0.2 g dextrose, 1 g HEPES (free acid); pH to 7.05, filter-sterilize, aliquot, and store at −20 °C.
14. Shock buffer: prepared fresh by mixing 2× HEPES with an equal volume of a sterile 40% dextrose solution (for 1× HEPES and 20% dextrose, final).
15. Neutral red solution: 3.330 g/l (Invitrogen, Carlsbad, CA, USA).
16. TNE buffer: 10 mM Tris (pH 7.4), 1 mM EDTA, 0.1 M NaCl.
17. Sterile, plugged Pasteur pipettes (Thermo Fisher Scientific).
18. 96 well flat-bottom tissue culture plates (Falcon).
19. Hybond-N nylon membrane (GE Life Sciences).

3 Methods

3.1 Design and Construction of Replication-Competent Controlled HSV-GS Viruses

The sections below outline in detail the construction and use of HSV-GS3, the prototype of the HSV-GS vectors. The HSV-GS3 vector contains two essential viral genes (ICP4 and ICP8) under control of an antiprogestin-activated transactivator that is expressed from a heat- and transactivator-induced gene. See Fig. 1a for an illustration of the operation of the regulation system. Placing two genes under control of the latter transactivator allows for a greater degree of safety. Engineering of this vector requires replacing the native HSV-1 promoters for these genes with transactivator-responsive (GAL4-responsive) promoters. This is achieved by constructing recombination plasmids that contain HSV-1 flanking sequences on both sides of the native promoter, and replacing the promoter with a GAL4-responsive promoter. These plasmids are then co-transfected with HSV-1 virion DNA into the appropriate cell line in order to allow recombination to occur. Viral progenies from these transfections are then screened for the presence of a GAL4-responsive promoter by dot blot hybridization. The construction of HSV-GS3 (as previously described in Ref. 27) is performed in two steps: (1) the construction of HSV-GS1, which contains the ICP4 gene under control of a GAL4-responsive promoter (Fig. 1b), and (2) HSV-GS3, which contains both ICP4 and ICP8 genes under transactivator control (Fig. 1c). It should be noted that in order for productive replication of the HSV-GS vectors to take place in culture, they need to be propagated either in the presence of an antiprogestin (either mifepristone or ulipristal) and a pulse of heat (43.5 °C for 30 min by placing the dishes on a stand in a waterbath) shortly after infection, or on a cell line that provides ICP4 and ICP8 in trans. While the construction of these vectors has been previously described in Ref. 27, the sections below give additional details regarding the methodologies employed.

For general molecular biology methods, the reader is referred to other volumes of this series or to other compilations, e.g., "Current Protocols in Molecular Biology". HSV-GS vectors are based on wild type HSV-1 strain 17syn+. This strain is fully virulent and is well characterized. Its complete genomic sequence is available. As mentioned above, viral recombinants were generated by homologous recombination of engineered plasmids along with purified virion DNA in rabbit skin cells (RS) transfected by the calcium phosphate precipitation method (detailed below). All recombination plasmids used to insert the transactivator cassette or the GAL4-responsive promoters comprised HSV-1 sequences originating from strain 17syn+.

3.1.1 Construction of HSV-GS1

1. A portion of HSV-1 DNA (17syn+) is amplified with primers DB112 (5′-GAGCTCATCACCGCAGGCGAGTCTCTT-3′) and DB113 (5′-GAGCTCGGTCTTCGGGAC TAATGCC TT-3′) to generate an upstream recombination arm (base pairs 95,441 to 96,090).
2. The PCR fragment is digested with SacI and then ligated into the SacI site of pBluescript. The resulting construct is named pUP.
3. To generate a downstream recombination arm, a portion of HSV-1 (17syn+) DNA is amplified using primers DB115-KpnI (5′-GGGGTACCGGTTTTG TTTTGTGTG AC-3′) and DB 120-KpnI(5′-GGGGTACCGGTGTGTGATGATTTCGC-3′)

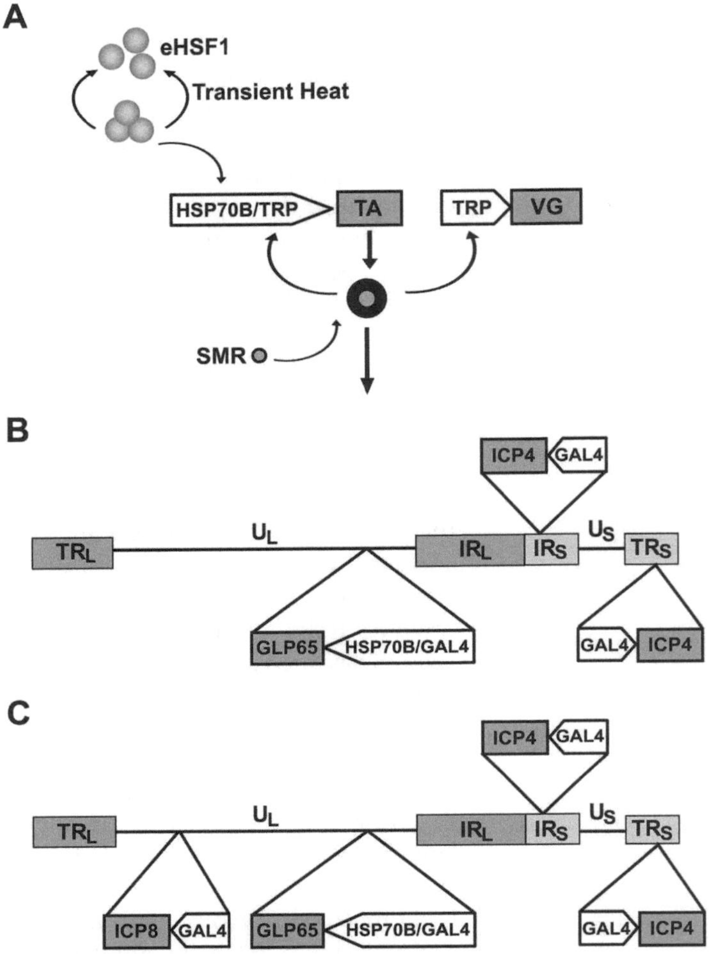

Fig. 1 (**a**) Scheme illustrating the operation of the type of gene switch utilized in the HSV-GS vectors. *eHSF1* endogenous heat shock transcription factor, *TRP* transactivator-responsive promoter, *TA* transactivator, *VG* replication-essential viral gene, *SMR* small-molecule regulator. In the particular gene switch employed in the HSV-GS vectors, TRP is a GAL4-responsive promoter, TA is GLP65, VG is ICP4 and/or ICP8, and SMR is an antiprogestin. Relevant aspects of the genomes of HSV-GS1 and HSV-GS3 are shown schematically in (**b**) and (**c**), respectively. *TRL , TRS* long and short terminal repeats, *UL , US* long and short unique regions, *IRL, IRS* long and short internal repeats, respectively

(base pairs 96,092 and 96,538). The PCR fragment is digested with KpnI and then ligated into the KpnI site of pUP. The resulting construct, named pIN994, is capable of recombining with HSV-1 at the UL43/44 intergenic region. In the following steps, a transactivator (TA) cassette containing a GLP65 gene under the control of a promoter cassette consisting of a functional assembly of a human HSP70B (HSPA7) promoter and a GAL4-responsive promoter is inserted into the multiple cloning site of plasmid pIN994. (The latter multiple cloning site is located between flanking sequences of the HSV-1 UL43 and UL44 genes). The TA cassette is isolated from plasmid HSP70/GAL4-GLP65 [31] and is subcloned by 3-piece ligation to minimize the region that is amplified by PCR.

4. To produce a left insert containing the HSP70/GAL4 promoter cassette as well as the GAL4 DNA-binding domain, the progesterone receptor ligand-binding domain and part of the P65 activation domain of GLP65, HSP70/GAL4-GLP65 is digested with BamHI and BstX1, and the resulting 2875-bp fragment is gel-purified.
5. To generate a right insert containing the 3′ end of the P65 activation domain and 3′ nontranslated sequences from a bovine growth hormone gene (BGH), a portion of pHSP70/GAL4-GLP65 is PCR-amplified with primers TA.2803–2823. fwd (5′-TCGACAACTCCGAGTTT CAGC-3′) and BGHpA. rev (5′-CTCCTCGCGGCCGCATCGATCCATAGAGCCCA CCGCATCC-3′). The resulting 763-bp fragment is digested with BstX1 and NotI, and the trimmed 676-bp fragment is gel-purified.
6. Vector pIN994 is digested with BamHI and NotI, and the resulting 4099-bp fragment is gel-purified and shrimp alkaline phosphatase (SAP)-treated. Left and right inserts are then simultaneously ligated into the latter vector fragment. Subsequent to transformation, a colony is expanded, and the plasmid, named pIN:TA1, is verified by restriction and sequence analysis.
7. One μg of pIN:TA1 and 2 μg of purified HSV-1 (17syn+) virion DNA are co-transfected into RS cells by calcium phosphate precipitation. Resulting viruses are screened for recombinants by the picking of plaques, amplification of these plaques on 96-well plates of RS cells, and dot-blot hybridization with a ^{32}P–labeled TA fragment (labeled by random-hexamer priming). A positive well is re-plaqued and re-probed several times, and the purified virus is demonstrated to contain the TA cassette by PCR and sequence analysis. This intermediate recombinant is named HSV-17GS43.
8. A second recombination plasmid, pBS-KS:GAL4-ICP4, is constructed by insertion of a GAL4-responsive promoter between the HSV-1 ICP4 recombination arms of plasmid pBS-KS:ICP4Δpromoter (*see* **Note 2**). The GAL4-responsive promoter is released from plasmid pGene/v5-HisA (Invitrogen Corp.) with AatII and HindIII, and the resulting 473-bp fragment is gel-purified.

9. Plasmid BS-KS:ICP4Δpromoter is digested with AatII and HindIII, and the resulting 3962-bp fragment is gel-purified and SAP-treated. This fragment is ligated to the fragment of step 8, placing the GAL4-responsive promoter in front of the ICP4 transcriptional start site. Subsequent to transformation, a colony is expanded, and pBS-KS:GAL4-ICP4 is identified by restriction enzyme digestion and sequencing.
10. One μg of pBS-KS:GAL4-ICP4 and 4 μg of purified HSV-17GS43 virion DNA are co-transfected by calcium phosphate precipitation into cells of the ICP4-complementing cell line E5. Resulting viruses are screened for recombinants by the picking of plaques, amplification of the plaques on 96-well plates of E5 cells, and dot blot hybridization with a ^{32}P–labeled GAL4-responsive promoter fragment (labeled by random-hexamer priming). A positive well is re-plaqued and re-probed several times, and the purified recombinant is verified to contain the GAL4-responsive promoter in both copies of the short repeat sequences by PCR analysis and sequencing. This recombinant is named HSV-GS1.

3.1.2 Construction of HSV-GS3

1. To construct ICP8 recombination plasmid pBS-KS:GAL4-ICP8, a 473-bp fragment containing the GAL4-responsive promoter is released from plasmid pGene/v5-HisA by digestion with AatII and HindIII. This fragment is gel-purified.
2. A 4588-bp fragment is obtained by digestion of pBS-KS:ICP8Δpromoter with AatII and HindIII (*see* **Note 3** for the construction of pBS-KS:ICP8Δpromoter). The latter fragment is gel-purified, SAP-treated and then ligated to the fragment of step 1, placing the GAL4-responsive promoter in front of the ICP8 transcriptional start-site. A transformant is expanded and its identity verified by restriction digestion and sequencing.
3. One μg of pBS-KS:GAL4-ICP8 and 10 μg of purified HSV-GS1 virion DNA are co-transfected into E5 cells by calcium phosphate precipitation. Mifepristone (10 nM) was added to the medium, and the transfected cells are exposed to 43.5 °C for 30 min and then incubated at 37 °C. This heat and mifepristone treatment is repeated on days 2 and 3. Plaques are picked and amplified on 96-well plates of E5 cells in medium supplemented with mifepristone. The plates are exposed to 43.5 °C heat for 30 min 1 h after infection and then post-incubated at 37 °C. The plates are subjected to the same heating and post-incubation protocol on days 2 and 3. At 90–100% cytopathic effect (CPE), the plates are dot-blotted, and the dot blot membrane is hybridized with a ^{32}P–labeled HSV-1 ICP8 promoter fragment (that has been deleted). A faintly positive well is re-plaqued and re-probed several times (using the above

protocol). The purified virus is shown by PCR and sequence analysis to have lost the ICP8 promoter and to contain the GAL4-responsive promoter in its stead. This recombinant is named HSV-GS3.

3.2 Detailed Methods for the Generation of HSV-GS Recombinants by Transfection

The above general strategy can be employed to regulate other genes of HSV-1, or genes of other DNA viruses (that make use of the host cell's transcription machinery). Once the desired recombination plasmids have been constructed, they can be introduced into cells by transfection along with the appropriate recipient viral DNA and the resulting progeny viruses from the transfection screened for recombinants. The following sections detail the transfection and screening processes.

3.2.1 Preparation of HSV Transfection DNA

1. Trypsinize five confluent T75 flasks of rabbit skin cells and resuspend each flask in a total of 15 mL of Modified Eagle's Medium (MEM). Seed ten 150-mm flasks with 7 mL of this cell suspension by adding the cells to 20 mL of (supplemented) medium in each dish. Incubate overnight at 37 °C.
2. The following day (the dishes should be approximately 90% confluent at this point), the medium is removed, and the cells are infected by adding 5 mL of medium containing 2×10^6 pfu of HSV. The virus is allowed to adsorb to the cells for 60 min at 37 °C. The dishes are rocked gently halfway through the incubation.
3. 25 mL of medium are added to the cells, and the dishes are incubated until all of the cells have rounded and detach easily when the dish is swirled. This usually takes 2–3 days.
4. Harvest the cells by pipeting the cells off the bottom of the dishes. Transfer the cell suspension to 250 mL centrifuge bottles, and pellet the cells and free virus by centrifugation at 10,000 × *g* for 40 min at 4 °C.
5. Pour off supernatant, resuspend the pellet in hypotonic lysis buffer (10 mL), and transfer the suspension to a conical 15 mL Falcon tube. Vortex vigorously and incubate for 5 min on ice. Vortex again briefly.
6. Centrifuge at 800 × *g* for 10 min at 4 °C. (This pellets the nuclei.)
7. Transfer the supernatant to a new conical tube and add 1 mL 10% SDS and 0.5 mL 20 mg/mL Pronase (or 10 mg/mL proteinase K).
8. Incubate for 1 h at 50 °C.
9. Add another 0.5 mL of 20 mg/mL pronase (or 10 mg/mL proteinase K) and incubate overnight at 37 °C.
10. Phenol-extract 2×.

11. Phenol/SEVAG (1:1)-extract 1×. (SEVAG is chloroform–isoamyl alcohol, 24:1.)
12. SEVAG-extract 1×.
13. Dialyze the DNA vs. 1× TE overnight at 4 °C (with 2 changes of buffer). Alternatively, the DNA can be precipitated by the addition of 2.5 vol of cold 100% ethanol and 1/10 vol of 5 M sodium acetate. Often this allows the precipitated DNA to be "spooled" or removed as a puff of precipitated material. At this point, the DNA can be washed with 70% ethanol, dried, and resuspended in 1× TE.
14. Determine the concentration of DNA spectrophotometrically by determining the absorbance (A_{260}).
15. Digest 1 μg of the DNA with HindIII and run the digest on a 0.8% agarose gel along with uncut DNA to determine the purity and quality of the preparation. There will be some cellular contamination as indicated by some very faint smearing in the digested sample and very high molecular weight DNA in the uncut sample, but the viral DNA as evidenced by distinct bands ranging in size from approximately 23,000–500 bp should be the predominant form.
16. For long-term storage of the DNA, it is advisable to aliquot the DNA into small fractions and freeze. Repeated freeze-thawing should be avoided.

3.2.2 Co-Transfection of HSV DNA and Recombination Vector

Transfections are performed in 60-mm dishes on subconfluent monolayers of rabbit skin (RS) cells (or another appropriate cell line). The RS cells are propagated in MEM supplemented with 5% calf serum, 292 μg/mL glutamine, 250 U penicillin and 2.5 μg/mL streptomycin. Full length HSV DNA is co-transfected with the desired plasmid at various ratios using a modified calcium phosphate precipitation procedure. The transfections are generally allowed to proceed until all cells are rounded, i.e., until 100% CPE is evident (usually 3–4 days), although the dishes may be harvested earlier if one wishes to prevent amplification of siblings.

1. 60-mm dishes are seeded from a flask of actively growing RS cells at a ratio that will produce a cell density of approximately 50% confluency the following day (typically 1/30th of a T75 flask/60-mm dish). The dishes are incubated overnight at 37 °C, 5% CO_2.
2. The following day, the medium is removed from the dishes (which should be at 50% confluency) and replaced with MEM supplemented with 1.5% fetal bovine serum. The dishes are then incubated overnight at 31.5 ° C, 5% CO_2. This is to serum-starve the cells.

3. The transfection mixture is prepared by diluting the desired amount of DNA (typically, 1–10 μg of HSV per dish and a tenfold molar excess of the linearized plasmid DNA) in a final volume of 225 μL TNE buffer. After the dilutions have been made, 25 μL of a 2.5 M $CaCl_2$ solution are added to each tube (*see* **Notes 4** and **5**).
4. The DNA is precipitated by adding 250 μL of 2× HEPES buffer to the above sample while bubbling air into the solution with a mouth aspirator connected to a sterile-plugged Pasteur pipette. The critical parameter here is to regulate the amount of air that you are blowing into the solution so that you generate rapid bubbles to facilitate mixing and the formation of DNA:calcium phosphate precipitation complexes that are of uniform small size.
5. The DNA precipitate is then incubated for 20 min at room temperature.
6. Aspirate the medium from the 60-mm dishes, and pour on the transfection mixture. Incubate the dishes for 20–30 min at room temperature.
7. Add 5 mL of MEM supplemented with 1.5% fetal bovine serum and incubate for 4 h at 37 °C. Do not remove the DNA solution.
8. After the 4 h, aspirate the medium and wash the monolayer with medium 2×, and then briefly hypertonically shock the cells (less than 1 min) by adding 1–2 mL of shock buffer.
9. Aspirate the shock buffer and wash 2× with medium. After the last wash, add 5 mL of MEM supplemented with 5% calf serum to the dishes, and incubate 3–4 days at 37 °C, 5% CO_2.
10. The transfections are harvested by scraping cells into the medium using a rubber policeman.
11. The contents of the dishes (transfections) are transferred to a 15 mL conical tube and frozen at −80 °C. The virus released is a mixture of wild-type virus and recombinants. The next step is to plate dilutions of this mixture onto cell monolayers in order to obtain well-isolated plaques, which are then screened to identify the recombinants.

3.2.3 Plaquing of Transfections

1. Transfections are subjected to two rounds of freeze-thaw (with vortexing in between the freezes) to release the virus from the cells.
2. The transfection mixes are diluted into unsupplemented MEM to concentrations of 10^{-5}, 10^{-6}, 10^{-7}, and 10^{-8}.
3. 0.5 mL of each dilution are plated onto each of three 60-mm dishes of confluent RS cells (media removed first).
4. The inoculum is allowed to adsorb for 1 h at 37 °C, 5% CO_2.

5. Infected monolayers are overlayed with 5 mL of 0.8% agarose mixed with 2× supplemented medium (note that the agarose is warmed to 45 °C and the medium to 37 °C, and the two are mixed immediately before pouring onto the dishes to prevent premature gelling), and incubated for 2 days.
6. On the morning of the third day, the dishes are stained with neutral red to aid in the visualization of the plaques. A 1:30 dilution of the Neutral red stock solution is made in unsupplemented medium. An equal volume of the neutral red overlay is then added to the dishes on top of the agar overlay (5 mL of diluted neutral red per 60-mm dish), and the dishes are incubated at 37 °C until the monolayers are stained red. For rabbit skin cells this is approximately 6 h. When staining with neutral red, it is important not to leave the neutral red on too long, as it will eventually kill the cells (rendering the plaques invisible).
7. After the monolayers are stained, the liquid overlay is aspirated, and the plaques are picked using a sterile Pasteur pipet. The plaques are picked by applying slight pressure to the bulb of the pipette, then coring the plaque straight down, and twisting the pipet. The bulb is then released, and the plaque aspirated partially into the pipet.
8. The plaque is then expelled into a well of a 96-well plate, the well having been filled with 2–3 drops of medium.
9. After all of the plaques are picked, the plate is frozen at −70 °C and then thawed in the incubator to release infectious virus from the cells.
10. 50 μL from each well of this plate is transferred to a 96-well plate containing confluent rabbit skins cells from which medium has been removed.
11. The virus is then allowed to adsorb for 1 h at 37 °C.
12. Two drops of supplemented medium are added to each well, and the dishes are incubated until the wells show 100% CPE (usually 3 days).

    For additional considerations, *see* **Note 6**.

3.2.4 Screening for Recombinants

1. After cells in the wells of the latter 96-well plate have reached full CPE, they are ready to be dot-blotted.
2. Set up the Millipore dot-blot apparatus with one piece of blotting paper underneath a piece of nylon membrane (Hybond-N or Nytrans). Wet the blotting paper and membrane completely with 2× SSPE before clamping the apparatus together.
3. After clamping the apparatus together, apply vacuum. Using a multichannel pipetter, transfer 50 μL of the infected cells (approximately ¼ of the suspension in the well) from each well of the 96-well plate to the apparatus (pipet the wells up and down several times to mix before transferring).

4. After the medium has filtered through the apparatus, add 200 μL of Solution A to each well of the apparatus.
5. Likewise, after Solution A has filtered through all of the wells, add 200 μL of Solution B.
6. Finally, after all of Solution B has filtered through the apparatus, add 200 μL of Solution C.
7. After Solution C has filtered through all of the wells, remove the membrane from the apparatus, label the membrane (remember to mark orientation), and bake it at 80 °C for 1 h. The blot is now ready for hybridization (*see* **Note 7**).
8. Freeze the 96-well plate at −70 °C for later use.

3.2.5 Confirmation of Viral Recombinants

After the recombinants identified as positive in the initial hybridization screen have been plaque-purified in at least three rounds to purity, small "master stocks" of several "clones" can be grown up for confirmation. Typically, the following tests are performed using the standard techniques of viral genome and RNA analysis presented elsewhere in this volume:

1. Southern blot analysis. The goal is to determine that the gene of interest is inserted into the proper location within the viral genome. If the recombination site is within the viral repeat sequences, it is important to determine that that the virus is "double-sided" or that two copies of the gene is present. This is critical in that single-sided viruses tend to be unstable and the inserted gene may recombine out. For example, if the recombinant is to contain a transgene inserted into the ICP4 locus, then one must make sure that the transgene has indeed been inserted stably into both copies of ICP4.
2. Northern blot analysis. This is performed in order to determine that the transgene or modified viral gene is transcribed properly in the context of the viral genome.

3.3 Propagation of HSV-GS Vectors

One of the major advantages of using HSV-1 as a vaccine vector is that high titer stocks can be easily produced. Once the HSV-GS vectors are constructed and master stocks have been produced, the following techniques are used to amplify and titrate the stocks.

3.3.1 Large-Scale Amplification of HSV-GS3 Stocks

1. For propagation of HSV-GS3, ten confluent T75 flasks of E5 cells (stably transfected Vero cells containing the HSV ICP4 gene under its native promoter) are transfected 24 h prior to infection with an expression plasmid for ICP8 using Lipofectamine 2000 (Life Technologies).
2. The flasks are infected with the viral vector at a multiplicity of infection (MOI) of 0.01.
3. Virus is allowed to adsorb for 1 h at 37 °C, and then the inoculum is removed, and the cells are overlayed with complete medium.

4. The flasks are then incubated for 72 h at 37 °C.
5. After the cells show 100% CPE and are no longer adherent, cells and medium are decanted into 250 mL centrifugation bottles.
6. The cells and aggregates of free virus are pelleted by centrifugation at 10,000 × *g* for 30 min.
7. The pellets are resuspended in a total volume of 2 mL medium by trituration with a pipet and then transferred to a 15 mL conical tube.
8. The vector stock is then subjected to two rounds of freeze-thaw at −80 ° C, with vortexing in between to release virus from the cells.
9. The stock is then divided into aliquots of 0.1 or 0.2 mL each in cryovials and stored at −80 °C.

3.3.2 Assay of Vector Titers

Infectious virus titers of stocks are determined by titrating the lysate of the above stocks on confluent E5 cells.

1. For titration of HSV-GS3, 24-well plates of confluent E5 cells are transfected 24 h prior to infection with an expression plasmid for ICP8 using Lipofectamine 2000 (Life Technologies). Note that typical titers of the HSV-GS stocks are in the range of 1×10^8 pfu/mL (as prepared above). Using bracketed dilutions, one 24-well plate is sufficient per stock.
2. The virus stock is diluted from 10^{-2} to 10^{-9} in 1 mL of medium.
3. The medium is removed from the wells of the 24-well plate, and 200 μL of each dilution is added in triplicate to the plate (three wells per dilution).
4. The virus is allowed to adsorb for 1 h at 37 °C.
5. The inoculum is removed and 1 mL of overlay medium is added to each well (complete medium + 50 μL/50 mL of human pooled IgG (Sigma). This neutralizes free HSV virus and prevents secondary plaques from forming.
6. The plates are incubated at 37 °C for 2 days.
7. The medium is removed from all wells, and the monolayers are fixed with cold 100% methanol for 20 min at 20 °C.
8. The monolayers are washed with phosphate-buffered saline (PBS).
9. 100 μL of a 1/1000 dilution of a polyclonal anti-HSV antiserum (rabbit anti-HSV HRP conjugate, DAKO labs) are added to the wells, and the plates are incubated for 1 h a room temperature.
10. The antiserum is aspirated, and the monolayers rinsed twice with PBS.

11. The plaques on the monolayers are visualized by adding to each well 200 μL of Immunopure DAB substrate (Pierce Chemicals), which is removed after approximately 10 min by rinsing with PBS.
12. The plaques are counted under a dissecting microscope and the averages of the three replicates are determined. After correcting for the dilution factor, the final titer of the stock is determined.

3.4 Use of HSV-GS Vectors for Vaccination

For immunization, the HSV-GS vectors are applied locally to the skin of mice. In order to induce one or two controlled rounds of replication in the skin, an antiprogestin is administered to the mice and local heat is applied to the vaccination site. The section below provides detailed methodology for how the HSV-GS vectors, specifically HSV-GS3, are used to vaccinate mice against HSV-1, and how efficacy is tested using an HSV-1 lethal challenge model.

Mice are first immunized with the HSV-GS vectors on the rear foot pads. The reason that this route of vaccination delivery is used is because (1) the footpad is a convenient epithelial surface to infect on the mouse that does not require shaving hair first, and (2) the foot is easily treated with local heat to activate the GS vector (in the presence of an antiprogestin).

3.4.1 Footpad Inoculation of Mice

Swiss Webster outbred female mice (4–6 weeks old) are anesthetized and inoculated with 5000 to 1×10^5 PFU of HSV-GS3 vector following saline pretreatment and light abrasion of both rear footpads as described below. Each treatment group may consist of 10–20 mice. Ulipristal (50 μg/kg) is administered intraperitoneally (IP) at the time of infection, and heat treatment is performed at 45 °C for 10 min (by immersion of hind feet in a water bath or using a heating pad) 3 h after virus administration. Mice are allowed to recover at 37 °C for 15 min and are then returned to their cages for at least 21 days, at which time they are challenged with wild type HSV-1 to determine the efficacy of the vaccination.

1. The mice (16–19 g) are anesthetized one at a time briefly with isoflurane (4% induction) using an anesthesia vaporizer (VetEquip) connected to a rodent chamber (just until heavy breathing ensues).
2. The mice are injected with a sterile 10% saline solution under the footpad of each foot with a 1 cc tuberculin syringe with a 28 G needle. Approximately 0.05 mL per foot are injected intradermally (just underneath the cornified epithelial layer). This injection facilitates removal of the cornified epithelial layer and makes the vector application to the epithelial cells more efficient.
3. The mice are returned to their cages and left for at least 4 h (but no longer than 6 h).

4. The mice are anesthetized by intramuscular (IM) injection of 0.010–0.020 mL of a cocktail of acepromazine (2.5–3.75 mg/kg), xylazine (7.5–11.5 mg/kg) and ketamine (30–45 mg/kg). The reason that the ketamine/xylazine/acepromazine cocktail is used for the vaccination step is that it is important to give the viral vector time to adsorb and enter the epithelial cells (30 min for 80–90% efficiency) before the mice recover and start moving around. The anesthesia time for the ketamine/xylazine/acepromazine is adequate for that requirement. The inclusion of the acepromazine prevents the mice from twitching their feet (and flicking off the vector). Also at this point, 0.1 mL of Ulipristal (50 μg/kg) are administered to the mice by IP injection.
5. Mice are removed from their cages and laid on their backs.
6. With an emery board, the feet are lightly abraded with 1–2 strokes only to remove the surface layer of skin.
7. With a pipetman, 25–50 μL of the vaccine vector are applied to each foot and rubbed over the surface with the side of the pipet tip. The animals are then arranged on their backs feet up and flat in the cage with the bedding material to prop them up.
8. An additional 25–50 μL is applied to each foot. Care should be taken so that the feet are level and the inoculum stays on the feet.
9. The vaccine vector is allowed to adsorb for 30–60 min (when the mice begin waking).
10. Watch the mice to ensure that they are awakening.
11. After 3 h, heat activation of the vector is performed. The mice are anesthetized with isoflurane (using a vaporizer and mouse nose cones) at 4% induction and 3% maintenance.
12. Heat is applied either with a heating pad or by immersing the hind feet in a 45 °C water bath for 10 min, after which time the feet are dried off, and the mice are held in a 37 °C incubator for 15 min to allow them to recover from the exposure to water (and not enter a hypothermic state).
13. The mice are then returned to the vivarium for 2–3 weeks.

3.4.2 Challenge Assays for Efficacy

To determine the efficacy of the vaccination, the mice are challenged with a lethal dose of wild type HSV-1 strain 17syn+. In BALB/c or Swiss-Webster mice, the footpad infection LD_{50} is approximately 500 pfu/mouse. Therefore, an inoculum of 10,000 pfu/mouse represents a robust challenge. The challenge assays are performed as follows:

1. The mice are infected with HSV-1 in a manner identical to the viral vector treatment. The feet are pretreated with saline and then infected with HSV-1 as outlined in Subheading 3.4.1.

2. For these studies, a modified LD_{50} endpoint assay is typically performed, where vaccinated and control groups are masked. Mice are observed daily for signs of HSV encephalitis. Typically, mice begin showing these signs around day 6. These signs include loss of activity, unilateral or bilateral hindlimb paralysis, reduced activity, ruffled fur, and dehydration. Mice that exhibit clinical signs of being moribund (failure to move when handled, and/or bilateral hindlimb paralysis) are euthanized by isofluorane overdose.
3. A daily tally of mice that die or must be euthanized is maintained for 25 days, at which time all remaining mice will have recovered from the challenge. Tissues (feet and DRG) can be analyzed by PCR for the presence of HSV-1 (challenge virus and/or viral vector), and blood and serum for immune markers.

4 Notes

1. Replication-competent controlled viruses were developed based on the premise that immune responses to a vaccine should be at least as strong and broad as those induced by the wild type virus targeted by the vaccine and that immune responses induced by replication-defective or even replication-attenuated viruses cannot be expected to attain the latter ambitious mark. Controlled viruses are intended to replicate with near wild type efficiency specifically in a region in which no significant organ damage can occur and for the time required to induce an optimal immune response. Hence, the viruses functionally resemble wild type viruses but are contained to prevent induction of disease. While generally beneficial, replication-competent controlled viruses are expected to be uniquely suited for the vaccination of immunocompromised persons. Such persons may be particularly at risk for various microbial infections and would more than others benefit from effective vaccination. Their condition calls for the administration of the most potent vaccines available, which arguably are live attenuated viruses. Unfortunately, attenuated viruses may replicate too well and cause disease in some of these patients and, therefore, are generally considered to represent an unacceptable risk. In contrast, there is no reason for believing that activation and de-activation of replication-competent controlled viruses will be affected by the status of the immune system.
2. Recombination plasmid pBS-KS:ICP4Δpromoter was constructed as follows: a 600-bp segment of cosmid COS48 (a gift of L. Feldman, UCLA) was PCR-amplified using primers

HSV1.131428–131,404 (5′-CTCCTCAAGCTTCTCGAG CACACGGAGCGCGGCTGCCGACACG-3′) and HSV1.13 0859–130,880 (5′-CTCCTCGGTACCCCATGGAGGCCA GCAGAGCCAGC-3′). The primers placed HindIII and XhoI sites on the 5′ end of the amplified fragment and NcoI and KpnI sites on the 3′ end, respectively. Digestion of the PCR fragment with HindIII and KpnI yielded a 598-bp fragment which was gel-purified. Vector pBS-KS:ΔSacI (derived from plasmid vector Bluescript-KS+ by deletion of the polylinker SacI site) was digested with HindIII and KpnI, the resulting 2914-bp fragment was gel-purified and SAP-treated, and the purified fragment was ligated to the above 598-bp fragment. The resulting intermediate vector was named pBS-KS:ICP4–3′ end. A 549-bp segment of cosmid COS48 was PCR-amplified using primers HSV1.132271–132,250 (5′- CTCCTCGCGG CCGCACTAGTTCCGCGTGTCCCTTTCCGATGC-3′) and HSV1.131779–131,800 (5′- CTCCTCCTCGAGAAGC TTATGCATGAGCTCGACGTCTCGGCGGTAAT GAGATACGAGC-3′). These primers placed NotI and SpeI sites on the 5′ end of the amplified fragment and AatII, SacI, NsiI, HindIII and XhoI sites on its 3′ end. Digestion of the PCR fragment with NotI and XhoI yielded a 530-bp fragment that was gel-purified. Plasmid BS-KS:ICP4–3′ end was digested with NotI and XhoI, and the resulting 3446-bp fragment was gel-purified and SAP-treated. Ligation of the 3446- bp and 530-bp fragments produced pBS-KS:ICP4Δpromoter. The identity of pBS-KS:ICP4Δpromoter was confirmed by sequence analysis.

3. Essentially the same approach that was used to generate pBS-KS:ICP4Δpromoter was employed to construct recombination plasmid BS-KS:ICP8Δpromoter: a fragment derived by PCR amplification from HSV-1 syn17+ virion DNA using primers HSV1.61841–61,865 (5′- CTCCTCAGAACCCAGGACCA GGGCCACGTTGG-3′) and HSV1.62053–62,027 (5′- CTC CTCATGGAGACAAAGCCCAAGACGGCAACC-3′) was subcloned into pBS-KS:ΔSacI to yield pBS-KS:ICP8–3′ end. A second fragment derived by PCR amplification from HSV-1 syn17+ virion DNA using primers HSV1.62173–62,203 (5′-CTCCTCGGAGACCGGGGTTGGGGAATGAAT CC CTCC-3′) and HSV1.62395–62,366 (5′- CTCCTCGC GGGGCGTGGGAGGGGCTGGGGCGGACC-3′) was subcloned into pBS-KS:ICP8–3′ end to generate pBS-KS:ICP8Δpromoter.

4. Probably the most important single parameter dictating the efficiency of transfection is the quality of the viral DNA for the transfection. In order to work, the HSV transfection DNA needs to be unit length—that is, not sheared or degraded.

Care should be taken at all steps after the SDS/Proteinase K digestion not to vortex or too vigorously pipet the DNA.

5. The exact amount of HSV DNA used per transfection is generally in the range of 1–10 μg per 60-mm dish of cells. The optimal amount for a given DNA preparation should be determined empirically by transfecting dilutions of the stock DNA and determining the concentration that yields the highest efficiency. Once this is determined for a particular stock of DNA, the proper amount of DNA should not vary appreciably from experiment to experiment.
6. On average, a single 96-well plate will yield 1 or 2 wells that are positive for a recombinant, so generally two 96-well plates are screened for any given construct. In addition, it is generally a good idea to plaque-purify 2 or 3 independent recombinants (from separate transfection plates, and individual wells on the 96-well plate). This helps guard against a false positive that will lead nowhere and provides a back-up in the event a recombinant is found to have genome rearrangements in later stages of characterization. Note that plaques can be screened by limiting dilution, but in our hands picking the plaques and screening them directly speeds up the screening process and has allowed us to identify some recombinants that we were unable to detect by limiting dilution. This may be due to the fact that wild type virus may have a significant growth advantage over some recombinants.
7. While the DNA can be cross-linked to nylon membranes by UV irradiation, we have found that the baking method is more efficient when performing dot blots.

References

1. Roizman B (1996) The family Herpesviridae. A brief introduction. In: Fields RN, Knipe DM, Howley PM (eds) Fields virology, 3rd edn. Philadelphia, PA, Lippincott, Williams & Wilkins
2. Looker KJ, Margaret AS, May MT et al (2015) Global and regional estimates of prevalent and incident herpes simplex virus type 1 infections in 2012. PLoS One 10:e0140765
3. Looker KJ, Margaret AS, Turner KME et al (2015) Global estimates of prevalent and incident herpes simplex virus type 2 infections in 2012. PLoS One 10:e0114989
4. Belshe RB, Leone PA, Bernstein DI et al (2012) Efficacy results of a trial of a herpes simplex vaccine. N Engl J Med 366:34–43
5. CDC (2013) Varicella (chickenpox) and herpes zoster (shingles): overview of VZV disease and vaccination for healthcare professionals. Revised Aug 2, 2013
6. Kinchington PR, St Leger AJ, Guedon JM et al (2012) Herpes simplex virus and varicella zoster virus, the house guests who never leave. Herpes 3:5
7. Luo C, Goshima F, Kamakura M et al (2012) Immunization with a highly attenuated replication-competent herpes simplex virus type1 mutant, HF10, protects mice from genital disease caused by herpes simplex virus type 2. Front Microbiol 3:158
8. Brans R, Akhrameyeva NV, Yao F (2009) Prevention of genital herpes simplex virus type 1 and 2 disease in mice immunized with a gD-expressing dominant-negative recombinant HSV-1. J Invest Dermatol 129:2470–2479
9. Stanfield BA, Stahl J, Chouljenko VN et al (2014) A single intramuscular vaccination of mice with the HSV-1 VC2 virus with mutations in the glycoprotein K and the membrane protein UL20 confers full protection against

lethal intravaginal challenge with virulent HSV-1 and HSV-2 strains. PLoS One 9:e109890

10. Da Costa X, Kramer MF, Zhu J et al (2000) Construction, phenotypic analysis, and immunogenicity of a UL5/UL29 double deletion mutant of herpes simplex virus 2. J Virol 74:7963–7971
11. Hoshino Y, Dalai SK, Wang K et al (2005) Comparative efficacy and immunogenicity of replication-defective, recombinant glycoprotein, and DNA vaccines for herpes simplex virus 2 infections in mice and guinea pigs. J Virol 79:410–418
12. Petro C, Gonzalez PA, Cheshenko N et al (2015) Herpes simplex type 2 virus deleted in glycoprotein D protects against vaginal, skin and neural disease. eLife 4:e06054
13. Bran R, Eriksson E, Yao F (2008) Immunization with a dominant-negative recombinant HSV type 1 protects against HSV-1 skin disease in guinea pigs. J Invest Dermatol 128:2825–2832
14. Akhrameyeva NV, Zhang P, Sugiyama N et al (2011) Development of a glycoprotein D-expressing dominant-negative and replication-defective herpes simplex virus 2 (HSV-2) recombinant viral vaccine against HSV-2 infection in mice. J Virol 85:5036–5047
15. Vagvala SP, Thebeau LG, Wilson SR et al (2009) Virus-encoded B7-2 costimulation molecules enhance the protective capacity of a replication-defective herpes simplex virus type 2 vaccine in immunocompetent mice. J Virol 83:953–960
16. Johnston C, Koelle DM, Wald A (2014) Current status and prospects for development of an HSV vaccine. Vaccine 32:1553–1560
17. Aurelian L, Kokuba H, Smith CC (1999) Vaccine potential of a herpes simplex virus type 2 mutant deleted in the PK domain of the large subunit of ribonucleotide reductase (ICP10). Vaccine 17:1951–1963
18. Aurelian L (2004) Herpes simplex virus type 2 vaccines: new ground for optimism? Clin Vaccine Immunol 11:437–445
19. Casanova G, Cancela R, Alonzo L et al (2002) A double-blind study of the efficacy and safety of the ICP10ΔPK vaccine against recurrent genital HSV-2 infections. Cutis 70:235–239
20. Prichard MN, Kaiwar R, Jackman WT et al (2005) Evaluation of AD472, a live attenuated recombinant herpes simplex virus type 2 vaccine in guinea pigs. Vaccine 23:5424–5431
21. Halford WP, Püschel R, Gershburg E et al (2011) A live-attenuated HSV-2 ICP0⁻ virus elicits 10 to 100 times greater protection against genital herpes than a glycoprotein D subunit vaccine. PLoS One 6:e17748
22. Halford WP, Geltz J, Messer RJ et al (2015) Antibodies are required for complete vaccine-induced protection against herpes simplex virus 2. PloS One 10:e0145228
23. Awasthi S, Zumbrun EE, Si H et al (2012) Live attenuated herpes simplex virus 2 glycoprotein E deletion mutant as a vaccine candidate defective in neural spread. J Virol 86:4586–4598
24. Shin H, Iwasaki A (2012) A vaccine strategy that protects against genital herpes by establishing local memory T cells. Nature 491:463–468
25. Jones CA, Taylor TJ, Knipe DM (2000) Biological properties of herpes simplex virus 2 replication-defective mutant strains in a murine nasal infection model. Virology 278:137–150
26. Voellmy R, Bloom DC, Vilaboa N (2015) A novel approach for addressing diseases not yielding to effective vaccination? Immunization by replication-competent controlled virus. Expert Rev Vaccines 14:637–651
27. Bloom DC, Feller J, McAnany P et al (2015) Replication-competent controlled herpes simplex virus. J Virol 89:10668–10679
28. Lauterbach H, Kerksiek KM, Busch DH et al (2004) Protection from bacterial infection by a single vaccination with replication-deficient mutant herpes simplex virus type 1. J Virol 78:4020–4028
29. Murphy CG, Lucas WT, Means RE et al (2000) Vaccine protection against simian immunodeficiency virus by recombinant strains of herpes simplex virus. J Virol 74:7745–7754
30. Kaur A, Sanford HB, Garry D et al (2007) Ability of herpes simplex virus vectors to boost immune responses to DNA vectors and to protect against challenge by simian immunodeficiency virus. Virology 357:199–214
31. Vilaboa N, Fenna M, Munson J et al (2005) Novel gene switches for targeted and timed expression of proteins of interest. Mol Ther 12:290–298

Chapter 5

Generating Recombinant Pseudorabies Virus for Use as a Vaccine Platform

Feifei Tan[\$], Xiangdong Li[\$], and Kegong Tian

Abstract

Pseudorabies virus (PRV) is a promising vaccine vector due to its distinctive features including many non-essential replication regions and a broad host range. Foreign genes of other viruses have been successfully inserted into and expressed in PRV and these recombinant viruses are very likely to induce humoral and/or cellular responses in immunized animals. This chapter offers an overview of methods for generating recombinant pseudorabies virus for use as a vaccine vector.

Key words Pseudorabies, Vaccine platform, Bacterial artificial chromosome, Recombination

1 Introduction

Pseudorabies virus (PRV) is a member of the *herpesviridae* family, *Alpha-herpesvirinae* subfamily [1]. While swine species are the naturally infected hosts of PRV, this virus can infect a wide range of hosts, including most mammals [2]. In pigs, PRV infection may cause signs of nervous system involvement and death in newborn pigs, respiratory disorders in fattening pigs, and reproductive failure in sows [3].

PRV has a linear double strand-DNA genome, with a length of about 145 kb, containing a unique long region (UL), a unique short region (US), a terminal repeat sequence (TRS), and internal repeat sequences (IRS) [4]. Nearly half of the PRV genome is nonessential for virus infectivity [5]; therefore, this large genome is able to accommodate foreign sequence insertions into several of these nonessential sites (e.g., TK, gE, gI, gG) [6]. The most commonly used attenuated pseudorabies vaccine strain (Bartha) has a deletion of the gE and gI genes, yet retains its infectivity and immunogenicity [7].

[\$]These authors contribute equally in this work.

Maureen C. Ferran and Gary R. Skuse (eds.), *Recombinant Virus Vaccines: Methods and Protocols*, Methods in Molecular Biology, vol. 1581, DOI 10.1007/978-1-4939-6869-5_5, © Springer Science+Business Media LLC 2017

Live attenuated PRV has proven to be an excellent vector for foreign gene expression including the E2 glycoprotein of classical swine fever virus (CSFV) [8], the ORF2 of porcine circovirus [9], and the capsid and 3C genes of foot and mouth disease virus [10]. These findings indicate that recombinant PRV viruses can be generated, and that these viruses may be used as multivalent vaccines to control animal diseases.

Genomic and functional analysis of PRV has been difficult due to the virus's large and complicated genome. Homologous recombination can be used for genome manipulation, however this method is time-consuming. Therefore manipulation of the PRV genome was challenging until the PRV genome was cloned into an infectious plasmid as bacterial artificial chromosomes (BACs) [11]. The first BAC-based PRV infectious clone was constructed in 1999 [12]. This technique enables the stable maintenance of the PRV genomes as BACs in *Escherichia coli* [13, 14] and facilitates mutagenesis of the viral genome using the bacterial recombination machinery. The recombinant virus can be rescued by transfection of the constructed BAC plasmid into permissive eukaryotic cells. This chapter will detail how recombinant PRV (rPRV) can be generated using the above technique. The well-established bacteriophage λ Red homologous recombination system is commonly used for genome manipulation in *E. coli*. Recombinants could be easily generated using very short homology sequences for recombination [15].

As shown in Fig. 1, generation of a PRV-BAC clone involves co-transfection of the PRV genome and the constructed BAC plasmid into permissive eukaryotic cells such as Vero cells. The Red system allows the recombination of linear DNA containing limited regions of homology with the *E. coli* chromosome, a process known as recombineering. During co-transfection recombination happens between the BAC cassette and one PRV nonessential gene such as TK gene, the most commonly targeted nonessential gene. The recombinant virus containing the BAC cassette (PRV-BAC) is then rescued by fluorescence-positive cell selection since BAC cassette contains the GFP gene. The circular DNA of PRV-BAC is next isolated and transformed into DH10B competent cells to generate the BAC-PRV plasmid [12]. Positive BAC-PRV plasmid clones are identified by digestion with the Bam HI restriction enzyme [16].

This BAC-PRV plasmid can now be used as a platform for PRV genome modification such as insertion of foreign genes or deletion of PRV genes. To insert foreign genes, PCR products containing a positive selection marker such as a kanamycin resistant gene and short sequences duplications flanking the target insertion site (some other PRV nonessential gene except TK gene) are transformed into competent cells that harbor recombinant BAC-PRV plasmid to obtain the mutant BAC plasmid [13]. This mutant plasmid is co-transfected with pBS185 CMV-Cre, expressing the Cre

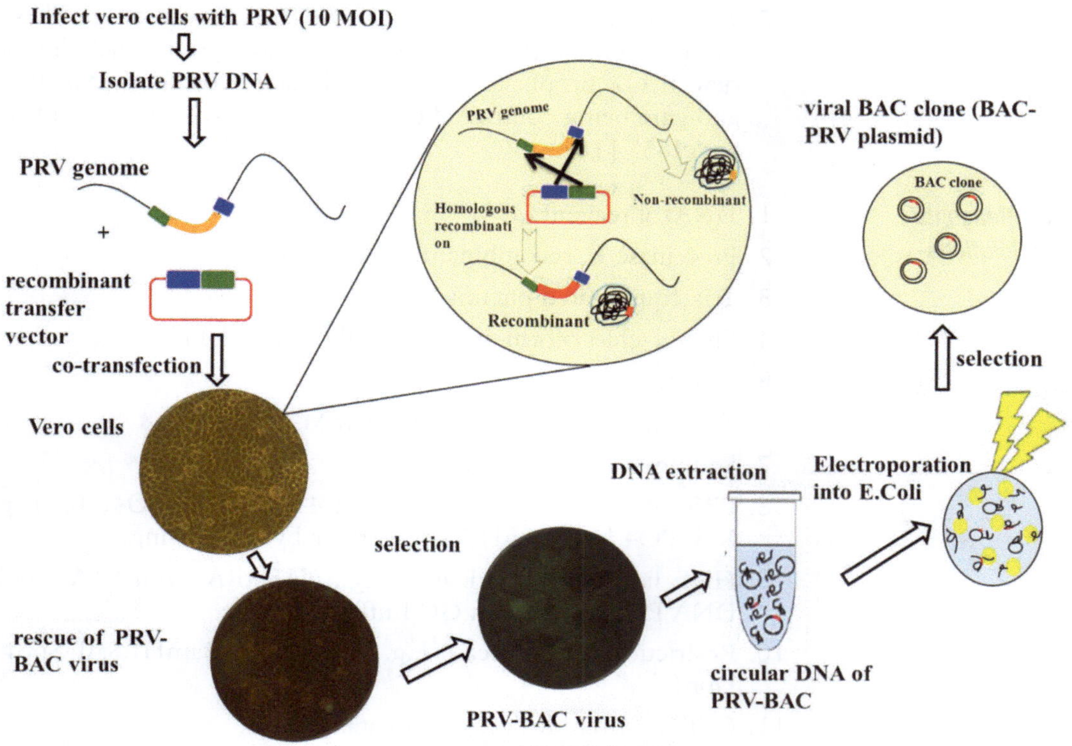

Fig. 1 Generation of a PRV-BAC clone in E. coli. Recombinant PRV-BAC is achieved by co-transfection of PRV genome and engineered BAC plasmid into Vero cells. The GFP positive virus colonies are selected and subject to plaque purification to get RPV-BAC. The circular DNA of PRV-BAC is next extracted and transformed into DH10B competent cells to get BAC-PRV plasmid. The BAC-PRV plasmid is verified by restriction enzymes Bam HI digestion

recombinant enzyme, into Vero cells. The mutant recombinant PRV (with exogenous gene inserted) is isolated after several rounds of plaque purification.

2 Materials

2.1 Plasmids and Bacterial Strains

1. pUC19: plasmid containing multiple cloning sites.
2. pAcGFP1-C1: plasmid containing GFP cassette used for recombinant virus screening.
3. BAC vector, e.g., pBeloBAC11.
4. pBS185 CMV-Cre, available from Addgene (Cambridge, MA).
5. DH-5α competent cells: containing gpt gene used for pressure selection.
6. DH10B Competent Cells.

7. *E. coli* strain DY380: the original DH10B-derived strain. These bacteria contain the full Red recombinase system, including a defective λ prophage with recombination proteins exo, bet, and gam being controlled by the temperature-sensitive repressor cI857 [18].

2.2 Reagents and Solutions

1. DNAzol reagent.
2. Proteinase K, recombinant, PCR grade.
3. Tris-equilibrated phenol.
4. Phenol–chloroform–isoamyl alcohol (25:24:1).
5. Ethanol.
6. TE buffer (10 mM Tris–HCl, 1 mM EDTA).
7. Sodium acetate (3 M, pH 5.2).
8. PBS (8 g NaCl, 0.2 g KCl, 1.44 g Na2HPO4, 0.24 g KH2PO4 in 1 L., pH 7.4). Sterilize by autoclaving.
9. High fidelity PCR enzyme, e.g., TAKARA PrimeSTAR HS DNA Polymerase with GC Buffer.
10. Restriction endonuclease, e.g., XbaI, XhoI, BamHI,SalI, SphI, DpnI.
11. Calf intestinal alkaline phosphatase (CIP).
12. T4 DNA ligase.
13. Lysis Buffer (0.5% M/V SDS; 10 mM Tris–HCl, pH 8.0;100 mM EDTA; pH 8.0,20 μg/ml RNase A) [17].
14. SOC medium(1 g yeast extract,4 g tryptone, 0.4 ml 5 N NaCl, 0.5 ml 1 N KCl, 2 ml 1 N MgCl2,2 ml 1 N MgSO4). Make up the total volume to 150 ml with ddH_2O and autoclave. Dissolve 0.72 g of glucose in 50 ml ddH_2O and filter sterilize the solution. Add the entire sterile glucose solution to the autoclaved solution once cooled.
15. Low-salt LB medium: 0.5% yeast extract, 1% tryptone, 0.5% NaCl.
16. Low-salt LB plates:1.0% tryptone, 0.5% yeast extract, 0.5% NaCl, 1.5% agar.
17. Antibiotic: 15 μg/ml chloramphenicol, 50 μg/ml kanamycin, 50 μg/ml ampicillin.
18. Plasmid mini Kit, e.g., QIAGEN plasmid mini Kit.
19. Commercial Kit for purifying BAC DNA or low-copy number plasmid, e.g., QIAGEN Large Construct Kit.

2.3 Tissue Culture Medium

1. Fetal bovine serum (FBS).
2. Dulbecco's modified Eagle's medium (DMEM): Dissolve the DMEM power (Invitrogen) in 10 liters of ddH_2O and filter sterilize the solution.

3. Maintenance medium (DMEM containing 2% FBS).
4. Growth medium (DMEM containing 10% FBS).
5. Screening medium: 100 ml DMEM containing 50 μg/ml mycophenolic acid, 65 μg/ml xanthine, 100 μg/ml hypoxanthine, pH 7.2.
6. Opti-MEM reduced serum medium.
7. Trypsin with 0.125% EDTA, tissue culture grade.
8. Lipofectamine 2000 transfection reagents.
9. Low-melting point agarose.

2.4 Equipment

1. Class II biological safety cabinet.
2. Cell culture incubator.
3. Incubators set at 32 and 37 °C
4. Electroporation system, e.g., Bio-Rad Gene Pulser X cell.
5. High-speed refrigerated centrifuge
6. 0.1 cm cuvette.
7. Inverted fluorescence microscope.
8. Water bath shaker
9. PCR thermocycler.
10. Tissue culture plates: 6-well, 10 cm cell culture dish, T75 flask.
11. Conical tubes: 15 and 50 ml.

3 Methods

3.1 Preparation of Recombination Transfer Vector

As shown in Fig. 2, core elements of the recombinant transfer vector include the homology sequence (TKA and TKB) to PRV genome, screening cassette (reporter gene GFP and gpt), and the BAC vector sequence (pBeloBAC11). In this chapter, UL23 (TK gene) is used as the recombination target site of BAC vector, so the homology fragments (TKA and TKB as shown in Fig. 2) lie in the upstream UL24 gene and the downstream UL22 gene separately.

3.1.1 Amplification and Cloning of Homology Fragments

To facilitate cloning, proper restriction sites should be added to the end of primers to facilitate insertion into the pUC19 vector, and primers amplifying TKB should contain the restriction site (e.g., SphI) the allows the BAC vector to be linearized and cloned into pUC19. One loxp recognition site (5′-ATAACTTCGTATA-GCATACAT–TAT ACGAAGTTAT-3′) is introduced downstream of the left homology fragment TKA. Total genome DNA extracted from PRV-infected cells is used as template to amplify TKA and TKB. The PCR products are then cloned into the pUC19 vector

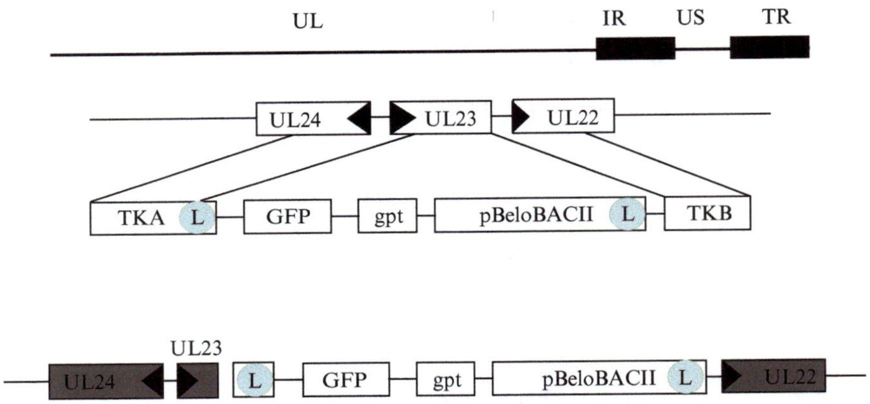

Fig. 2 Schematic illustration for preparation of recombination transfer vector. Core elements of recombinant vector include homology fragments (TKA and TKB), screen cassette (GFP and gpt), and BAC vector sequence (pBelBAC11). Two loxp sites (L) lie in downstream of TKA and upstream of TKB respectively. This figure was cited from Ref. 21

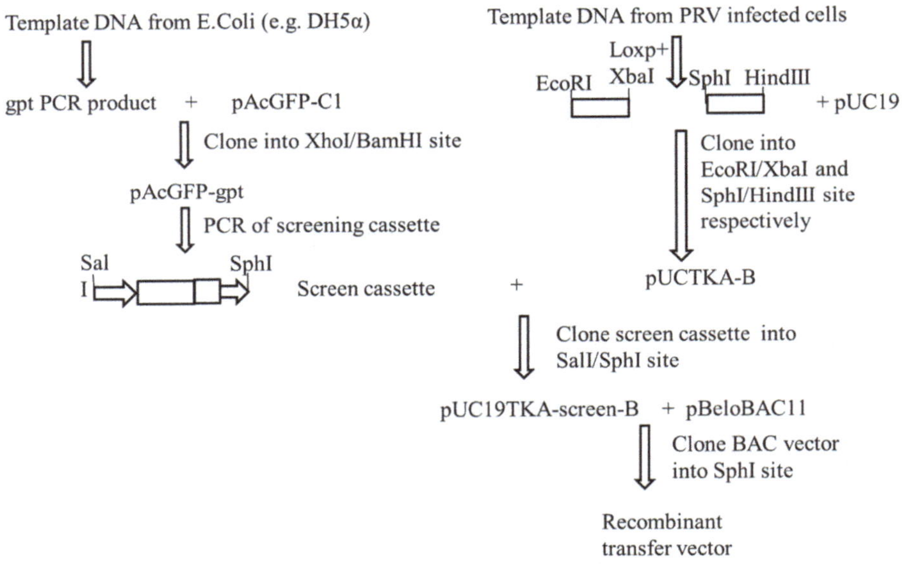

Fig. 3 Cloning strategy of recombinant transfer vector

successively through digestion and ligation (named pUC19TKA-B in Fig. 3) (*see* **Notes 1–3**).

3.1.2 Cloning of Screening Cassette

Two screening genes (GFP and gpt) are employed in this chapter. Firstly, the gpt gene from DH-5α *E. coli* is amplified and cloned into the XhoI/BamHI sites downstream of the GFP expression cassette of the pAcGFP-C1 vector. Then, the full screening cassette, including GFP and gpt, is amplified by PCR using the previous cloning product pAcGFP-gpt as template. The primer pairs used for PCR lie in the Human cytomegalovirus (CMV) immediate early promoter and SV40 early mRNA polyadenylation signal of pAcGFP-C1 respectively. The PCR product is cloned into SalI/SphI sites of the plasmid created in Subheading 3.1.1 (named pUC19TKA-screen-B in Fig. 3).

3.1.3 Generation of Final Recombinant Transfer Vector

Plasmid pUC19TKA-screen-B, created in Subheading 3.1.2, is dephosphorylated by CIP treatment after digestion with SphI. Vector pBeloBAC11 is also linearized by SphI digestion. After T4 DNA ligation, 10 μl ligation products are transformed into 100 μl *E. coli* DH10B and selected for colonies by growing on LB plates containing 50 μg/ml Ampicillin and 15 μg/ml chloromycetin. Isolate the recombinant transfer vector plasmid using QIAGEN plasmid mini Kit. Identify clones by Bam HI digestion analysis and sequencing analysis (*see* **Note 4**).

3.1.4 Preparing Large-Quantity of Transfer Vector by Electroporation and Midiprep

Electroporate the recombinant transfer vector into DH10B competent cells as follow:

1. Prepare the following materials: 50 μl competent cells on ice, 0.1 cm cuvette on ice, 1 ml SOC medium at room temperature.
2. Add 1 μl (about 0.5–1 μg) plasmid to the competent cells, mix gently by stirring with a pipette tip and incubate for 10 min on ice.
3. Turn on the electroporation machine, choose 0.1 cm cuvette, enter the preset program: bacterial -*E. coli*, 1.75kv,25 μF,200Ω-Enter.
4. Insert the cuvette and pipette the mixture prepared in **step 2** into it, avoid introduction of bubbles, close the lid and press the pulse button.
5. Observe the time constant, which should be about 4.5–5.0 ms.
6. Remove the cuvette and add 1 ml SOC medium immediately, then transfer the contents to a sterilize 1.5 ml centrifuge tube.
7. Incubate the tube at 37 °C for 1 h with shaking at 220 rpm. Concentrate the culture by centrifuging at 3000 × *g* for 4 min, resuspend the pellet in 100 μl LB medium and plate the entire culture onto LB plate containing ampicillin and chloromycetin.
8. Incubate in 37 °C overnight.
9. Pick single colonies into 3 ml LB medium containing ampicillin and chloromycetin and grow for 10 h in a shaking incubator. Use 1 ml starter culture to inoculate 200 ml LB medium containing Ampicillin and chloromycetin and culture overnight in shaking incubator at 37 °C.
10. Extract transfer vector DNA using a commercially available kit for BAC DNA extraction, such as the QIAGEN Large-Construct kit.

11. Resupend the high-quality plasmid DNA at 0.5–5 μg/μl in deionized water or TE buffer.

3.2 Rescue of PRV-BAC: Prepare PRV Genomic DNA

1. Infect a monolayer of Vero cells in a 10 cm dish at a multiplicity of infection (MOI) of 10.
2. To make the adsorption mix, dilute the appropriate amount of virus stock with DMEM without FBS to a final volume of 2 ml per dish.
3. Add adsorption mix to a dish.
4. After a 1 hour (h) incubation in a 37 °C incubator with 5% CO_2,the adsorption mix is removed and 15 ml DMEM with 2% FBS is added per plate.
5. Incubate in tissue culture incubator for 24 h.
6. Isolate PRV genomic DNA by DNAzol reagent following instruction manual.
7. Collected DNA is quantified and about 3 μg DNA is sufficient per transfection.

3.3 Rescue of PRV-BAC: Co-Transfection of PRV Genomic DNA with Transfer Vector

1. Trypsinize and dilute Vero cells to a density so that the monolayers will be 80–90% confluent on the following day. Cells are usually seeded into 6-well plates for transfection (*see* **Note 5**).
2. Shake cells constantly for a while (about 5–10 s) after seeding to allow even distribution of the cells. Incubate the cells at 37 °C, 5% CO_2 in a tissue culture incubator.
3. To co-transfect PRV genomic DNA with transfer vector, add the proper ratio of genomic DNA and transfer vector DNA into 150 μl Opti-MEM per transfection sample, and mix thoroughly and incubate for 5 min are room temperature. A ratio of 5 μg genomic DNA: 3 μg of transfer vector DNA per transfection sample is commonly used (*see* **Note 6**).
4. Dilute optimal amount (usually 10 μl) of Lipofectamine 2000 with 150 μl Opti-MEM per transfection sample. Incubate for 5 min at room temperature.
5. Mix the diluted DNA and diluted Lipofectamine 2000 reagent at a 1:1 ratio. Mix thoroughly and incubate for 20 min at room temperature.
6. During this period, remove the growth medium from the cells and wash the monolayer with PBS two times.
7. After incubation in **step 5**, add DNA-reagent complex to cells and mix gently.
8. Prepare three wells as controls: genomic DNA control, transfer vector DNA control, Lipofectamine reagent control, respectively.

9. After incubation in a tissue cell culture incubator for 4–6 h, replace the transfection solution with maintenance medium.
10. Visualize possible PRV-induced cytopathic effects (CPE). Look for enlarged and rounded cells and syncitium formation after 1–3 days
11. When cells exhibited 80% CPE, harvest virus culture supernatants by pipetting. This virus will be screened in the next section.

3.4 Rescue of PRV-BAC: Screening by Pressure Selection

1. Seed fresh Vero cells (80–90% confluent) in six-well plate, change the growth medium to screening medium 2 h before inoculate virus supernatants.
2. Make tenfold serial dilutions (from 10^{-1} to 10^{-8}) of virus supernatants in screening medium to a final volume of 1 ml in each dilution.
3. Infect Vero cells with 500 μl viral dilutions per well. After 1 h adsorption, wash cells twice with PBS and supply cells with 2 ml of screening medium containing 2% FBS per well.
4. When obvious CPE and green fluorescence under microscope appears, freeze the cells at −80 °C and thaw at room temperature for three times.
5. Repeat the selection procedure from **steps 2** to **5** until most cells showed CPE and harbors green fluorescence under the microscope. In this case, the relatively pure PRV-BAC will be achieved by several rounds of such virus purification. Normally, at least three rounds of screening are required.

3.5 Recue of PRV-BAC: Screening by Plaque Purification

1. 500ul supernatants harvested after above screening are used to infect 90% confluent fresh Vero cells to in six-well plates with serial dilution (from 10^{-1} to 10^{-8}).
2. At the end of 1 h–absorption, remove the medium and wash each well with 2 ml of pre-warmed PBS.
3. Overlay cells with 1% low-melting point agarose containing 2% FBS in DMEM.
4. 48–72 h after infection, when visible plaques have formed, pick several single plaques harboring green fluorescence with pipetting tips into 200 μl DMEM medium.
5. Freeze thaw at −80 °C three times, inoculate the medium on fresh cells.
6. Repeat passaging and picking plaques until all cells exhibit CPE and also express green fluorescent protein, this process might require three to five passages.
7. Centrifuge the cell culture at 3000 × *g* for 10mins and remove the cell debris, extract viral DNA from cell supernatants. The

viral DNA is confirmed by PCR and BamH I restriction enzyme digestion to ensure the purified virus carries the BAC vector sequence, correct screening cassette and correct genomic locus. Purified recombinant virus is referred to as PRV-BAC.

3.6 Preparation of BAC-PRV Plasmid from PRV-BAC DNA

Infect Vero cells in 10 cm dish with PRV-BAC at a MOI of 10. Collect cell debris after 3, 6, 9, 12, 15 h post-infection (hpi) by scraping cells off the dish and centrifuge at 3000 × *g* for 10 min and remove the supernatant (*see* **Note 7**). Isolate viral circular DNA by the Hirt method [19] with minor changes as follows:

1. Resuspend cells from each 10 cm dish in 300 μl PBS.
2. Add 1 ml lysis buffer to each resuspended sample and incubate at 37 for 1 h;
3. Add Proteinase K to a final concentration of 200 μg/ml to each lysed sample and incubate for 3 h at 50 °C, shake every 30 min for better digestion.
4. Extract the supernatant with an equal volume of Tris-equilibrated phenol twice and phenol–chloroform–isoamyl alcohol (25:24:1) twice. Centrifuge at 6500 × *g* for 15 min at 4 °C each time and collect the top aqueous layer using wide-orifice pipette tips.
5. Precipitate DNA with two volumes of ethanol and 0.4 vol of sodium acetate; wash pelleted DNA twice with 1 ml 70% ethanol.
6. Gently dissolve the DNA in 30 μl–50 μl TE buffer and determine DNA concentration.
7. Electroporate the DNA into *DH10B* electrocompetent cells using 0.1 cm cuvette with the preset procedure as described in Subheading 3.1.4.
8. Plate 100 μl culture on LB agar plate containing 15 μg/ml chloromycetin.
9. The next day pick a single colony into 5 ml liquid LB medium containing 15 μg/ml chloramphenicol and incubate at 37 °C overnight.
10. Extract plasmid using QIAGEN plasmid mini kit. Finally dissolve DNA in 50 μl TE buffer.
11. Analyze the plasmid by BamHI (most commonly used enzyme for PRV) digestion, and compare the restriction pattern to the predicted pattern of the parental virus. Figure 4 shows the restriction patterns of BAC-PRV plasmid by BamHI digestion.

3.7 Reconstitution of Infectious PRV from BAC Clones

The BAC-PRV plasmid must be transfected back to Vero cells to determine whether it can recover infectious virus in tissue culture.

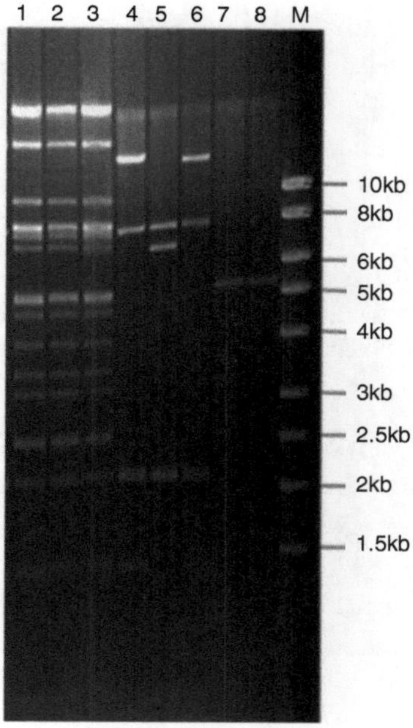

Fig. 4 Analysis of restriction patterns of PRV-BAC DNA by BamHI digestion. *Lanes 1–3* have the similar pattern with the predicted pattern of parental virus. *Lanes 4–8* contains only a few bands that cannot constitute integral genome of PRV

1. Transfect BAC-RPV plasmid into Vero cells. The transfection procedure is the same as described above; however, use BAC-PRV plasmid instead.
2. After transfection, examine the 6-well plate under the inverted fluorescence microscope, monitor cells exhibiting signs of CPE that also harbor green fluorescence (GFP expression) (Fig. 5a). Visible CPE and GFP expression means the BAC-RPV plasmid can reconstitute infectious virus in tissue culture, and non-CPE and fluorescence in single cell illustrates the failure of reconstitution, as shown in Fig. 5b. It is optional to compare the biological characters of the reconstituted virus to parental virus such as virus one-step growth curve or plaque assay.

3.8 Overview: Rescue of Recombinant PRV

A pseudorabies gene deleted vaccine that is highly attenuated has been used for many years all around the world. This attenuated PRV can be used as a promising vector for multivalent vaccines by inserting foreign genes into a replication nonessential region. The Virus-BAC system allows almost unlimited genetic manipulation, including gene-deletion and insertion [13].

The methods used to modify virus-BAC genome include transposon mutagenesis, RecA-based mutagenesis, Red and RecE/T based recombineering, I-SceI homing enzyme based *en passant* mutagenesis, and so on [20]. Among these methods, the well-established Red recombination system is commonly used. The

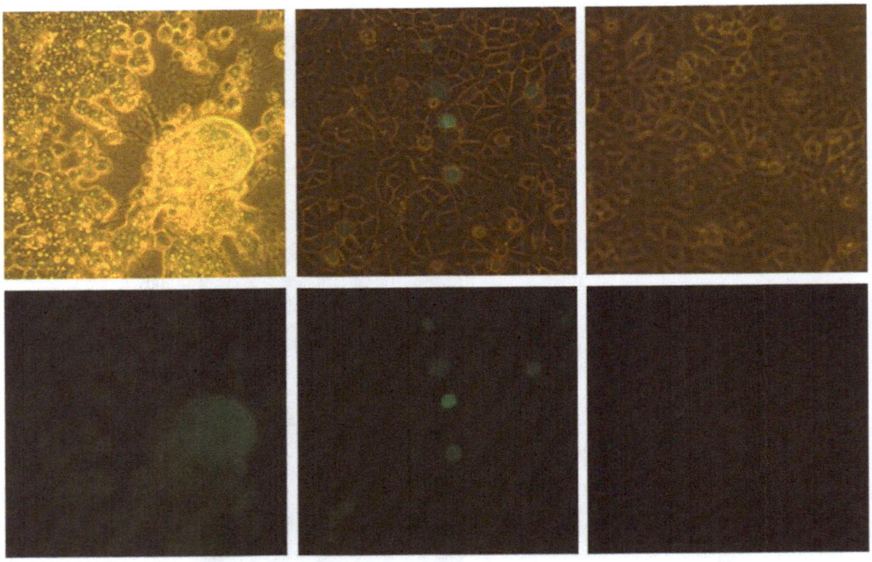

Fig. 5 Reconstitution of infectious PRV from BAC clones. The *top row* shows the CPE or normal cell under white light, and the *bottom row* shows the corresponding view under the fluorescent microscope. (**a**) successfully reconstitution, cell displays CPE with green fluorescence; (**b**) Failure of reconstitution, single cell containing green fluorescence represent the replication of incomplete BAC-DNA in eukaryotic cells; (**c**) Normal cell

major advantage of this system is allowing only 30–50 bp of homologous sequences which that for the recombination. The removal of resistance gene that contained in the recombinant cassette can be achieved by Cre-loxp or FLP/FRT system through induction of the Cre or FLP recombinase subsequently but retaining a single loxP or FRT site. *En passant* mutagenesis combines Red recombination with homing endonuclease I-SceI cleavage, and allows the introduction of a mutation without retaining any foreign sequence. The strategies for the Red-mediated sequence deletion and sequence insertion is illustrated in Fig. 6. The procedure of *en passant* mutagenesis is described in this section.

3.9 Rescue of Recombinant PRV: Preparation of the Recombinant Cassette

A PCR product containing a positive selection gene (e.g., kanamycin) together with an I-SceI site flanked by a 50 bp duplicated sequence is used as the recombination cassette. Short homologous sequences at either end of the marker cassette allow the first Red recombination, and the duplication allows the removal of entire marker in a second Red recombination after I-SceI digestion. As shown in Fig. 6. For gene-insertion, it is necessary to construct a transfer vector containing the gene of interest flanked by homologous sequences for Red recombination [13]. The gene of interest is inserted into a plasmid containing a resistant gene, I-SceI site, and a unique restriction site for sequence duplication.

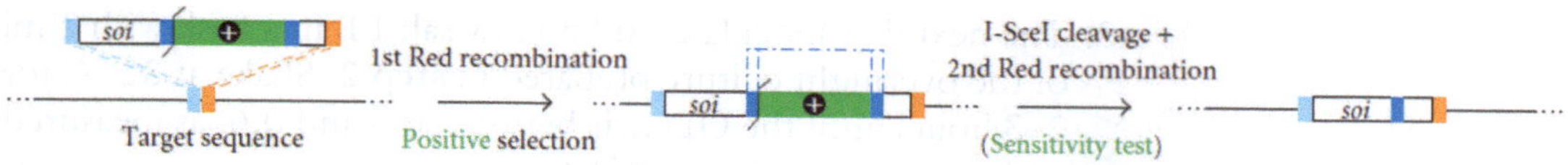

Fig. 6 General strategy for the Red-mediated sequence. This figure was cited from Ref. 13. *Light blue* and *orange boxes* represent the homologous sequence target to the PRV-BAC DNA. *Green box* represent the resistance gene cassette. Soi means sequence of interest (*deep blue box* lies upstream of the unique restriction site); represent the sequence need to be insertion. Soi containing positive marker is inserted into the targeted site through the first Red recombination by terminal homology sequence. Upon insertion of the transfer cassette, linearize the BAC construct by I-SceI endonuclease. The sequence duplications flanking the selection marker allow a second Red recombination resulting in the removal of all operational sequence

1. Select one unique restriction site in interested gene for insertion of selection marker.
2. Amplify the selection marker gene (such as kanamycin) from plasmid pAcGFP-C1 by PCR using a pair of primers described below. The 5′ primer contains unique restriction site, I-SceI site, 20–25 bp sequence that anneals the template pAcGFP-C1. The 3′ primer contains 30–50 bp duplication sequence upstream of unique restriction site gene, 20–25 bp sequence that anneals the template pAcGFP-C1, and unique restriction site.
3. Amplify the sequence of interested and clone it into a cloning vector. Then clone the PCR product in **step 2** into the interested gene by the unique restriction site.
4. To achieve the final recombinant cassette, amplify the intact cassette from the cloning product in **step 3** by PCR using a pairs of primers containing duplication sequences flanking targeted insertion site and interested gene terminal sequences.
5. Add 1–2 μl DpnI directly to the PCR reaction (works well in PCR buffer), and incubate for 1 hour at 37 °C, followed by gel purification.

3.10 Rescue of Recombinant PRV: Preparation of Recombination-Competent Cells that Harbor BAC-PRV Plasmid

Transform the BAC-PRV plasmid identified in **step 1** of Subheading 3.3 into DY380 *E. coli*, which contains a chromosomally encoded λ prophage. The DY380 cells transformed with the BAC-PRV plasmid strain are induced in a temperature-dependent manner and made competent for electroporation as follow:

1. Streak the original DY380 bacterial culture out for single colony isolation on a low salt LB plate containing 15 g/ml chloromycetin. Incubate for 18–20 h at 32 °C until single colonies are visible (*see* **Note 8**).
2. Pick a single colony into 3 ml low salt LB medium containing 15 g/ml chloromycetin. Grow the cells overnight (about 18–20 h) at 32 °C with shaking at 240 rpm.

3. The next day, inoculate 100 ml low salt LB in a flask with 2 ml of the overnight culture prepared in **step 2**. Shake at 32 °C for 2–3 hours until the OD_{600} is between 0.5 and 0.6, as measured with a spectrophotometer.
4. Transfer 50 ml of this culture to a sterile 50 ml conical tube and place on ice for the preparation of uninduced electroporation competent cells.
5. The remaining 50 ml of culture is used for preparation of induced competent cells. Quickly transfer this flask to a water shaker set to 42 °C. Shake the cells at 220 rpm for 15 min to induce the expression of the Red recombinase enzyme.
6. Incubate both the uninduced and induced cultures on ice for 20–30 min. Keep these cells on ice for the following steps and prechill 50 ml centrifuge tubes, and the 10% glycerol needed for the subsequent steps.
7. Transfer the cultures to the labeled, prechilled 50 ml centrifuge tube and centrifuge at 3000 × *g* for 5 min at 4 °C. Carefully discard the supernatant and resuspend the pelleted cells in 40 ml prechilled 10% glycerol.
8. Centrifuge at 3000 × *g* for 5 min at 4 °C. Carefully discard the supernatant and resuspend the pelleted cells in 20 ml prechilled 10% glycerol.
9. Centrifuge at 3000 × *g* for 5 min at 4 °C. Carefully discard the supernatant and resuspend the pelleted cells in 10 ml prechilled 10% glycerol.
10. Centrifuge at 3000 × *g* for 5 min at 4 °C.
11. Add 2% of initial culture volume (100 ml in **step 3**) of prechilled 10% glycerol to the cell pellet, resuspend and aliquot (50 μl/tube). Use each tube for one electroporation immediately (*see* **Note 9**).

3.11 Rescue of Recombinant PRV: Electroporation (Using BioRad Gene Pulser Xcell) into Freshly Prepared Competent Cells

1. For each sample to be electroporated, these following materials should be prepared: 50 μl competent cells, one 0.1 cm cuvette, 1 ml SOC medium at room temperature.
2. Add 100–500 ng linearized DNA fragment (purified PCR product of recombinant cassette after DpnI digestion) to the induced competent cells on ice. Also add an equal amount of this DNA to the uninduced competent cells as a control. Mix gently by stirring with a pipette tip and incubate for 10 min on ice.
3. Turn on the electroporation machine, choose 0.1 cm cuvette, and set up the preset program: bacterial—*E. coli*, 1.75kv, 25 μF,200Ω-"Enter".
4. Insert the cuvette and pipette the mixture in **step 2** to the bottom of the cuvette, close the lid and press the "Pulse" button.

5. Observe the time constant, which should be about 4.5–5.0 ms.
6. Take out the cuvette and add 1 ml SOC medium immediately, then transfer to a sterilize 1.5 ml centrifuge tube.
7. Incubate at 32 °C for 1 h with shaking at 220 rpm. Plate the entire culture on LB plate containing 15 μg/ml chloramphenicol and 50 μg/ml kanamycin. Incubate at 32 °C for 24 h.

3.12 Rescue of Recombinant PRV: Screening of PRV Mutant Containing the Gene of Interest

1. Inoculate a single colony into 5 ml LB medium containing chloramphenicol and kanamycin. Repeat this process with several other single colonies. Incubate at 32 °C overnight.
2. To extract the recombinant mutant DNA using the Qiagen Plasmid Mini Kit, harvest the bacterial cells by centrifugation at 12000 × *g* for 2 min at 4 °C.
3. Resuspend the cell pellet with 0.2 ml Buffer P1.
4. Add 0.2 ml Buffer P2 to cell lysis, and mix thoroughly by inverting the tubes 4–6 times.
5. Add 0.2 ml Buffer P3, mix immediately and thoroughly by inverting the tubes 4–6 times. Incubate for 5 min on ice.
6. Centrifuge at 12,000 × *g* for 10 min at 4 °C, and transfer the supernatant to a new tube.
7. Extract the supernatant with an equal volume of phenol–chloroform–isoamyl alcohol (25:24:1), and centrifuge at 6500 × *g* for 10 min at 4 °C.
8. Precipitate DNA with two volumes of ethanol and 0.4 volume of Sodium acetate. To wash pellet add 1 ml 70% ethanol. Repeat twice. Remove as much ethanol as possible.
9. Gently dissolve the DNA in 30 μl~50 μl TE buffer.
10. Confirm the correct recombinant mutant by PCR amplification and restriction enzyme BamHI digestion (*see* **Note 10**).

3.13 Rescue of Recombinant PRV: Removal of the Resistance Gene (Such as Kanamycin) from Constructed DNA

1. Linearize the recombinant DNA confirmed in Subheading 3.15 with homing enzyme I-SceI and incubate at 37 °C for about 12 h.
2. The next day, add ddH_20 to a final volume of 200 μl, and extract DNA using the phenol–chloroform–isoamyl alcohol (25:24:1) method as described in **step 4** of Subheading 3.4.
3. The purified linearized DNA is used for the second-recombination as following **steps 4–8**:
4. Prepare induced DY380 competent cells without any DNA, as protocols described in **step 2** of Subheading 3.4.
5. Electroporate the linearized DNA into DY380 competent cells as described in step 4 of Subheaidng 3.4.

6. After incubation in a 32 °C shaker for 1 h, plate the bacterial cells on LB plates containing15 μg/ml chloromycetin. Use a plate containing chloromycetin and kanamycin resistance as controls. Zero to very few colonies should grow on this control plate.
7. Pick at least 20–30 colonies from the chloromycetin resistance plate and screen for deletion of the resistance gene using the methods described in **step 1** of Subheading 3.3; including PCR amplification and BamHI restriction analysis (*see* **Note 10**).
8. Innoculate the candidate positive clone without the resistance gene into a large volume (at least 200 ml) of bacterial culture. Extract plasmid DNA using QIAGEN Large Construct Kit that can be used for transfection.

3.14 Rescue of Recombinant PRV that Expressed Foreign Genes

1. To recover the recombinant deletion/insertion mutant virus without removing the BAC vector, transfect Vero cells with the verified plasmid DNA only as described in **step 2** of Subheading 3.3. The transfection procedure is as described above.
2. When visible CPE appears, gather supernatants as recombinant mutant virus stock. Titration of virus is optional.

3.15 Remove the Screening Cassette and BAC Gene from the Recombinant PRV

As previously described, the two loxp sites in the transfer vector make the sequences between them easy to remove using the Cre recombinase. This is useful if removal of the screening cassette and BAC gene is desired. Removal of GFP is sometimes desirable because the exogenous genes, other than the gene of interest, are not allowed to be included in recombinant viruses during vaccine registration in some countries. Upon co-transfection of BAC-PRV and pBS185 plasmid, the Cre recombinase expressed by pBS185 in cells will recognize the two loxp sites in the recombinant deletion/insertion PRV genome and produce virus without GFP and BAC gene. It is worth noting that the mutant virus obtained by this strategy still contains a 34 bp loxp recognition site which cannot be removed.

1. Co-transfect Vero cells with the pBS185 CMV-Cre plasmid with the extracted BAC-PRV as described above.
2. Use a ratio of 3 μg recombinant genomic DNA and 5 μg of pBS185 CMV-Cre plasmid per transfection sample.
3. 2–3 rounds of plaque purification are required to isolate purified virus without foreign sequence.

3.16 Growth and Harvesting of Recombinant PRV Stocks

1. Grow Vero cells in a T75 or larger flask so they will be 90–95% confluence at time of infection.
2. Infect Vero cells with recombinant PRV at an MOI of 0.01.

3. When visible CPE appears after 48–72 h after infection, transfer the supernatants to 50 ml centrifuge tube and centrifuge at 4000 × *g* for 10 min at 4 °C. Aliquot the supernatants into sterile tubes and freeze at −80 for long-term storage.

4 Notes

1. Preferably, the length of the homology arms should be longer than 1000 bp.
2. Using a high-fidelity PCR polymerase to avoid introduction of random mutations.
3. The recombinant transfer vector should be verified by sequencing to ensure that it encodes the correct sequence of the homology arm, loxp sites, and screening cassette. This will ensure the value of continuing on with the recombination and gene manipulation procedures.
4. Plasmid pBeloBAC11 contains a loxp site at its 3′-terminal, so the transfer vector contains two loxp sites flanking the screening cassette with BAC vector, which is convenient for removing BAC vector from the recombinant virus ultimately [21].
5. Other cell lines suitable for PRV propagation can also be used, such as Marc-145 and BHK.
6. Optimize the ratio of genomic DNA to transfer vector at first operation.
7. To maximize collection of circular DNA (a replicative intermediate), samples are collected during several time points post infection. This ensures sample collection during optimal viral replication.
8. Low salt LB is preferred during preparation of competent cells. Residual salt may affect efficiency of electroporation and/or result in arching.
9. It is better to prepare fresh competent cells for each electroporation, otherwise freeze the cells at −80° for long-term storage.
10. PCR product should be able to distinguish recombinant and non-recombinant mutant, primers usually locates in both sides of the target deletion/insertion site. BamHI analysis could ensure the genomic integrity of recombinant DNA.

Acknowledgments

This work was supported by grant from Innovation Scientists and Technicians Troop Construction Projects of Henan Province (Grant No.142101510001), Talents Plan for Scientific and

Technological Innovation in Henan Province (Grant No.144200510002), Science and Technology Innovation team in Henan Province (Team No. C20130005), and Luoyang Heluo Talent Plan (Kegong Tian).

References

1. Kaplan AS, Vatter AE (1959) A comparison of herpes simplex and pseudorabies viruses. Virology 7(4):394–407
2. Klupp BG, Hengartner CJ, Mettenleiter TC, Enquist LW (2004) Complete, annotated sequence of the pseudorabies virus genome. J Virol 78(1):424–440
3. Oliver RE (1989) Aujeszky's disease. Aust Vet J 66(12):432–433
4. Ben-Porat T, Kaplan AS (1985) Molecular biology of pseudorabies virus. In: Roizman B (ed) The herpesviruses. Plenum Press, New York, pp 105–173
5. Song, YF, Jin, ML, Zhang, SL, Xu, XJ, Xiao, SB, Cao, SB, and Chen.CH (2007) Generation and immunogenicity of a recombinant pseudorabies virus expressing cap protein of porcine circovirus type 2. Vet Microbiol 119 (2–4), 97–104.
6. Dong B, Zarlenga DS, Ren XF (2014) An overview of live attenuated recombinant pseudorabies viruses for use as novel vaccines. J Immunol Res. doi:10.1155/2014/824630
7. Klupp BG, Lomniczi B, Visser N, Fuchs W, Mettenleiter TC (1995) Mutations affecting the UL21 gene contribute to avirulence of pseudorabies virus vaccine strain Bartha. Virology 212(2):466–473
8. Peeters B, Bienkowska-Szewczyk K, Hulst M, Gielkens A, Kimman T (1997) Biologically safe, non-transmissible pseudorabies virus vector vaccine protects pigs against both Aujeszky's disease and classical swine fever. J Gen Virol 78(12):3311–3315
9. Ju C, Fan H, Tan Y, Liu Z, Xi X, Cao S, Wu B, Chen H (2005) Immunogenicity of a recombinant pseudorabies virus expressing ORF1-ORF2 fusion protein of porcine circovirus type 2. Vet Microbiol 109(3–4):179–190
10. Qian P, Li XM, Jin ML, Peng GQ, Chen HC (2004) An approach to a FMD vaccine based on genetic engineered attenuated pseudorabies virus: one experiment using VP1 gene alone generates an antibody responds on FMD and pseudorabies in swine. Vaccine 22(17–18):2129–2136
11. Messerle M, Crnkovic I, Hammerschmidt W, Ziegler H, Koszinowski UH (1997) Cloning and mutagenesis of a herpesvirus genome as an infectious bacterial artificial chromosome. Proc Natl Acad Sci 94(26):14759–14763
12. Smith GA, Enquist LW (1999) Construction and transposon mutagenesis in *Escherichia coli* of a full-length infectious clone of Pseudorabies virus, an Alpha herpes virus. J Virol 73(8):6405–6414
13. Tischer BK, Kaufer BB (2012) Viral bacterial artificial chromosomes: generation, mutagenesis, and removal of Mini-F sequences. J Biomed Biotechnol. doi:10.1155/2012/472537
14. Narayanan K, Chen Q (2011) Bacterial artificial chromosome mutagenesis using recombineering. J Biomed Biotechnol. doi:10.1155/2011/971296
15. Tischer BK, Smith GA, and Osterrieder N (2010) En passant mutagenesis: a two step markerless red recombination system. In: Jeff Braman (ed) In vitro mutagenesis protocols, 3rd edn, Methods in molecular biology, vol 634, Chapter 30. pp 421–430
16. Paul PS, Mengeling WL, Pirtle EC (1982) Differentiation of pseudorabies (Aujeszky's disease) virus strains by restriction endonuelease analysis. Arch Virol 73(2):193–198
17. Warden C, Tang Q, Zhu H (2011) Herpesvirus BACs: past, present, and future. J Biomed Biotechnol. doi:10.1155/2011/124595
18. Maniatis T, Fritsch EF, Sambrook J (1989) Molecular cloning: a laboratory manual. Cold Spring Harbor Laboratory Press, New York
19. Hirt B (1967) Selective extraction of polyoma DNA from infected mouse cell cultures. J Mol Biol 26(2):365–369
20. Tischer BK, Einem JV, Kaufer B, Osterrieder N (2006) Two-step Red-mediated recombination for versatile high-efficiency markerless DNA manipulation in *Escherichia coli*. BioTechniques 40(2):191–197
21. Zhang CL, Guo LH, Jia XR, Wang TY, Wang J, Sun Z, Wang LL, Li XD, Tan FF, Tian KG (2015) Construction of a triple gene-deleted Chinese Pseudorabies virus variant and its efficacy study as a vaccine candidate on suckling piglets. Vaccine 33:2432–2437

Chapter 6

Generation and Production of Modified Vaccinia Virus Ankara (MVA) as a Vaccine Vector

Vincent Pavot*, Sarah Sebastian*, Alison V. Turner, Jake Matthews, and Sarah C. Gilbert

Abstract

The smallpox vaccine based on the vaccinia virus was successfully used to eradicate smallpox, but although very effective, it was a very reactogenic vaccine and responsible for the deaths of one to two people per million vaccinated. Modified Vaccinia virus Ankara (MVA) is an attenuated derivative, also used in the smallpox eradication campaign and now being developed as a recombinant viral vector to produce vaccines against infectious diseases and cancer. MVA can encode one or more foreign antigens and thus can function as a multivalent vaccine. The vector can be used at biosafety level 1, has intrinsic adjuvant properties, and induces humoral and cellular immune responses. Many clinical trials of these new vaccines have been conducted, and the safety of MVA is now well documented. Immunogenicity is influenced by the dose and vaccination regimen, and information on the efficacy of MVA-vectored vaccines is now beginning to accumulate. In this chapter, we provide protocols for generation, isolation, amplification, and purification of recombinant MVA for preclinical and clinical evaluation.

Key words Modified vaccinia virus Ankara, Non-replicative viral vector, Recombinant vaccines, Large-scale production, Clinical trials

1 Introduction

1.1 Overview of the Process and General Considerations

Recombinant MVA (rMVA) is a promising vaccine vector being assessed in clinical trials against infectious diseases such as malaria, tuberculosis, and HIV, and as therapeutic cancer vaccines (reviewed in [1]). MVA is a highly attenuated derivative of vaccinia virus and, in its unmodified form, is licensed as a smallpox virus vaccine in Europe and Canada (Imvamune®/Imvanex®, Bavarian Nordic). Unable to replicate in humans and most mammalian cell lines, MVA has an excellent safety record as a vaccine vector [2], and has been shown to be highly immunogenic for induction of antigen-specific T-cells as well as antibodies [1].

*These authors contributed equally in this work.

Maureen C. Ferran and Gary R. Skuse (eds.), *Recombinant Virus Vaccines: Methods and Protocols*, Methods in Molecular Biology, vol. 1581, DOI 10.1007/978-1-4939-6869-5_6, © Springer Science+Business Media LLC 2017

Unlike many other viral genomes, MVA genomic DNA is not infectious by itself; transfection of genomic DNA alone into permissive cells does not result in the production of virus. This is due to the fact that MVA relies on its own (and not the host's) transcription and replication machinery to initiate a productive infection. Therefore, generation of recombinant MVA generally requires intracellular homologous recombination of a shuttle vector plasmid (containing the desired antigen cassette) with an infectious parent virus, in the form of a concurrent infection/transfection procedure. Successfully recombined viruses are then selected using (removable) markers and clonally isolated.

1.2 MVA Shuttle Vector Plasmid

Shuttle vectors are multicopy bacterial plasmids containing an antigen cassette flanked by homology arms for recombination into the MVA genome, as well as a marker cassette (Fig. 1). The antigen cassette consists of a vaccinia virus promoter upstream of the coding sequence for the antigen of choice (Table 1). Following the stop codon, a termination signal sequence for early transcripts (TTTTTNT) may be inserted. The choice of promoter which drives the antigen will depend on the vaccine aim: for the induction of antigen-specific T-cells, strong expression of antigen early in infection seems to be crucial (i.e. during the first 2 h), and several MVA promoters have been identified for this purpose [3, 4]. For antibody induction, strong overall antigen expression seems to be required; examples for commonly used strong constitutive promoters are p7.5, SSP, and mH5 (Table 1 and [5–7]). Antigen coding sequences should be devoid of the previously mentioned termination sequence (T_5NT), stretches of four or more G or C nucleotides, and can be codon-optimized for the vaccine host (i.e., human or mouse). Recombinant viruses are most easily identified and selected using a fluorescent marker cassette (e.g. eGFP), which is present on the shuttle vector plasmid and therefore integrated into the viral genome alongside the antigen cassette. The MVA genome tolerates large insertions of foreign DNA (up to 30 kb), and several insertion sites have been identified (e.g. thymidine kinase gene, major genomic deletions, F11 locus). The 5′ and 3′ homology arms on either side of the antigen cassette in the shuttle vector contain approximately 500–1000 bp of viral sequence identical to the sequence flanking the chosen insertion site in the MVA genome.

1.3 Homologous Recombination

Homologous recombination between the viral sequences in the shuttle vector plasmid and the MVA genome is facilitated by viral enzymes during viral DNA replication [8], and takes place between the flanking sequences in the shuttle vector and identical endogenous sequences at the chosen insertion site. The efficiency of homologous recombination for vaccinia virus is relatively low, and only about 0.1% of progeny viruses contain the inserted foreign

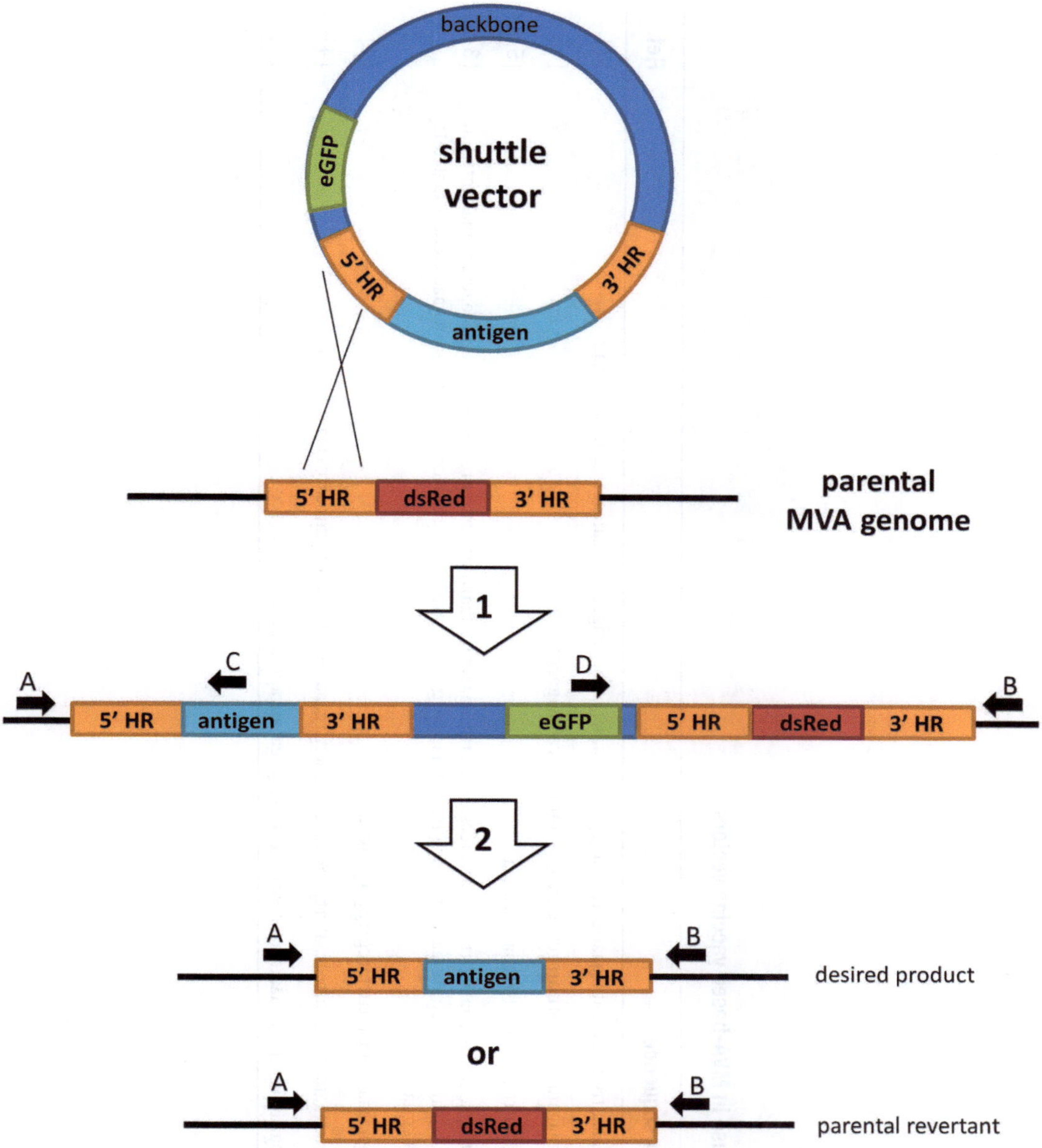

Fig. 1 Schematic diagram of recombination events. In *step 1* (*arrow 1*), single-crossover between the circular MVA shuttle vector plasmid and the MVA genome results in the integration of the entire shuttle vector. Multiple passages of this virus (*step 2*) will result in spontaneous intramolecular recombination between homology regions (3′HR or 5′HR), giving rise to one of two possible end products: antigen insertion (desired product) or parental revertant. *HR* homology region. *Black arrows* indicate location of primers

DNA [9]. The method described here pertains to a single crossover event which (in the first instance) leads to the integration of the entire shuttle vector into the viral genome. Alternatively, using a linearized shuttle vector, a double-crossover event involving both flanking sequences will lead to the integration of the antigen

Table 1

Selection of vaccinia promoters for use in MVA-based vaccine vectors

Promoter	Expression	Promoter sequence	Ref.
mH5	early/late	tcgacattaaaaattgaaaataaatacaaaggttcttgagggttgtgttaaattgaaagcgagaaataatcataaatatgattcaggtgac	[7]
p7.5	early/late	taaaagtagaaaatatattctaatttattgcacggtaaggaagtagaatcataaagaacagt	[6]
SSP	early/late	taaaaattgaaattttatttttttttttttgaatataaataa	[5]
pHyb	early/late	acgcgtgtttaaacgttttgaaaatttttttataataaatatccggtaaaattgaaaaactattctaatttattgcacggtccggtaaaaattgaaaaactattctaatttattgcacgg tccggtaaaaattgaaaaactattctaatttattgcacggtccggtaaaaattgaaaaactattctaatttattgcacggtccggtaaaaattgaaaaactattctaatttattg cacggtccgga	[3]
F11	early	aaaaaagtgaaaaacaatattatttttatcgttggttgtttcact	[4]
C11	early	atattactgaattaataatataaaattcccaatcttgtcataaacacacactgagaaacagcataaacacaaaatccatcaaaa	[4]
B8	early	atattattcaaaatatgatttttaaaatttaaaatatattatcacttcagtgacagtagtcaaataacaaacaacacc	[4]

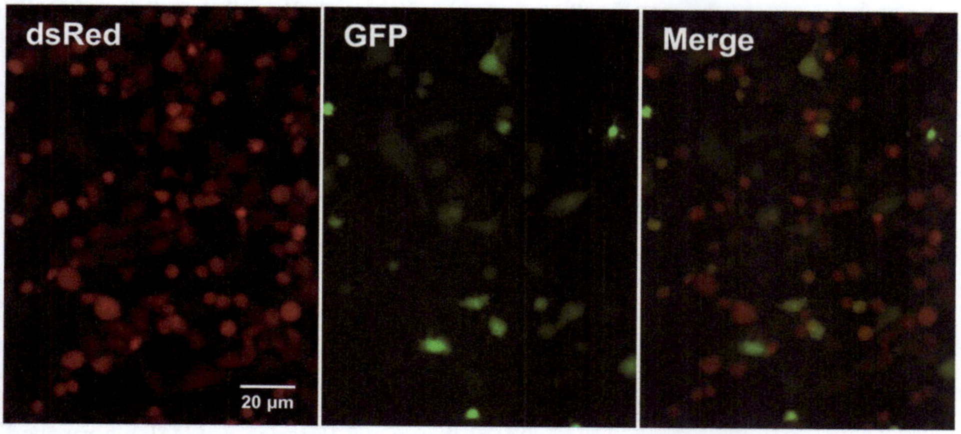

Fig. 2 Observation of DF-1 cells 48 h after homologous recombination between a parental MVA-dsRed and an MVA shuttle vector plasmid containing the GFP cassette. A single-crossover integration of the GFP-containing vector plasmid in one of the homology regions results in doubly positive (dsRed$^+$ and GFP$^+$) infected cells, which can be sorted by FACS

cassette only (*see* **Note 1**). The single-crossover approach is preferred since it facilitates the subsequent removal of the fluorescent marker cassette as well as the shuttle vector backbone by intramolecular recombination during successive virus passages, to generate a markerless recombinant virus as the end product (Fig. 1).

1.4 Selection of Recombined Virus

In the approach described here, the parental MVA carries a fluorescent marker at the target integration site (e.g. dsRed). A single-crossover integration of the GFP-containing shuttle vector in one of the homology regions will therefore result in doubly positive (dsRed and GFP) infected cells, which can be sorted by fluorescence-activated cell sorting (FACS: selection of dsRed-positive, GFP-positive infected cells) (Fig. 2). After PCR-based verification of the correct insertion of the shuttle vector, the virus is passaged several times to facilitate a second recombination event: the intramolecular recombination between identical flanking sequences. This event can have one of two results: the removal of the plasmid backbone and both fluorescent markers (desired), or the removal of the entire shuttle vector sequence, leaving the parental dsRed cassette intact (not desired). The desired product can be isolated by plaque-purification of markerless (dsRed- and GFP-negative) virus. For generation of MVA without removal of the fluorescent marker, *see* **Note 1**.

2 Materials

2.1 Cell Culture

1. CEF cells: primary chicken embryo fibroblasts, freshly prepared: method reviewed in [10] or from supplier (e.g., Institute for Animal Health, Compton, UK)

2. DF-1 cells: chicken embryonic fibroblast cell line (*Gallus gallus*, chicken) UMNSAH/DF-1 (ATCC® CRL-12203™). Use as an alternative to CEF
3. BHK-21 cells: baby hamster kidney cells (ATCC® CCL-10™)
4. Cell culture plates: T-75 and T-175 flasks, 6-well and 96-well plates
5. 15- and 50-mL tubes
6. Trypsin: TrypLE™ (GIBCO)
7. Trypan blue
8. DPBS: Sterile Dulbecco's phosphate buffered saline
9. Fetal bovine serum (FBS): for clinical trial evaluation, use current Good Manufacturing Practice (cGMP) approved FBS (e.g., FBS F2442 SIGMA)
10. Cell growth medium: Minimum Essential Medium with Earle's salts (E-MEM) for CEF or Dulbecco's Modified Eagle Medium (DMEM) for DF-1 and BHK-21 cells, supplemented with 10% heat-inactivated FBS, 1% antibiotics (100 units penicillin/mL and 0.1 mg streptomycin/mL final concentration), 4 mM L-glutamine

2.2 Generation of Recombinant MVA: Homologous Recombination

1. 2 μg shuttle vector plasmid (*see* Subheading 1.2)
2. Parental MVA (with fluorescent marker at desired insertion site, e.g. dsRed)
3. Virus growth medium: E-MEM (CEF, *see* **Note 2**) or DMEM (DF-1 and BHK-21) supplemented with 2% heat-inactivated FBS (*see* **Note 3**), 1% antibiotics (100 units penicillin/mL and 0.1 mg streptomycin/mL final concentration), 4 mM L-glutamine
4. Effectene® Transfection Reagent (QIAGEN) (*see* **Note 4**)
5. 1.5-mL microcentrifuge vials
6. Inverted fluorescence microscope with relevant filter cubes

2.3 Isolation of Recombinant MVA

2.3.1 Fluorescence-Activated Cell Sorting (FACS)

1. Flow cytometer
2. DPBS
3. Trypsin: TrypLETM (GIBCO)
4. 96-well plate
5. Sterile water

2.3.2 Plaque Picking

1. Cell culture reagents (*see* Subheading 2.1)
2. Carboxymethylcellulose (CMC) high viscosity (Sigma) made up to 1.6% w/v in ultrapure water

2.4 Virus Bulk-Up and Purification from a Single-Plaque Isolate

1. Virus growth medium (*see* Subheading 2.2)
2. Virus strain: vaccinia virus strain MVA (from ATCC)
3. Confluent monolayers of CEF, DF-1 or BHK-21 cells grown in T-75 and T-175 cell culture flasks
4. Sterile cell scrapers
5. 10 mM Tris–HCl, pH 9.0, autoclaved
6. Ultrasonic bath sonicator
7. Corning® 250-mL PP conical centrifuge tubes, sterile
8. 250-mL flat-bottomed ultracentrifuge bottles (autoclaved)
9. Thickwall Polycarbonate Ultracentrifuge Tubes (e.g., Beckman Coulter)
10. Optima™ L-80 XP ultracentrifuge (Beckman Coulter)
11. 36% w/v sucrose in 10 mM Tris–HCl pH 9.0: sucrose (Fluka—Sigma—84097), 18.2 MΩ/cm ultrapure water, 1 M Tris–HCl pH 9.0, 1000-mL autoclavable glass bottle

2.5 Titration of MVA

1. Cell culture reagents (*see* Subheading 2.1)
2. Virus growth medium (*see* Subheading 2.2)
3. Carboxymethylcellulose (CMC) high viscosity (Sigma) made up to 1.6% w/v in ultrapure water
4. 0.2% Triton X-100 in PBS
5. ImmPACT DAB (3,3′-Diaminobenzidine) plus Liquid Chromogen Stain & Diluent (Vector Labs)
6. Primary antibody: Rabbit anti-Vaccinia Virus (e.g., Abcam)
7. Secondary antibody: Donkey Anti-Rabbit HRP Conjugated (GE Healthcare, NA934V)
8. 4% paraformaldehyde (PFA)

2.6 Quality Control of Recombinant MVA

2.6.1 Confirmation of Recombinant MVA Genomes by PCR

1. Infected cells (GFP/dsRed positive) from 96-well plate post-FACS
2. DNAreleasy (Anachem)
3. Viral genomic DNA (as described in Subheading 3.6.1)
4. PCR primers (as described in Subheading 3.6.1)
5. PCR reagents (e.g., Phusion mastermix, NEB)
6. Thermocycler
7. Equipment and reagents for running agarose DNA gels

2.6.2 Sterility Test

1. BD BBL™ Trypticase™ Soy Broth, Tube, 5 mL (BD #221715)

2.6.3 Assay for Expression of Recombinant Gene by Immunofluorescence and Western Blot

1. Coverslips (autoclaved)
2. Six-well plates
3. 4% PFA

4. DPBS
5. Triton X-100
6. Blocking buffer (e.g., PBS-BSA 2%)
7. Primary antibody (directed against the protein of interest)
8. Secondary antibody (directed against the primary antibody)
9. Microscope slides
10. VECTASHIELD HardSet Antifade Mounting Medium, with or without DAPI (Vector Laboratories)
11. Fluorescence microscope
12. RIPA buffer (R0278 SIGMA)

3 Methods

3.1 Cell Culture

Currently, MVA-based vaccines for clinical evaluation are produced in primary CEF cells using cGMP approved reagents. However, DF-1 and BHK-21 cells can alternatively be used for virus amplification for preclinical evaluation, although growth in CEF cells produces higher yields of virus (*see* **Note 5**).

The usefulness of DF-1 cells exceeds primary CEF as they are an immortalized cell line and therefore can be stored in liquid nitrogen and passaged many times more than primary cells. MVA also forms more compact and uniform plaques on this cell line than on CEF, and therefore DF-1 cells allow more precise titer measurements.

3.2 Generation of Recombinant MVA: Homologous Recombination

rMVA can be easily generated in CEF cells that are prepared with cGMP approved reagents for clinical trials, or alternatively in DF-1 or BHK-21 cells for preclinical batches only. The use of selecting agents such as drugs may be undesirable, and therefore the most convenient method is the use of fluorescent reporters to screen for rMVA without requirement for other additives in the culture medium. This protocol should result in the production of rMVA expressing the recombinant antigen and transiently co-expressing a fluorescent marker (rMVA-GFP, rMVA-dsRed) that is isolated by FACS. For screening, green or red fluorescent cell foci (plaques) are visualized by microscopy. The shuttle plasmid containing the fluorescent reporter cassette is designed to contain flanking DNA sequences that allow for its deletion from the rMVA genome (*see* Fig. 1). Thus, to remove the reporter gene from rMVA, additional rounds of plaque purification are carried out, screening for non-fluorescent foci of virus-infected cells.

1. The day before transfection, seed 1×10^6 CEF, DF-1 or BHK-21 cells per well (6-well plate) in 2-mL growth medium. Incubate the cells at 37 °C and 5% CO_2. The well should be 80% confluent on the day of transfection (*see* **Notes 6** and **7**).

2. Discard the medium and overlay cells with virus growth medium containing the parental MVA at a multiplicity of infection (MOI) between 0.5 and 2.5 (in 1-mL medium per well). Incubate at 37 °C; 5% CO_2 for 90 min.
3. Approximately 75 min into the above incubation period, begin preparing transfection complexes of Effectene® Transfection Reagent/DNA as described by the manufacturer. Prepare 1–2 μg of plasmid DNA per well to transfect (*see* **Notes 8** and **9**).
4. Prepare the DNA-Enhancer solution: dilute 1 μg plasmid DNA with the DNA-condensation buffer (Buffer EC) and add the Enhancer and mix by vortexing (*see* **Note 10**).
5. Incubate at room temperature (RT) for 2–5 min.
6. Add Effectene® Reagent to the DNA–Enhancer solution. Mix by pipetting up and down or by vortexing (*see* **Note 11**).
7. Incubate the samples for 5–10 min at RT to allow transfection-complex formation.
8. During incubation, replace media from the well of cells to be transfected with 1 mL fresh, warm virus growth medium.
9. Make final volume of transfection mix up to 750 μL using warm virus growth medium and mix gently ten times to ensure the complexes are thoroughly resuspended.
10. Add 500 μL of the transfection complex mix to each well (*see* **Note 12**). Incubate 48 h at 37 °C; 5% CO_2.
11. Observe fluorescence 1–2 days post-transfection—GFP/dsRed positive cells should be visible (Fig. 2).
12. Harvest cells and media 2–3 days post-transfection by scraping, transfer to a sterile 2-mL screw-capped tube and store at −20 to −80 °C until required.

3.3 Isolation of Recombinant MVA

3.3.1 Fluorescence Activated Cell Sorting (FACS)

Selection of fluorescent rMVA can be accelerated by FACS whereby infected cells are single-cell sorted into a 96-well plate based on their fluorescence. This method is superior to that of plaque picking as none of the cells surrounding the plaque are co-transferred to the well. The resultant single cells are lysed by sorting them into wells containing sterile water. Cells are then added to the wells to permit virus propagation. Wells containing the desired virus are identified by fluorescence microscopy, and the entire well is harvested and screened by PCR.

1. CEF, DF-1, or BHK-21 cells are grown to 80% confluence in a T-75 flask.
2. Freeze/thaw three times the cells harvested from the recombination between MVA and the shuttle vector (*see* Subheading 3.2).

3. Add 10 μL of test sample cell lysate to 15-mL virus growth medium in a 50-mL tube and vortex (*see* **Note 13**).
4. Remove the cell growth medium from the T-75 flask of cells and replace with 15 mL of virus suspension in virus growth medium. Incubate infected cells for up to 3 days at 37 °C with 5% CO_2.
5. Observe the flask using the fluorescence microscope to check for GFP/dsRed positive cells.
6. Prepare one 96-well plate per virus to be sorted by adding 50 μL sterile water to each well.
7. Discard the medium from one T-75 flask and wash cells once with PBS.
8. Trypsinise cells and incubate at 37 °C until the cells are detached.
9. Add 10-mL PBS, then pipette cells up and down gently, transfer to a 50-mL tube, and centrifuge at 200 × *g* for 3 min at RT.
10. Aspirate the supernatant and resuspend the cells gently by tapping the tube.
11. Add 20-mL PBS and centrifuge at 200 × *g* for 3 min at RT.
12. Aspirate the supernatant (leaving approximately 200-μL residual volume) and then flick the tube gently in the liquid to get a single cell suspension to take to FACS.
13. Cell sort double positive GFP/dsRed fluorescent cells and put one double positive cell per well into the 96-well plate prepared in **step 6**.
14. Add cells (CEF, DF-1, or BHK-21) in the 96-well plate: 50,000 cells per well in 200 μL virus growth medium. Place the plate in an incubator (37 °C, 5% CO_2) for 2–4 days until recombinant virus can be observed (*see* **Note 14**).
15. The entire wells containing recombinant virus (as visualized by fluorescence microscopy) are harvested by scraping with a P1000 pipette, transferred into a 2-mL screw capped tube and frozen/thawed three times (*see* **Note 15**).
16. 20 μL of lysate is taken and viral DNA is extracted for confirmation of recombinant MVA genomes by PCR (*see* Subheading 3.6.1). The remaining lysate is stored at −20 to −80 °C for subsequent plaque purification and amplification.

3.3.2 Plaque Picking

Purify rMVA from parental virus by plaque picking following infection of CEF, DF-1, or BHK-21 cells with a serial dilution of plaque lysate. After each round of purification, identity, purity, and flank PCR are performed to screen for the presence of the desired recombinant gene and to check for the presence of parental MVA (e.g., MVA-dsRed) (*see* Subheading 3.6.1). When one round of plaque picking is confirmed as free of parental virus by PCR, a plaque from the next round of plaque picking is used to infect a T-175. This T-175 is then also screened by ID, flank, and purity PCR and is used as a premaster for subsequent master seed virus (MSV) infection, if found to be correct and pure (*see* **Note 16**).

1. Prepare one 6-well plate of 90% confluent cells per virus plaque to be plaque picked. Standard procedure is to purify one plaque.
2. Prepare serial dilutions of the cell lysate obtained after FACS: take 10 μL and put it in 990 μL of virus growth medium (1:100). Then 1:10 dilutions twice. Vortex well between each dilution.
3. Discard the media in the 6-well plates and replace with 1 mL of the three dilutions. Tilt the plate side to side and front to back five times to ensure mixing (*see* **Note 17**). Incubate for 90 ± 30 min at 37 °C with 5% CO_2.
4. During the incubation mix sufficient virus growth medium and CMC in a ratio 2/3 virus growth medium: 1/3 CMC for 2 mL per well required.
5. Aspirate media containing virus and replace with 2-mL virus growth medium/CMC overlay per well and incubate for 2–4 days.
6. Prepare 2-mL screw capped tubes containing 100 μL of 10 mM Tris–HCl pH 9.0 for the plaques to be picked into.
7. Using the microscope, identify a well-isolated plaque of desired fluorescence and use the objective cell dotter to mark a ring around the plaque.
8. Transfer the plate to a class 2 biosafety cabinet and use a P10 pipette to remove the plaque from the monolayer and transfer contents to the tube containing 100 μL of 10 mM Tris–HCl. Pick 5 to 15 plaques, using separate tips and placing contents into separate tubes.
9. Check, using the microscope, that the correct region has been harvested.
10. Freeze-thaw and vortex tubes three times (*see* **Note 18**).
11. Use PCR analysis of viral DNA to monitor for absence of parental MVA and presence of the desired recombinant gene (*see* Subheading 3.6.1).
12. Marker gene deletion: continue plaque purification now selecting for nonfluorescent plaques. Repeat **steps 1–11** until all viral isolates fail to produce any fluorescent plaques.
13. Proceed to PCR to confirm insert and purity (*see* Subheading 3.6.1).

3.4 Virus Bulk-Up and Purification from a Single-Plaque Isolate

Large-scale preparation of MVA requires the infection of cells, the extraction of virus from the cell lysate, and crude purification to remove cell debris from the sample. This protocol describes the preparation of a premaster stock of virus and infection of CEF with premaster lysate to form a master stock virus prep.

Premaster lysate: cells and media from a T-75 flask infected with material confirmed free from parental MVA by PCR. If this is the first time the virus has been made, the premaster will have been prepared from a plaque pick one round on from a plaque that passed quality control (QC) PCR (for example plaque 1.1 is usually used if plaque 1 passed QC PCR). If this is a re-bulk prep, the premaster is prepared by infection of cells in a T-75 flask with cell lysate from the original premaster.

3.4.1 Premaster Seed Virus Stock

1. Prepare one T-75 flask per virus with cells such that they are 90–100% confluent at the time of infection. One T-75 is required for each set of five T-175 flasks required for the Master Seed Virus prep (MSV).
2. The source material may either be a plaque pick or a previous premaster cell lysate (if performing a re-bulk):
   - Plaque pick: pipette 50 μL of prepared plaque pick (three times freeze-thaw and vortexed) into 15 mL of virus growth medium in a 50-mL tube and vortex thoroughly.
   - Premaster cell lysate: transfer 50 μL of prepared premaster (thawed and vortexed) into 15 mL of virus growth medium in a 50-mL tube and vortex thoroughly.
3. Discard the cell growth medium from the T-75 flask of CEF and replace with the virus growth medium containing the rMVA. Incubate at 37 °C, 5% CO_2 and monitor appearance of cytopathic effects (CPE) (*see* **Note 19**).
4. Scrape off the virus-infected cells from the T-75 flask into a 50-mL tube.
5. Freeze-thaw the 50-mL tube three times and vortex very hard: this is the premaster lysate.
6. Take 1 mL of the premaster lysate and transfer to a 1.5-mL O-ring tube and store this at −80 °C as a premaster for future preps.
7. Take a 20-μL aliquot and add to 30-μL DNAreleasy in a PCR tube for DNA extraction and QC PCRs. Store the remaining lysate at −80 °C until needed for MSV infection.

3.4.2 Master Seed Virus (MSV)

1. Prepare five T-175 flasks of cells per rMVA for a standard prep (adjust if a large prep is to be made) until 90–100% confluent.
2. Thaw premaster cell lysate using water bath at 37 °C (*see* **Note 20**).

3. To infect five T-175 flasks, prepare virus growth medium containing virus lysate by pipetting 161 mL of virus growth medium + 14 mL of the premaster lysate into a 250-mL conical tube and mix by inverting bottle gently five times (*see* **Note 21**).
4. Aspirate the cell growth medium from the five T-175 flasks and replace with 35 mL of virus growth medium/virus suspension. Incubate at 37 °C, 5% CO_2 until all cells are infected and beginning to show signs of CPE (3–5 days).

3.4.3 Harvesting Virus

1. Harvest the virus-infected cells with the cell scraper and transfer cells and supernatants into a 250-mL conical bottomed tube (~175 mL) (*see* **Note 22**).
2. Centrifuge the 250-mL conical bottomed tube at 670 × *g* for 10 min to pellet the cells.
3. Retain cell pellets and carefully pipette supernatants to an autoclaved 250-mL flat-bottom ultracentrifuge bottle. Keep on ice.
4. Resuspend cell pellets from the 250-mL conical bottomed tubes in 2 mL of 10 mM Tris–HCl (pH 9.0) and transfer to a 15-mL tube. Lyse the cells in three freeze-thaw cycles, vortex strongly, and sonicate for 1 min at 57 Hz using an ultrasonic bath sonicator. Centrifuge the 15-mL tube at 670 × *g* for 5 min.
5. Carefully take the supernatant and add to the previous supernatant in the 250-mL flat-bottom ultracentrifuge tube and centrifuge 60 min at 33,000 × *g* and 4 °C to pellet the virus particles.
6. Discard the supernatant and resuspend the pellet in 2 mL 10 mM Tris–HCl (pH 9.0). Mix by hard vortexing and transfer to a 15-mL tube (*see* **Note 23**).

3.4.4 Sucrose Cushion Purification of rMVA

Large-scale preparation of rMVA requires the infection of cells, the extraction of virus from the cell lysate, and crude purification to remove cell debris from the sample. This protocol describes the purification through a sucrose cushion to separate the viral particles from the cell lysate.

1. If previously frozen: thaw the impure virus from Subheading 3.4.3 at 37 °C in a water bath and vortex.
2. Ensure no clumps are present in the virus suspension and centrifuge samples at 950 × *g* for 3 min at 4 °C.
3. Prepare 2 vol. of sterile 36% sucrose cushions (in 10 mM Tris–HCl [pH 9.0]) in an ultracentrifuge tube and overlay with 1 vol. of virus suspension slowly and carefully with a sterile transfer pipette without disturbing the sucrose layer (*see* **Note 24**).

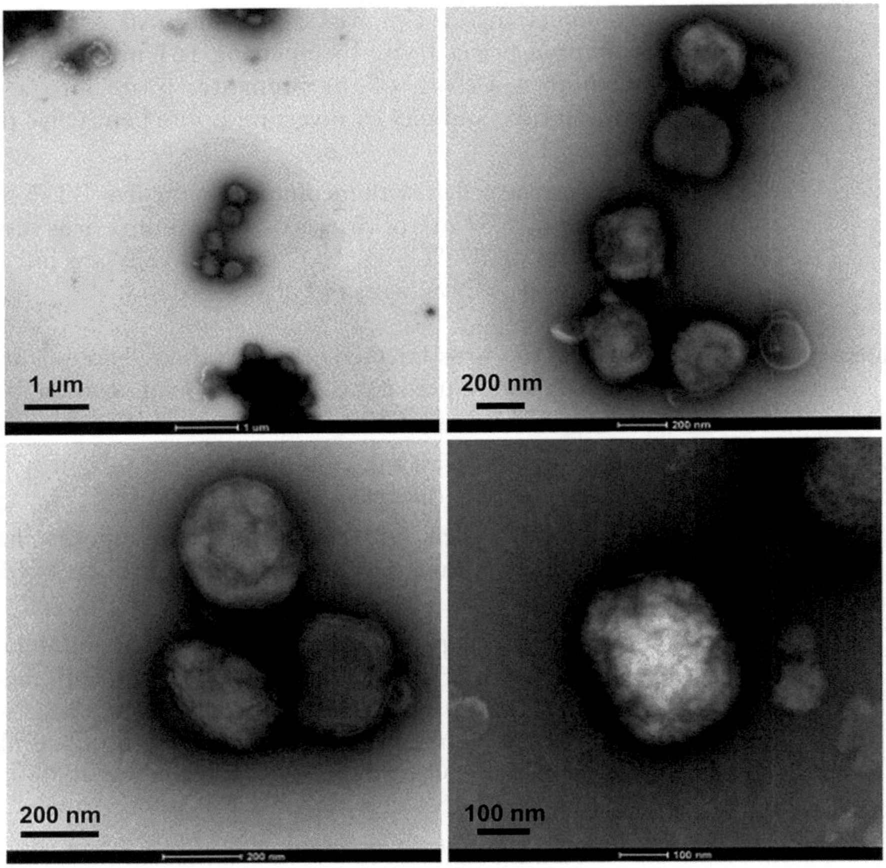

Fig. 3 Transmission electron microscopy of purified rMVA

4. Spin 2 h at 30,000 × *g* and 4 °C.
5. Discard the supernatant carefully. Remove the top of the upper layer first to ensure this does not contact the purified pellet at the base of the tube.
6. Resuspend the pellet in 10 mM Tris–HCl (pH 9.0) in a total volume of 400 μL per five cell culture flasks. Virus is stored at −80 °C (*see* **Note 25** and Fig. 3).

3.5 Titration of rMVA: Determining the Amount of Plaque Forming Units per mL (PFU/mL)

Plaque morphology of MVA differs in CEF and DF-1 cells. MVA plaques in CEF cells appear as large comet-shopped structures while in DF-1 cells MVA forms small round foci of infected cells.

The following method details the titration of a markerless MVA using DF-1 cells in 24-well plates by immunostaining (if the MVA contains a fluorescent marker, plaques can also be counted using the fluorescence microscope instead of immunostaining). Each virus is tested in quadruplicate: four separate 3-point serial dilutions are titrated. A negative control and a reference virus should be added to the plate at the same time.

3.5.1 *Cell Infection*

1. Cell seeding: per virus to be titrated, seed 1 × 24-well plate with 4 × 10^5 DF-1 cells/well in a volume of 500 μL of cell growth medium. Incubate the cells at 37 °C with 5% CO_2 for 16–28 h.
2. The next day, remove the medium from the cells and replace with 200 μL of fresh virus growth medium. Place cells back in an incubator until required for virus infection.
3. Thaw the virus to be titrated and homogenize by strong vortexing.
4. Make tenfold serial dilutions ranging from 10^{-2} to 10^{-8} of virus material in 1 mL virus growth medium.
5. Infection: add 100 μL of the appropriate viral dilutions to the relevant columns across the 24-well plate (final volume: 300 μL/well). Only use the last three dilutions from each dilution series, in quadruplicate.
6. Disperse the virus throughout the medium by rocking the plate backward and forward and side to side (*see* **Note 17**) and incubate at 37 °C, 5% CO_2 for 2 h.
7. Aspirate the media containing virus and add 400 μL of pre-warmed virus growth medium: CMC overlay per well (2 vol. virus growth medium + 1 vol. CMC 1.6%).
8. Place plates at 37 °C + 5% CO_2 for 48 h.

3.5.2 *Immunostaining*

1. Remove the medium/CMC from the wells and fix the cells with 200 μL per well of fresh paraformaldehyde (4% in PBS) for 5 min at RT.
2. Remove the fixative with a pipette to a formaldehyde waste bottle and wash once with 500 μL per well of PBS. Remove waste with a pipette to a formaldehyde waste bottle.
3. Permeabilise cells with 200 μL per well of 0.2% Triton X-100 in PBS. Incubate for 5 min at RT.
4. Wash cells twice with PBS.
5. Block with 300 μL per well of blocking solution (e.g. PBS + 3% FBS) and incubate for 1 h at RT.
6. Remove the blocking solution and put 200 μL per well of primary antibody diluted at 1:1000 in blocking solution. Place on a rocking platform and incubate for 1 h at RT.
7. Wash twice with PBS.
8. Prepare the secondary HRP-conjugated antibody (1:300 in blocking solution) and add 200 μL per well. Place on a rocking platform for 45 min at RT.
9. Wash twice with PBS.

10. Make up the DAB Liquid Chromagen developing solution (6 mL per plate): add one drop of Chromogen liquid to every 1 mL of DAB Liquid buffer solution that is required and mix well (always make up this solution fresh).
11. Add 200 μL of developing solution per well and leave for ~10 min at RT with rocking. Plaques will stain a distinct brown color.
12. Discard solution into a glass bottle (marked DAB waste) containing one Pre-Sept tablet (leave bottle overnight and discard contents with plenty of water down sink the next day).
13. Wash plates gently with approximately 1 mL tap water per well.
14. Allow plates to air-dry for half an hour. Ideally leave upside down on a paper towel.
15. Count the number of plaques in quadruplicate: wells with 20–70 plaques generate the most accurate results.

    To determine the titer (PFU/mL), count the number of plaques in quadruplicate wells and calculate the mean. Multiply the counted number by the dilution and the conversion factor (here: 10—*see* **Note 26**):

"geometric mean of plaque counts" x "conversion factor" x "serial dilution" = "x" PFU/mL

3.6 Quality Control of Recombinant MVA

3.6.1 Confirmation of Recombinant MVA Genome by PCR

Extraction of Viral DNA from Infected Cells

This protocol allows lysis of infected cells and release of the rMVA. DNA from the virus is then extracted using DNAreleasy reagent.

Cells are lysed and centrifuged before treatment with the DNAreleasy reagent such that the samples to be extracted are suspensions of virus particles in media with minimal cell debris.

1. Harvest cells and media using a P1000 pipette or a cell scraper, transfer to a tube, and freeze-thaw three times (*see* **Note 27**).
2. Pellet cell debris by centrifugation 1500 × *g* for 1 min and transfer a 20 μL of supernatant (containing the virus) to a PCR tube.
3. Add 30 μL DNAreleasy to sample, mix gently by flicking the tube.
4. Run the following program on the PCR machine:

   65 °C for 15 min (may be left longer if necessary); 96 °C for 2 min; 65 °C for 4 min; 96 °C for 1 min; 65 °C for 1 min; 96 °C for 30 s; 20 °C hold (*see* **Notes 28** and **29**).

3.6.2 PCR to Confirm Insert and Purity

Use 1 μL of the previously extracted viral DNA as a template in the quality control PCR to confirm the correct insertion of the shuttle vector into the target locus. The primer sequences will depend on the insertion locus in the MVA genome. In the first instance, two reactions are performed to ensure the correct insertion of the

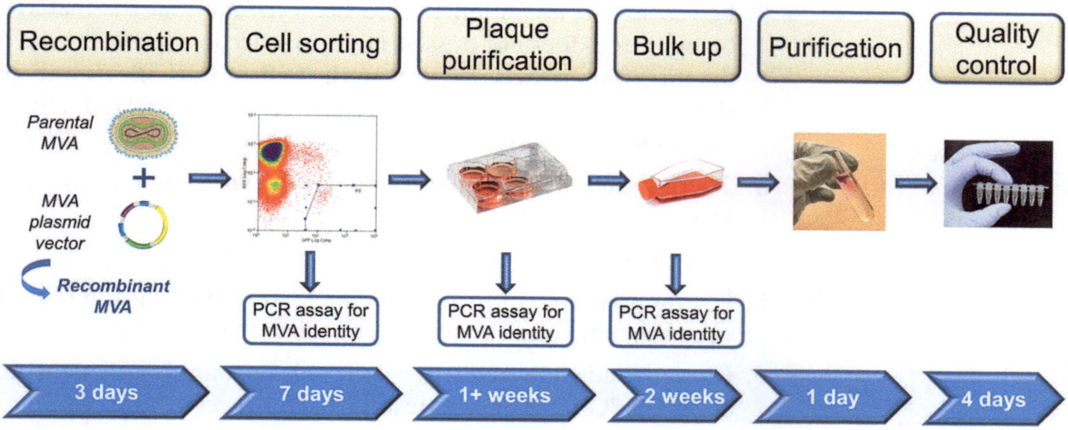

Fig. 4 Summary of workflow for the production of recombinant MVA

foreign sequences into the viral genome: two flanking PCRs (5′ and 3′), with one primer in the MVA genome and the other in the inserted sequence (primer set A/C and B/D). After passaging of the virus to remove the fluorescent markers (step 2 in Fig. 1), a purity PCR is performed using two primers outside of the flanking regions (primers A/B) to amplify the entire antigen cassette and to distinguish between the two possible outcomes (parental revertant or desired antigen insertion). *See* Fig. 1 for location of primers, *see* Fig. 4 for an overview of the process to generate modified MVA.

3.6.3 Sterility Test

This protocol describes a method for confirmation of sterility of a biological sample. This protocol is suitable for testing for the presence of aerobic bacteria or fungus; it does not test for the presence of anaerobic bacteria.

Tryptic Soy Broth (TSB) is a general-purpose liquid enrichment medium used in qualitative procedures for the sterility test and for the enrichment and cultivation of aerobic microorganisms that are not excessively fastidious. TSB is a nutritious medium that will support the growth of a wide variety of microorganisms, especially common aerobic and facultative anaerobic bacteria (common facultative anaerobic bacteria are Staphylococcus (Gram positive), *E. coli* (Gram negative), Corynebacterium (Gram positive), and Listeria (Gram positive)). Because of its capacity for growth promotion, this formulation was adopted by The United States Pharmacopeia (USP) and the European Pharmacopeia (EP) as a sterility test medium. EP stipulates that the volume of test material does not exceed 10% of the culture volume.

1. Place required amount of TSB-containing tubes in a wire rack and place in the biological safety cabinet.

2. For each test, it is important to demonstrate that the material being tested does not possess any anti-microbial properties. To do this, four vessels are prepared: TSB only, TSB + swab of shoe sole, TSB + test sample + swab of shoe sole, and TSB + test sample (*see* **Note 30**).
3. There should be two tubes of one of the virus samples to serve as a control as well.
4. Add the samples to the TSB tubes (*see* **Note 31**).
5. For the positive control, scrape a pipette tip along the sole of your shoe and add the tip to the relevant vial of TSB.
6. Close the lids fully and shake each vial thoroughly and incubate at 30–35 °C for 3 days to test for bacterial contamination.
7. Inspect the tubes for signs of microbial growth (cloudy media). The batch only passes if the positive controls have microbial growth evident by visual inspection.

3.6.4 Assay for Expression of Recombinant Gene by Immunofluorescence

1. Put autoclaved coverslips in wells of a 6-well plate (one coverslip per well) and add CEF or DF-1 cells to wells to obtain a subconfluent cell layer on the coverslips on the day of infection.
2. Infect subconfluent (80–90%) cell layer of the 6-well plate with the rMVA at an MOI of 0.01 in 1 mL virus growth medium (*see* **Note 32**).
3. Incubate for 2 h at 37 °C, remove inoculum, and add 2 mL fresh virus growth medium.
4. Incubate for 24 to 48 h.
5. Wash cells once with PBS and fix with 4% PFA for 10 min at RT (~1 mL per well).
6. Wash three times with PBS.
7. If necessary, permeabilize cells with 0.1–0.2% Triton X-100 for 10–15 min at RT.
8. Wash three times with PBS.
9. Block with 2-mL blocking buffer per well and incubate 1 h at RT (*see* **Note 33**).
10. Dilute the primary antibody (directed against the protein of interest) in blocking buffer.
11. Replace the blocking buffer in each well with 1 mL of the antibody solution and incubate for 1 h at RT (rocking gently) or overnight at 4 °C.
12. Remove primary antibody solution and wash cells three times with PBS or blocking solution.
13. Dilute the fluorescent secondary antibody (directed against the primary antibody) in blocking buffer and add 1 mL per

well and incubate for 30–60 min at RT in the dark (rocking gently).

14. Remove secondary antibody solution and wash cells three times with 2 mL PBS or blocking buffer. Leave washing solution in the well after the last wash.
15. Remove the coverslip from the wells using a tweezer and a needle and mount on a slide using a drop of VECTASHIELD HardSet Antifade Mounting Medium (with or without DAPI).
16. Assess antigen-specific staining by fluorescence microscopy.

3.6.5 Assay for Expression of Recombinant Gene by Western Blot

1. Infect subconfluent (80–90%) CEF or DF-1 cells layer or BHK-21 cells of a 6-well plate with the rMVA at an MOI of 5 in 1 mL virus medium (*see* **Note 32**).
2. Incubate for 2 h at 37 °C, remove inoculum, and add 2 mL fresh virus growth medium.
3. Incubate for 24 to 72 h.
4. Wash cells twice with PBS.
5. After the removal of the final wash solution from the cells, add an appropriate volume of RIPA Buffer (1 mL for 0.5–5 × 10^7 cells). Incubate on ice or in a refrigerator (2–8 °C) for 5 min.
6. Rapidly scrape the plate with a cell scraper to remove and lyse residual cells. Transfer the cell lysate to a tube on ice (*see* **Note 34**).
7. Clarify the lysate by centrifugation at 8000 × *g* for 10 min at 4 °C to pellet the cell debris (*see* **Note 35**).
8. Carefully transfer the supernatant containing the soluble protein to a tube on ice.
9. Proceed with western blot analysis of the lysates for the recombinant protein. Generally, 1/10 of the supernatant should provide enough protein for one lane on a protein gel.

3.6.6 Assay for Stability of Recombinant Gene Expression

Occasionally, expression of a recombinant gene product can hamper the replication of the rMVA. Strong suppressive effects on virus growth will result in the occurrence of nonexpressing virus mutants that may outgrow the rMVA upon amplification.

To test for the stability of recombinant gene expression, primary stocks of rMVA should be evaluated for maintained target protein synthesis after serial cell culture passage at low MOI.

1. Infect subconfluent (80–90%) CEF or DF-1 cells in a 6-well plate with the recombinant MVA at an MOI of 0.05 in 1-ml virus growth medium.
2. Incubate for 48 h and harvest cells and supernatant together.
3. Freeze–thaw and vortex three times.

4. Sonicate three times (vortex in between).
5. Dilute virus suspension 1:1000 by tenfold serial dilutions at a final volume of 1 mL.
6. Infect new subconfluent CEF or DF-1 cells of a well of a 6-well plate with 1 mL of the 1:1000-diluted virus material.
7. Incubate for 48 h at 37 °C and repeat **steps 3–6** three additional times.
8. Check genetic stability by comparing DNA from the starting material and DNA from the fifth passage in PCR assay for MVA identity (*see* Subheading 3.6.1).
9. Monitor for recombinant gene product by immunofluorescence and Western blot of infected cells (*see* Subheadings 3.6.3 and 3.6.4).

4 Notes

1. The approach described here was developed for the generation of MVA-based vaccines for use in humans, where a markerless virus is required. In those instances where an MVA-based vaccine is generated for preclinical use only (e.g. in mice), a markerless recombinant virus is not mandatory. In this case, when designing the shuttle vector, the GFP cassette should be placed between the homology arms, along with the antigen cassette, and double-crossover recombination between the linearized shuttle vector and the viral genome will result in a recombinant virus that constitutively expresses GFP.
2. For clinical evaluation, recombinant MVAs must be generated and amplified on CEF cultures prepared from embryonated eggs from specific pathogen-free chickens and use cGMP approved reagents.
3. 2% FBS is used for virus growth medium to slow down cell growth.
4. Other transfection reagents such as Lipofectamine® 2000 (Thermo Fisher Scientific) can also be used for transfection according to the manufacturer's protocol.
5. DF-1 cells are not validated for the generation of vaccines for GMP manufacture. Therefore, they must only be used for virus titration (not plaque picking or any stage of bulk up) during routine production of clinical batches. DF-1 cells can be used for virus amplification for preclinical evaluation.
6. A specific GMP FBS has to be used to prepare GMP batches.
7. One plate is needed for each virus to be made—multiple recombinations must not be performed on the same plate to avoid cross-contamination.

8. DNA used should be high-quality plasmid DNA, purified using a plasmid purification kit.
9. Effect of serum: in contrast to many liposome-based transfection reagents, Effectene® Reagent enables transfection in the presence of serum without lowering transfection efficiencies. Therefore, serum can be included in medium when incubating cells with transfection complexes, and during subsequent incubation for gene expression.
10. Always keep the ratio of DNA to Enhancer constant according to manufacturer's instructions.
11. It is not necessary to keep Effectene reagent on ice at all times. 10–15 min at RT will not alter its stability.
12. Ensure equal distribution by rocking the plate backward, forward, and side to side, avoiding circular motion, as this will concentrate the transfection mix in the center of the well.
13. It is important that the cell culture does not contain a large amount of virus as although the cells are sorted based on fluorescence, if there are virus particles attached to the outside of the cell membrane they will be co-transferred to the wells where they can then replicate.
14. Alternatively, the 96-well plates can be placed at −20 °C and the cells added later.
15. Where possible, at least five wells should be harvested in the first instance. In cases where FACS sorting has previously failed for a particular virus it may be worth harvesting as many candidate wells as possible for PCR screening to maximize the chance of obtaining correct virus.
16. Ensure cells infected with different viruses are handled separately in the biological safety cabinet, wiping the surface down and changing gloves between different vectors.
17. Do not move the plate in circles as this forces the virus to the edge of the well.
18. Virus may be frozen at −20 to −80 °C for storage.
19. 100% infected cells should be evident after approximately 3 to 4 days.
20. Ensure material is only just thawed – do not leave in water bath longer than necessary as prolonged incubation will lead to proteolytic degradation of the virus particles.
21. Avoid bubble formation as this will potentially denature proteins on the virus surface and reduce infectivity.
22. For all the next steps, keep the tubes on ice.
23. The viruses can be stored at −20 to −80 °C at this step.
24. If preparing many viruses, seal the tubes, wipe down the surfaces, and change gloves before loading the second virus.

25. If band purified virus is required, **step 4** can be centrifuged through a 25–40% sucrose gradient for 50 min at 28000 × *g* and 4 °C. Harvest virus band that appears at the lower middle of the tube. To concentrate the virus in the band and to remove remaining sucrose, fill an ultracentrifuge tube with >3× volume of 1 mM Tris–HCl, pH 9.0, and pellet virus material at 38000 × *g* for 1 h at 4 °C. Resuspend the pellet in this Tris–HCl buffer and store at −80 °C.
26. The "conversion factor" allows expression of the number of PFUs in 1 mL.
27. Cell lysate samples must be freeze-thawed to completely lyse cells and release the virus particles. If the cells are not lysed, the virus will remain in the cells and will be removed in the centrifugation step. If the cell debris is not completely removed, it can be transferred to the PCR reaction mix. The template DNA is sequestered in the cell debris and can then get stuck in the wells of the agarose gel.
28. The DNA extract can be stored at −20 °C for future use.
29. For purified virus, 10 μL of virus is added to 30 μL DNAreleasy and then heat-treated as described.
30. The swab of shoe sole and one of the test samples is to control for any factors within the samples that may inhibit microbial growth (e.g., antibiotics carried through during purification).
31. Add the samples to the neck of the glass tubes; do not put the micropipette down into the tubes.
32. Controls should be infected cells with wild-type MVA and uninfected cells.
33. To minimize unspecific staining, blocking can be performed at 37 °C for 1 h.
34. The lysate can either be used immediately or quick-frozen in liquid nitrogen and stored at −70 °C for future use. It is best to freeze the lysate before clarification, since the freeze-thaw cycle may cause some denatured protein aggregates.
35. If a mucoid aggregate of denatured nucleic acids is present, carefully remove it with a micropipette before centrifugation.

References

1. Gilbert SC (2013) Clinical development of modified vaccinia virus Ankara vaccines. Vaccine 31:4241–4246
2. Overton ET, Stapleton J, Frank I, Hassler S, Goepfert PA, Barker D, Wagner E, vonKrempelhuber A, Virgin G, Meyer TP, Muller J, Badeker N, Grunert R, Young P, Rosch S, Maclennan J, Arndtz-Wiedemann N, Chaplin P (2015) Safety and immunogenicity of modified vaccinia Ankara-Bavarian nordic smallpox vaccine in vaccinia-naive and experienced human immunodeficiency virus-infected individuals: an open-label, controlled clinical phase II Trial. Open Forum Infect Dis 2 ofv040
3. Baur K, Brinkmann KI, Schweneker M, Patzold J, Meisinger-Henschel C, Hermann J,

Steigerwald R, Chaplin P, Suter M, Hausmann J (2010) Immediate-early expression of a recombinant antigen by modified vaccinia virus ankara breaks the immunodominance of strong vector-specific B8R antigen in acute and memory CD8 T-cell responses. J Virol 84:8743–84852

4. Orubu T, Alharbi NK, Lambe T, Gilbert SC, Cottingham MG (2012) Expression and cellular immunogenicity of a transgenic antigen driven by endogenous poxviral early promoters at their authentic loci in MVA. PLoS One 7:e40167
5. Chakrabarti S, Sisler JR, Moss B (1997) Compact, synthetic, vaccinia virus early/late promoter for protein expression. Biotechniques 23:1094–1097
6. Cochran MA, Puckett C, Moss B (1985) In vitro mutagenesis of the promoter region for a vaccinia virus gene: evidence for tandem early and late regulatory signals. J Virol 54:30–37
7. Wyatt LS, Shors ST, Murphy BR, Moss B (1996) Development of a replication-deficient recombinant vaccinia virus vaccine effective against parainfluenza virus 3 infection in an animal model. Vaccine 14:1451–1458
8. Yao XD, Evans DH (2001) Effects of DNA structure and homology length on vaccinia virus recombination. J Virol 75:6923–6932
9. Moss B (1991) Vaccinia virus: a tool for research and vaccine development. Science 252:1662–1667
10. Hernandez R, Brown DT (2010) Growth and maintenance of chick embryo fibroblasts (CEF). Curr Protoc Microbiol Appendix 4: pp 4I

Chapter 7

Poxvirus Safety Analysis in the Pregnant Mouse Model, Vaccinia, and Raccoonpox Viruses

Rachel L. Roper

Abstract

Poxviruses cause many diseases in humans and animals worldwide, and there is a need for vaccines with improved safety and good efficacy. In addition, poxvirus vectors are widely used as recombinant vaccines for various infectious diseases and as recombinant and oncolytic vaccines for cancer. One concern with poxvirus vaccine vectors is that some poxviruses can infect a developing fetus and cause fetal loss or congenital disease. This can be an issue both for patients receiving a vaccine and for pregnant health care providers, including doctors, nurses, and veterinarians, who might receive accidental exposure to the poxvirus by injection or during patient care. We describe here a method for analyzing the safety of virus exposure in pregnant mammals using a mouse model testing vaccinia, canarypox, and raccoonpox virus vectors.

Key words Pregnant mouse, Virus, Vaccine, Poxvirus safety, Raccoonpox, Canarypox

1 Introduction

Poxviruses cause disease in humans and animals worldwide. Smallpox is estimated to have killed ~500 million people during the twentieth century, but it was eradicated from nature by 1980 by a worldwide vaccination program headed by the World Health Organization [1]. Vaccination of civilian populations has ceased due to the poor safety record of this vaccine, but lab workers, first responders, and US military personnel are vaccinated due to biowarfare/bioterrorism concerns. Most extant human-infecting poxviruses are zoonotic, transmitted mostly via rodents, including monkeypox, which caused an outbreak in the US Midwest in 2003 with more than 80 cases reported [2, 3]. Monkeypox virus (MPXV) is endemic in Africa and has a case fatality rate that can reach approximately 10% [2, 4]. Cowpox and Orf viruses also infect humans, but these infections are rarely fatal [5]. Molluscum contagiosum virus is only known to infect humans, is common worldwide and is emerging as a sexually transmitted disease [6, 7].

Maureen C. Ferran and Gary R. Skuse (eds.), *Recombinant Virus Vaccines: Methods and Protocols*, Methods in Molecular Biology, vol. 1581, DOI 10.1007/978-1-4939-6869-5_7, © Springer Science+Business Media LLC 2017

New poxviruses are identified each year in animal populations, and several zoonotic poxviruses appear to be emerging worldwide in humans [8], such as Cantagalo in South America [9, 10], Tanapox, in Africa (and also detected in Europe and the US among travelers) [11, 12], and buffalopox in India [13]. Thus, development of safe and effective poxvirus vaccines remains desirable.

Poxviruses are often used as recombinant vaccine vectors for infectious diseases and cancer therapies [14–16]. The only HIV vaccine with demonstrated efficacy in humans thus far employs a canarypox vector, and this is entering NIH-sponsored Phase 2b/3 trials in 2016 [17]. Poxviruses such as vaccinia virus (VACV) are suitable as vectors because they are easily grown to high titer in a wide variety of animals and cell types, can accommodate insertions of large pieces of DNA into their genomes, are very stable even when dried, and induce robust B and T cell immunity [18]. VACV is the most commonly used poxvirus vaccine vector, however its use is limited by its potential virulence, especially in immunocompromised hosts. The Modified Vaccinia Ankara (VACV-MVA) strain is much more attenuated, but its replicative capacity and immunogenicity are limiting [18–25]. Raccoonpox virus (RCNV) is a naturally occurring attenuated North American poxvirus that is of interest evolutionary, as a vaccine vector platform, and for its oncolytic therapy potential [26, 27].

The RCNV strain Herman was originally isolated from an apparently healthy raccoon [28], and has been successfully employed as a safe recombinant vaccine in numerous animal models [29–34]. We have recently reported that RCNV is less virulent and much safer than VACV in immunocompromised or pregnant mouse models [27, 35, 36]. This is important because VACV infection can be fatal, especially in immunocompromised or pregnant humans, and its use is contraindicated for such individuals. We compared canarypox and several VACV and RCNV mutants and showed that 8×10^6 plaque forming units per mouse of VACV strain Western Reserve reduced viable pup counts to 1–2 pups per mouse, while uninfected mice deliver 5–6 pups normally [27]. The RCNV wild type Herman strain reduced pups to about 4 per litter, similar to a thymidine kinase knock out mutant virus (TK-). Canarypox and a recombinant RCNV with deletions in both the TK and hemagglutinin genes and containing the gene for rabies G2 protein (RCNV-G2) did not cause any loss of pups. Interestingly, the highly attenuated VACV A35 gene deletion mutant [37–40] caused pup loss equal to the virulent WR strain [35], indicating that safety in pregnant mammals may not be easily predicted from other measures of attenuation. These data underscore the need for testing of mutant strains in pregnant mammals. RCNV has the advantage that it is far safer than VACV but can still replicate and amplify in mammalian cells, forming plaques that are just slightly smaller than the VACV WR strain (Fig. 1). This is a significant

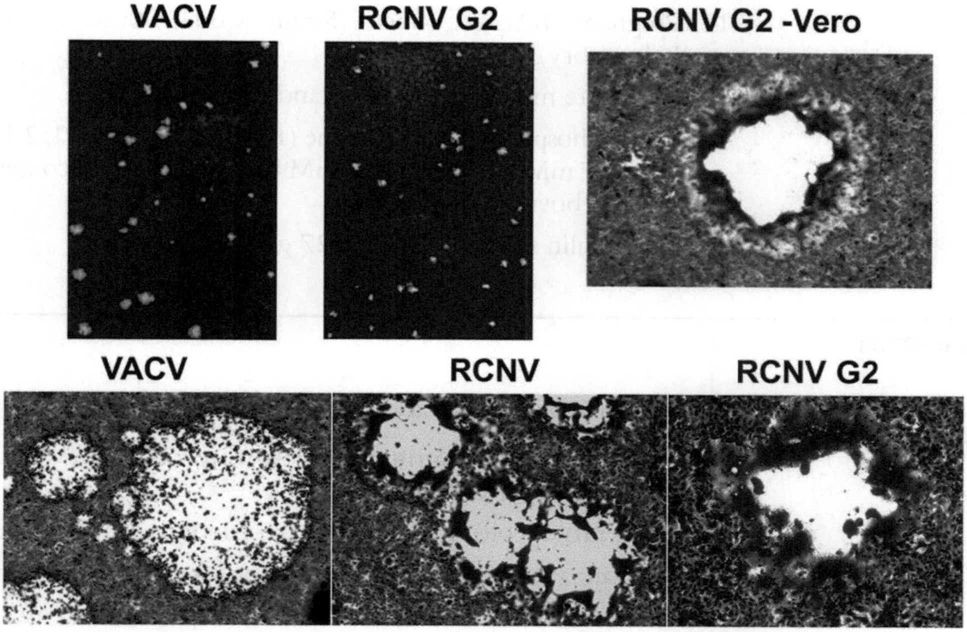

Fig. 1 VACV and RCNV grown on BS-C-1 and VERO cells. (*Top left*) VACV and RCNV-G2 grown on BS-C-1 cells for 40 h and stained with crystal violet (no magnification). (*Top right*) RCNV plaque on VERO cells, 40× magnification. (*Bottom row*) plaques on BS-C-1 cells, VACV, RCNV, and RCNV-G2

advantage compared to MVA, which does not replicate well in most mammalian cells. In this chapter, we describe methods for analyzing poxvirus exposure and safety in pregnant mammals.

2 Materials

Use only sterile reagents and materials. Keep virus on ice.

1. Crude virus stock.
2. Pasteur pipettes.
3. 36% sucrose in 10 mM Tris, pH 9.
4. Ultracentrifuge, SW-40 rotor and buckets.
5. Ultracentrifuge tube (Ultra Tube, Nalgene, stock number 3140-1495).
6. Complete media -MEM/10% FBS: MEM containing 10% FBS, 2 mM glutamine, 100 μg/mL, streptomycin, 100 U/mL penicillin.
7. BS-C-1 African green monkey kidney cells.
8. Six well tissue culture plates.
9. 0.1% crystal violet solution in 20% ethanol.
10. Approved Animal Use Protocol.

11. Pregnant BALB/c mice (Strain Code 000651, Jackson Laboratory).
12. Complete mouse cages with standard bedding.
13. Sterile Phosphate Buffered Saline (PBS, 110 mM NaCl, 2.1 mM KCl, 6.7 mM Na_2HPO_4, 1.1 mM KH_2PO_4) pH 7.4 containing 2% fetal bovine serum (FBS).
14. 1 cc insulin syringes with 25–27 gauge needles.

3 Methods

3.1 Purification of Crude Virus

Purified virus is normally used for infecting animals.

1. Precool the ultracentrifuge, SW-40 rotor, and buckets. Keep all samples on ice.
2. Put 3 mL of cold, sterile 36% sucrose in ultracentrifuge tubes.
3. Sonicate a crude virus preparation for 30 s, 500 μl at a time.
4. Carefully layer 3 mL of crude virus on top of the sucrose using Pasteur pipettes.
5. Add complete MEM medium to bring the liquid to the top of the tube, approximately 6 mL.
6. Weigh tubes and balance before placing in rotor (pairs of tubes should be the same weight, ±0.01 g).
7. Centrifuge at 30,000 rpm (114,000 × *g*) for 40 min.
8. Carefully remove all liquid from the tube and discard.
9. Resuspend the purified virus pellet(s) in 500 μl PBS with 2% FBS. The FBS is important for virus stability.
10. Combine like virus pellets and aliquot into 20, 40, and 100 μl tubes, store in −80 °C freezer.
11. Titer virus after making aliquots and freezing at −80 °C. Do not sonicate purified virus before titering or use.
12. Three milliliters of crude virus will yield approximately 500 μl of purified virus with a titer of approximately 1×10^9 pfu/mL.

3.2 Titer Purified Virus

Infectious virus quantities are measured by counting formation of plaques (cleared spaces or holes) on a cell monolayer and expressed as plaque forming units (pfu).

1. Grow confluent monolayers of BS-C-1 cells in a six well plate overnight, one plate per virus to be titered. Check for confluency using a microscope. Cells should be touching but not overly confluent or plaques will be very small.
2. Remove growth media and replace with 1 mL fresh complete media per well, place plate in a 37 °C incubator with (5% CO_2) while virus is prepared.

3. Remove a vial of purified virus from the −80 °C freezer, thaw quickly, centrifuge enough to make all liquid move to the bottom of the tube, and mix to ensure a homogenous mixture. Place on ice immediately. Do not sonicate or trypsinize purified virus before use in titering or infections.
4. Make a 1:1000 dilution of purified virus, add 1 μl of this dilution to the first well of the top row and swirl the plate immediately to mix. If the titer of the purified virus is ~1×10^9 pfu/mL, this dilution will results in a solution of 1×10^6 pfu/mL and 1 μl of virus will contain 1000 pfu in the first well. If the titer was actually 10^8 pfu/mL, this first well will have 100 plaques.
5. Make a 1:10 dilution from the 1:1000 dilution above, resulting in a 1:10,000 dilution. Place 1 μl of this in the second well of the top row and swirl. This should result in approximately 100 plaques if the original virus solution contains 1×10^9 pfu/mL.
6. Make another 1:10 dilution from the 1:10,000 dilution above, resulting in a 1:100,000 dilution. Place 1 μl of this in the third well of the top row and swirl. This should result in approximately ten plaques if the original virus solution contains 1×10^9 pfu/mL. In this way, there should be one or two countable wells (those containing between 1 and ~80 plaques) in each row on which to base titer calculations.
7. Repeat **steps 4** through **6** in the bottom three wells of the plate to create duplicates.
8. Check that the cell monolayer is intact and healthy using a microscope, and place the plate in a 37 °C (5% CO_2). Record the time of infection.
9. Swirl the plate every 20 min for the first hour.
10. After approximately 1 h, add an additional 500 μl of media per well to ensure adequate volume.
11. Incubate for 40–48 h. 40 h is ideal for VACV, but longer incubation times may be required if the virus used has a small plaque phenotype.
12. Using a microscope, check the wells for plaques and note the health of the cells.
13. Aspirate the media from each well of the six-well plate.
14. Quickly add 1 mL per well of 0.1% crystal violet solution. Do not let wells dry out. Do one plate at a time.
15. Allow plate to stain at room temperature for 5 min.
16. Aspirate the crystal violet and allow the plate to dry. Plaques should be visible at this point.
17. Count plaques in each countable well and calculate the pfu/mL of the original virus solution. To determine if a hole in the monolayer is a plaque or a space between cells, check

under the microscope. Plaques have a darker purple ring around them and show cells with cytopathic effects, usually with long thin cellular extensions.

3.3 Ordering and Receiving Pregnant Mice

1. Call the company at least 1 month prior to beginning experiments and speak with an animal technician about placing this special order (*see* **Note 1**). Order mice to be shipped overnight on gestational day 11, for arrival and infection on gestational day 12. The technician can advise you on when the mice are available for shipping.
2. Order 7–8 mice per experimental group (*see* **Note 2**).
3. Coordinate mouse arrival with your animal care technicians.
4. Once received, animals should be observed for health checks and placed into individual cages.
5. Cages should be labeled and organized according to experimental design: (e.g., saline controls, virulent wild type virus, and experimental virus groups).

3.4 Intraperitoneal Virus Injection

Mice are injected the same day they arrive on gestational day 12. There is an instructional video on intraperitoneal (i.p.) injections available at: http:www.procedureswithcare.org.uk/intraperitoneal-injection-in-the-mouse.

1. Determine the number of plaque forming units (pfu) per mouse needed to obtain desired results: typically 8×10^6 plaque forming units per mouse of VACV strain Western Reserve are used in order to reduce pup count to around 1 pup per mouse. Virus amounts will vary based on experimental design (*see* **Note 3**).
2. On day 12 of gestation, immediately before use, dilute virus in PBS containing 2% FBS for 50 μl injection final volume per mouse. Once diluted, virus should be stored on ice and used quickly.
3. Consider the order of injection. Diluted virus may lose titer over time so negative control groups (i.e., PBS) should be injected last.
4. Mix unsonicated, purified virus and draw up 50 μl in an insulin syringe.
5. Mice are not anesthetized prior to injection. Grasp the base of the mouse-tail with your thumb and forefinger.
6. Lift the mouse from floor of the cage onto cage lid while maintaining a firm grip onto the base of its tail.
7. Using the forefinger and thumb of your second hand, draw up the loose skin between mouse head and shoulders and hold securely.

8. Maintaining the grip, lift the mouse so that its body rests in the palm of your hand. Transfer the grip of the mouse tail to your pinky finger.
9. Position the mouse so that its head is facing slightly downward and its abdomen is exposed.
10. Intraperitoneal injection is made into the lower left or right portion of the abdomen. Be careful to avoid injection of organs. Insert the needle ½ to 1 cm into the abdomen.
11. Aspirate gently to ensure you are not in a blood vessel, bladder or intestine (*see* **Note 4**).
12. Inject 50 μl of virus and withdraw the needle.
13. Place the mouse back into the cage and release. Watch for activity/health.

3.5 Labor, Delivery and Pup Counts

1. Check mice daily for health and arrival of pups.
2. When pups arrive, document the number of pups and the health status of the pups post-delivery (e.g., live, healthy, sick, or dead).
3. Remove any carcasses from cages.
4. From gestational day 17 until day 24 mice should be checked for pups twice daily (*see* **Note 5**).
5. Pups should be monitored for health for 2 weeks post-delivery.
6. Report numbers of healthy pups after deliveries have stopped and when the number of surviving pups has stabilized (*see* **Note 6**).

4 Notes

1. Pregnant BALB/c mice may be obtained through The Jackson Laboratory https://www.jax.org/jax-mice-and-services (or other reputable companies).
2. Animal technicians from the company from which you procure the mice assess mouse pregnancy via the presence of a mucous plug. This requires specialized skill, and mice have been received that were not pregnant that were supposed to be pregnant. Pregnancy cannot be easily detected upon arrival. For this reason, it is recommended that 7–8 mice be used per experimental group.
3. Virus amounts: Uninfected mice deliver 5–6 viable pups normally, and 8×10^6 plaque forming units per mouse of VACV WR will reduce numbers to about 1 pup per mouse. A titration series of virus amounts may be done to show the relative virulence of

different strains. For example, 1000 times as much of a mutant virus may be required to equal the virulence of VACV WR.

4. If aspiration shows blood, urine, or feces, discard the needle and repeat the procedure with a clean needle and inoculum.
5. It is very important to count pups twice a day after gestational day 17. Mice could deliver pups up to 2 days after initial pups are seen. Animals in labor should be monitored closely and a veterinarian should be notified if the animal is unable to deliver or seems unable to complete delivery. Infected mice sometimes have difficulty delivering and may deliver still born pups, deformed pups, or pups that die post delivery.
6. Control mice injected with PBS delivered five or six viable pups. Infection with either VACV-WR or the attenuated VACV-A35Del mutant virus [37] reduced live pup survival significantly ($p < 0.01$) compared to PBS injected mice to about 1 per litter. Because mice were born from days 17–20 and sometimes died shortly after delivery, live pups may be counted on day 26 post gestation as the time point to report and graph data. As the time may vary by experiment, researchers should analyze their data for a stable time point to report.

Acknowledgments

The author wishes to thank Gwendolyn JB Jones and Rishita Yeduri for assistance with the manuscript preparation and to acknowledge funding from Boehringer Ingelheim, Inc. and the National Institutes of Health (1R01AI110542 and R15AT006122).

References

1. Mahalingam S, Damon IK, Lidbury BA (2004) 25 years since the eradication of smallpox: why poxvirus research is still relevant. Trends Immunol 25:636–639
2. Chen N, Li G, Liszewski MK et al (2005) Virulence differences between monkeypox virus isolates from West Africa and the Congo basin. Virology 340:46–63
3. McCollum AM, Damon IK (2014) Human monkeypox. Clin Infect Dis 58:260–267
4. Lederman ER, Reynolds MG, Karem K et al (2007) Prevalence of antibodies against orthopoxviruses among residents of Likouala region, Republic of Congo: evidence for monkeypox virus exposure. Am J Trop Med Hyg 77:1150–1156
5. Lewis-Jones S (2004) Zoonotic poxvirus infections in humans. Curr Opin Infect Dis 17:81–89
6. Molino AC, Fleischer AB Jr, Feldman SR (2004) Patient demographics and utilization of health care services for molluscum contagiosum. Pediatr Dermatol 21:628–632
7. Senkevich TG, Koonin EV, Bugert JJ et al (1997) The genome of molluscum contagiosum virus: analysis and comparison with other poxviruses. Virology 233:19–42
8. Shchelkunov SN (2013) An increasing danger of zoonotic orthopoxvirus infections. PLoS Pathog 9:e1003756
9. Damaso CR, Esposito JJ, Condit RC et al (2000) An emergent poxvirus from humans and cattle in Rio de Janeiro State: Cantagalo virus may derive from Brazilian smallpox vaccine. Virology 277:439–449
10. Oliveira DB, Assis FL, Ferreira PC et al (2013) Group 1 Vaccinia virus zoonotic outbreak in Maranhao State, Brazil. Am J Trop Med Hyg 89:1142–1145
11. Dhar AD, Werchniak AE, Li Y et al (2004) Tanapox infection in a college student. N Engl J Med 350:361–366
12. Stich A, Meyer H, Kohler B et al (2002) Tanapox: first report in a European traveller

and identification by PCR. Trans R Soc Trop Med Hyg 96:178–179
13. Kolhapure RM, Deolankar RP, Tupe CD et al (1997) Investigation of buffalopox outbreaks in Maharashtra State during 1992–1996. Indian J Med Res 106:441–446
14. Campbell CT, Gulley JL, Oyelaran O et al (2013) Serum antibodies to blood group A predict survival on PROSTVAC-VF. Clin Cancer Res 19:1290–1299
15. Hui EP, Taylor GS, Jia H et al (2013) Phase I trial of recombinant modified vaccinia ankara encoding Epstein-Barr viral tumor antigens in nasopharyngeal carcinoma patients. Cancer Res 73:1676–1688
16. Gomez CE, Najera JL, Krupa M et al (2008) The poxvirus vectors MVA and NYVAC as gene delivery systems for vaccination against infectious diseases and cancer. Curr Gene Ther 8:97–120
17. Rerks-Ngarm S, Pitisuttithum P, Nitayaphan S et al (2009) Vaccination with ALVAC and AIDSVAX to prevent HIV-1 infection in Thailand. N Engl J Med 361:2209–2220
18. Tscharke DC, Karupiah G, Zhou J et al (2005) Identification of poxvirus CD8+ T cell determinants to enable rational design and characterization of smallpox vaccines. J Exp Med 201:95–104
19. Jones-Trower A, Garcia A, Meseda CA et al (2005) Identification and preliminary characterization of vaccinia virus (Dryvax) antigens recognized by vaccinia immune globulin. Virology 343:128–140
20. Hersperger AR, Siciliano NA, DeHaven BC et al (2014) Epithelial immunization induces polyfunctional CD8+ T cells and optimal mousepox protection. J Virol 88:9472–9475
21. Guzman E, Cubillos-Zapata C, Cottingham MG et al (2012) Modified vaccinia virus Ankara-based vaccine vectors induce apoptosis in dendritic cells draining from the skin via both the extrinsic and intrinsic caspase pathways, preventing efficient antigen presentation. J Virol 86:5452–5466
22. Weltzin R, Liu J, Pugachev KV et al (2003) Clonal vaccinia virus grown in cell culture as a new smallpox vaccine. Nat Med 9:1125–1130
23. Hatch GJ, Graham VA, Bewley KR et al (2013) Assessment of the protective effect of Imvamune and Acam2000 vaccines against aerosolized monkeypox virus in cynomolgus macaques. J Virol 87:7805–7815
24. Belyakov IM, Earl P, Dzutsev A et al (2003) Shared modes of protection against poxvirus infection by attenuated and conventional smallpox vaccine viruses. Proc Natl Acad Sci U S A 100:9458–9463
25. Earl PL, Americo JL, Wyatt LS et al (2004) Immunogenicity of a highly attenuated MVA smallpox vaccine and protection against monkeypox. Nature 428:182–185
26. Evgin L, Vaha-Koskela M, Rintoul J et al (2010) Potent oncolytic activity of raccoonpox virus in the absence of natural pathogenicity. Mol Ther 18:896–902
27. Jones GJ, Boles C, Roper RL (2014) Raccoonpoxvirus safety in immunocompromised and pregnant mouse models. Vaccine 32:3977–3981
28. Herman YF (1964) Isolation and characterization of a naturally occurring poxvirus in racoons. Bacteriol Proc 64th Annu Meeting Am Soc Microbiol, 17.
29. DeMartini JC, Bickle HM, Brodie SJ et al (1993) Raccoon poxvirus rabies virus glycoprotein recombinant vaccine in sheep. Arch Virol 133:211–222
30. Esposito JJ (1989) Live poxvirus-vectored vaccines in wildlife immunization programmes, the rabies paradigm. Res Virol 140:480–491
31. Fekadu M, Shaddock JH, Sumner JW et al (1991) Oral vaccination of skunks with raccoon poxvirus recombinants expressing the rabies glycoprotein or the nucleoprotein. J Wildl Dis 27:681–684
32. Hu L, Ngichabe C, Trimarchi CV et al (1997) Raccoon poxvirus live recombinant feline panleukopenia virus VP2 and rabies virus glycoprotein bivalent vaccine. Vaccine 15:1466–1472
33. Lodmell DL, Sumner JW, Esposito JJ et al (1991) Raccoon poxvirus recombinants expressing the rabies virus nucleoprotein protect mice against lethal rabies virus infection. J Virol 65:3400–3405
34. Osorio JE, Frank RS, Moss K et al (2003) Raccoon poxvirus as a mucosal vaccine vector for domestic cats. J Drug Target 11:463–470
35. Fleischauer C, Upton C, Victoria J et al (2015) Genome sequence and comparative virulence of raccoonpox virus: the first north American poxvirus sequence. J Gen Virol 96:2806–2821
36. Benning N, Hassett DE (2004) Vaccinia virus infection during murine pregnancy: a new pathogenesis model for vaccinia fetalis. J Virol 78:3133–3139
37. Roper RL (2006) Characterization of the vaccinia virus A35R protein and its role in virulence. J Virol 80:306–313
38. Rehm KE, Connor RF, Jones GJ et al (2010) Vaccinia virus A35R inhibits MHC class II antigen presentation. Virology 397:176–186
39. Rehm KE, Jones GJ, Tripp AA et al (2010) The poxvirus A35 protein is an immunoregulator. J Virol 84:418–425
40. Rehm KE, Roper RL (2011) Deletion of the A35 gene from Modified Vaccinia Virus Ankara increases immunogenicity and isotype switching. Vaccine 29:3276–3283

Part II

Negative Sense Single-Stranded RNA Viruses

Chapter 8

Development of Recombinant Arenavirus-Based Vaccines

Luis Martínez-Sobrido and Juan Carlos de la Torre

Abstract

The development of arenavirus reverse genetics has provided investigators with a novel and powerful approach for the investigation of the arenavirus molecular and cell biology. The use of cell-based minigenome systems has allowed examining the *cis*- and *trans*-acting factors involved in arenavirus replication and transcription, and the identification of novel anti-arenaviral drug targets without requiring the use of live forms of arenaviruses. Likewise, it is now feasible to rescue infectious arenaviruses entirely from cloned cDNAs containing predetermined mutations in their genomes to investigate virus-host interactions and mechanisms of pathogenesis. These advances in arenavirus genetics have also facilitated screens to identify anti-arenaviral drugs and the pursuit of novel strategies to generate live-attenuated arenavirus vaccine candidates. Moreover, the generation of tri-segmented (r3) arenaviruses expressing foreign genes of interest (GOI) has opened the possibility of implementing live-attenuated arenaviruses-based vaccine vector approaches. In this chapter, we will summarize the implementation of plasmid-based reverse genetics techniques for the development of r3 arenaviruses expressing foreign GOI for their implementation as vaccine vectors.

Key words Recombinant arenavirus, Arenavirus rescue systems, Arenavirus reverse genetics, Recombinant trisegmented (r3) arenavirus, Virus vectors

1 Introduction

1.1 Arenavirus Virion Structure and Genome Organization

Arenaviruses are enveloped viruses with a bisegmented negative-sense, single-stranded, RNA genome [1]. Each arenaviral genome segment encodes, using an ambisense coding strategy, two viral proteins in opposite orientations separated by a noncoding intergenic region (IGR) (Fig. 1a) [1]. The large (L) segment encodes the viral RdRp or L polymerase protein (Fig. 1a, blue) involved in viral replication and gene transcription [2], and the small really interesting new gene (RING) finger protein Z (Fig. 1a, orange) that is the counterpart of the matrix (M) protein present in other negative-stranded (NS) RNA viruses and the major driving force of arenavirus assembly and budding [3–5]. The small (S) segment encodes the viral glycoprotein precursor (GPC) (Fig. 1a, green) that is posttranslationally cleaved to form the two mature virion glycoproteins (GP1 and GP2) involved in receptor binding, cell

Maureen C. Ferran and Gary R. Skuse (eds.), *Recombinant Virus Vaccines: Methods and Protocols*, Methods in Molecular Biology, vol. 1581, DOI 10.1007/978-1-4939-6869-5_8, © Springer Science+Business Media LLC 2017

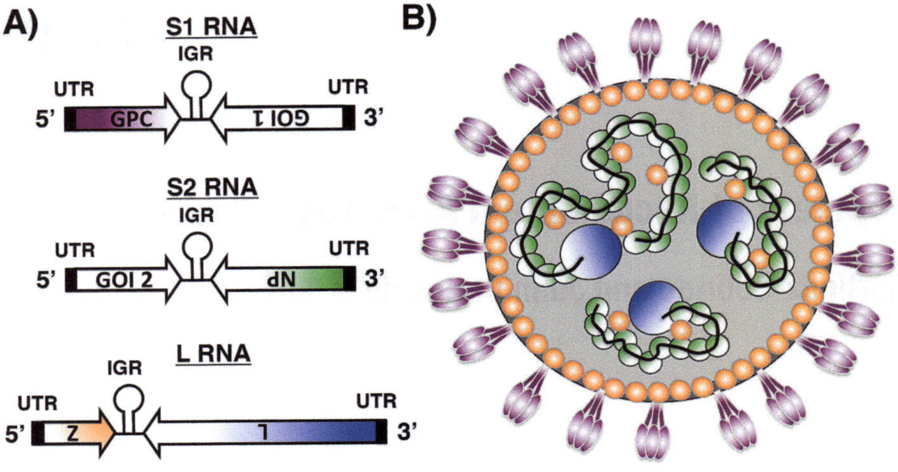

Fig. 1 Arenavirus genome organization and virion structure. (**a**) Genome organization: Arenaviruses are enveloped viruses with a single-stranded, bi-segmented RNA genome of negative polarity. Each of the two viral RNA genome segments uses an ambisense coding strategy to direct the synthesis of two viral polypeptides in opposite orientation. The Small (S) RNA segment (3.5 kb, *top*) encodes the viral glycoprotein precursor (GPC, *purple*) and nucleoprotein (NP, *green*). The Large (L) RNA segment (7.2 kb, *bottom*) encodes the RNA-dependent RNA polymerase (L, *blue*) and the small RING finger protein (Z, *orange*). (**b**) Virion structure: Arenaviruses are surrounded by a lipid bilayer containing the posttranslationally processed viral glycoprotein involved in receptor binding (GP1) and viral cell entry (GP2). Underneath the lipid bilayer is a protein layer composed of the Z protein (*orange*), which plays a major role in viral assembly and budding, and is the arenavirus counterpart of the matrix protein present in other enveloped NS RNA viruses. The core of the virus is made of a viral ribonucleoprotein (vRNP) complex, composed of the viral genome segments encapsidated by the viral NP (*red*). Incorporation of the vRNPs into newly nascent virions is mediated by NP-Z interaction. Associated with the vRNPs is the L polymerase protein (*blue*) that, together with NP, are the minimal components for viral genome replication and gene transcription. Indicated are also host cell ribosomes incorporated into the virus particle

entry, and fusion [6–8]; and the viral nucleoprotein (NP) (Fig. 1a, red), which encapsidates the viral RNA and, together with the L polymerase, constitute the viral ribonucleoproteins (vRNPs) that are the minimal functional unit to direct arenavirus genome replication and gene expression [1, 9, 10]. NP mediates the incorporation of the vRNPs into mature infectious virions by interacting with Z [11]. In addition, NP has also been shown to counteract the cellular host type-I interferon (IFN-I) [12–17] and inflammatory [16, 18] responses during viral infection.

1.2 Arenavirus Life Cycle

The arenavirus replication cycle takes place entirely in the cytoplasm of infected cells [1]. Homo-trimer complexes, consisting of the GP1 globular head and GP2 stalk region, form the spikes that decorate the surface of the arenavirus envelope [1, 19] (Fig. 1b). GP1, located at the top of the spike, mediates attachment of the virus particle to receptors located on the surface of the cell [20]. Alpha-dystroglycan (αDG) has been described as the main receptor for OW and NW clade C arenaviruses [21–23]. However, clade A, B,

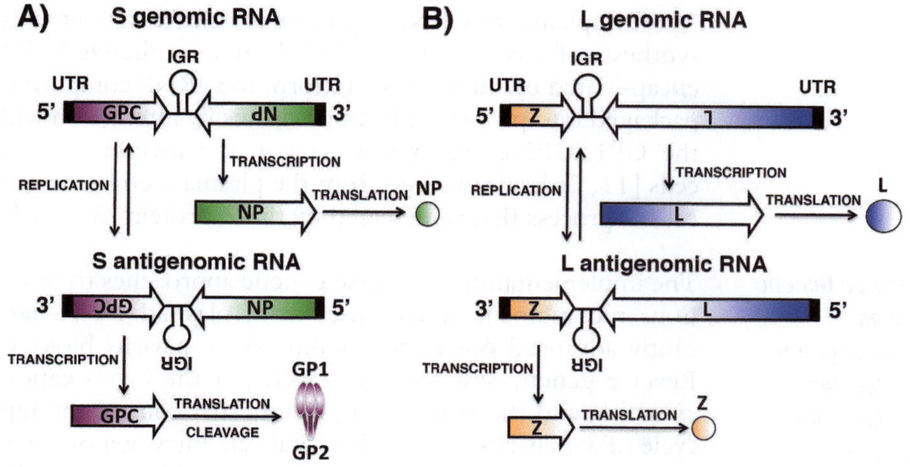

Fig. 2 Arenavirus genome replication and gene transcription: The arenavirus replication cycle takes place entirely in the cytoplasm of infected cells. The L polymerase associated with the vRNPs initiates transcription from the viral promoter located within the untranslated region (UTR, *black boxes*) at the 3′ termini of the vRNAs. Primary transcription results in the synthesis of NP (**a**) and L (**b**) mRNAs from the S and L segments, respectively. Transcription termination is mediated by a secondary stem-loop structure formed by the intergenic region (IGR) found in both vRNA segments between each of the two viral genes. Subsequently, the virus polymerase L adopts a replicase mode and moves across the IGR to generate a copy of the full-length antigenome S and L vRNAs. The antigenomic RNA S and L segments serve as templates for the synthesis of GPC (**a**, S segment) and Z (**b**, L segment) mRNAs. The antigenomic RNA S and L segments also serve as templates for the amplification of the corresponding viral RNA genome species. For more details see the text

and A/B NW arenaviruses were found to use the human transferrin receptor I as the cellular receptor for viral entry [24]. Upon viral attachment, arenavirus virions enter the cell via receptor-mediated endocytosis [20, 25]. The acidic environment of the endosome induces a conformational change in the viral GP1/GP2 complex that promotes fusion of the virion and cell membranes [25]. This in turn releases the vRNPs into the cytoplasm of infected cells where viral RNA replication and gene transcription occur (Fig. 1b) [1].

Arenavirus gene transcription is mediated by the viral promoters located within the untranslated regions (UTRs) at the 3′ termini of viral (v)RNA and complementary (c)RNA species [1] (Fig. 2). NP and L proteins, located at the 3′ end of the S and L viral segments, respectively, are translated from mRNAs with antigenomic sense polarity transcribed directly from the vRNAs and, therefore, are the first arenaviral proteins encoded upon infection [1] (Fig. 2). Transcription termination is mediated by a secondary stem-loop structure formed by the IGR found in both vRNA segments [1] (Fig. 2). GPC and Z proteins are located, respectively, at the 5′ end of the S and L genome segments and are not translated from mRNA derived from the vRNAs but from antigenome complementary RNA species after replication of the vRNAs [1] (Fig. 2).

Complementary RNA segments also serve as templates for the synthesis of nascent vRNAs [1]. Newly synthesized vRNAs are encapsidated by the viral NP to form the vRNP complexes and are packaged into progeny infectious virions by interaction with Z and the GP1/GP2 complexes present in the membrane of infected cells [11, 26]. Virions bud from the plasma membrane of infected cells, a process that is mediated by the Z protein [3, 4, 27, 28].

1.3 Reverse Genetic Approaches for the Investigation of the Molecular and Cellular Biology of Arenavirus

The implementation of reverse genetic approaches to rescue infectious recombinant arenaviruses from plasmid DNA has significantly advanced our understanding of arenavirus biology [1, 2]. Reverse genetic systems have facilitated the investigation of the *cis*-acting and the *trans*-acting factors that control the replication cycle of arenaviruses, including viral cell entry, genome viral replication and gene transcription, virion assembly, and budding [29–32]. Reverse techniques have also allowed the generation of recombinant arenaviruses with mutations in their genomes to examine their contribution to viral replication using cell cultures as well as in viral pathogenesis and associated disease using validated animal models of infection [13, 33–36]. Likewise, implementation of arenavirus reverse genetics has allowed researchers to study arenavirus-host interactions [31, 37, 38], and facilitated the generation of novel candidate live-attenuated arenavirus vaccines [32, 37–41], as well as the development of screening methods to identify and evaluate novel anti-arenaviral drugs targeting specific steps of the virus life-cycle [37, 40].

1.4 Recombinant Trisegmented (r3) Arenavirus as Vaccine Vectors

The generation of recombinant tri-segmented (r3) arenavirus expressing additional genes of interest (GOI) [32, 37, 38, 41, 42] has facilitated studies aimed at the identification of antiviral drugs that inhibit the replication cycle of arenaviruses [43], as well as the implementation of arenaviruses as vaccine vector candidates [32, 37, 38, 42]. The rationale behind the generation of r3 arenaviruses is that physical separation of arenavirus GPC and NP loci into two different S segments imposes a strong selective pressure to package and maintain the three (1L + 2S) segments to provide all necessary viral proteins. Accordantly, a variety of r3 arenaviruses expressing different GOI, including reporter genes, have been documented and shown to be genetically very stable [32, 37, 38, 41, 42]. These findings support the feasibility of generating r3 arenaviruses expressing GOI as vaccine vectors. In this chapter, we will focus on arenavirus reverse genetic techniques for the generation of r3 arenaviruses using the prototype member in the family, LCMV [11, 32, 37, 38, 44]. Generation of r3LCM viruses can be performed under biosafety level (BSL) 2 conditions. Rescue of other r3 arenaviruses may require higher levels of biocontainment [45].

2 Materials

2.1 Tissue Culture Media and Reagents

1. Cell Culture Medium: 10% Dulbecco's modified Eagle's medium (DMEM), 50 ml of Fetal Bovine Serum (FBS), and 1% Penicillin/Streptomycin (PS).
2. OptiMEM: OptiMEM is used in the transfection protocol for the rescue of r3 arenaviruses.
3. Infection and post-infection Media: Mix (2:1) OptiMEM and cell culture medium.
4. 10× Phosphate buffered saline (PBS): 80 g of NaCl, 2 g of KCl, 11.5 g of $Na_2HPO_4{\bullet}7H_2O$, 2 g of KH_2PO_4. Add ddH_2O up to 1 L. Adjust pH to 7.3. Sterilize by autoclaving.
5. 1× PBS: Dilute 10× PBS 1:10 with ddH_2O. Autoclave to sterilize.
6. 2.5% Albumin bovine serum (BSA): 2.5 g of BSA in 97.5 ml of 1× PBS.
7. Lipofectamine 2000 (LPF2000): LPF2000 is used for plasmid DNA transfection in BHK-21, HEK293T, or Vero cells. We recommend a LPF2000:DNA ratio of 2.5:1 for r3 arenavirus rescue approaches (*see* Table 1).
8. Trypsin-EDTA: Trypsin-EDTA is used to detach cell monolayer from the tissue culture plate, prior to DNA transfection or for the passaging of transfected cells.

Table 1
Plasmid DNA and LPF2000 conditions to generate r3 arenaviruses: Amounts of plasmid DNA and LPF2000 recommended to generate r3 arenaviruses using 6-well (1.0–1.2 × 10^6 cells/well) plates are indicated

Plasmid	6-well plates (μg)
pCAGGS NP	0.8
pCAGGS L	1.0
pPol-I S1(GPC/GOI 1)	0.8
pPol-I S2 (GOI 2/NP)	0.8
pPol-I L	1.4
Total DNA	4.8
LPF2000	12
Cells	~1.0–1.2 × 10^6/well

2.2 Cell Lines for the Generation of r3 Arenaviruses

1. Vero cells: African green monkey kidney epithelial cells available from the American Type Culture Collection (ATCC).
2. Human HEK293T cells: Human embryonic kidney cells available from the ATCC.
3. BHK-21 cells: Baby hamster kidney cells available from the ATCC.

2.3 Immuno-fluorescence Media and Reagents

1. 96-well plates.
2. Fixation and permeabilization solution: 4% formaldehyde, 0.1% Triton X-100 diluted in 1× PBS.

3 Methods

3.1 Generation of r3 Arenaviruses

Several approaches have been used to successfully generate recombinant negative-stranded (NS) RNA viruses expressing foreign genes. These include the use of the self-cleavage 2A protease of picornaviruses [46], dicistronic genome segments containing internal promoters [47, 48], internal ribosome entry sites (IRES) [49, 50], and virus-specific packaging signals within vRNA segments [51, 52]. Although viable strategies in other NS segmented RNA viruses, these approaches were unsuccessful in yielding recombinant arenaviruses encoding foreign GOI [41]. However, more recently, it has been possible to rescue a rLCMV expressing GFP from a bicistronic NP mRNA via the use of the small 2A peptide sequence derived from porcine teschovirus (PVT1) [53]. Successful rescue of r3 arenavirus packaging two S segments into mature, infectious virions have been described for the OW arenavirus LCMV [32, 37, 38, 41, 42] and the NW arenavirus JUNV [37, 38, 41]. Within this approach, the S segment is altered to replace one of the viral-encoded proteins (e.g., GPC and NP) by a foreign GOI [32, 37, 38, 41, 42]. The physical separation of the GPC and NP proteins into two different S segments (S1 and S2) presents a strong selective pressure to maintain a virus capable of packaging one L segment and two S segments. The ability of arenavirus to package two S segments has been previously suggested based on genetic [54] and structural [55, 56] analyses. Moreover, because of the stability of the r3LCM viruses, these findings suggest that production of infectious arenavirus particles containing two S and one L segments is a common event [1, 41]. Importantly, each of the S segments can direct expression of a GOI and therefore, two foreign proteins can be expressed within the same virus, contrary to the situation observed with other NS-segmented RNA viruses. Notably, regulation of foreign protein expression depended on the location in the S segment [32]. Expression levels of a GOI in the NP locus are higher than that observed when the GOI was located in the GPC locus, similar to the situation observed during viral infection [32]. Moreover, results obtained with the generation of r3 arenaviruses suggest that, unlike the situation observed with other NS segmented RNA viruses [57] but similar to members in the bunyamwera family [58], the arenavirus NP and GPC coding regions do not appear to play a critical role in the packaging of the viral S segment [41]. Several r3 arenaviruses have been generated that express one or two additional GOI [32, 37, 38, 41, 42]. Depending on the GOI expressed, these r3 arenaviruses showed little or no attenuation in cultured cells and they exhibited long-term genetic stability as reflected by unaltered expression levels during serial virus passages of the GOI incorporated into the S segments [41]. However, compared to WT arenaviruses, r3 arenaviruses have consistently exhibited attenuation in vivo [41]. Since r3 arenaviruses are not attenuated in vitro (ideal for vaccine production) but are attenuated in vivo, these r3 arenaviruses represent a promising approach for their implementation not only as arenavirus vaccines but also as vaccine vectors [32, 37, 38, 42]. In addition, the use of r3 arenaviruses expressing appropriate GOI (e.g., reporter genes) could be used to facilitate the development of cell-based infection assays amenable for the development of HT chemical and genetic screens to identify antiviral compounds and host cell genes involved in the arenavirus life cycle, respectively [53]. So far, several r3 arenaviruses expressing CAT, fluorescent, and luciferase genes have been described [32, 37, 38, 41, 42].

To generate r3 arenaviruses, susceptible cells (e.g., murine or human cells) are co-transfected with the pCAGGS protein expression plasmids encoding NP and L (Fig. 3a) (*see* **Note 1**) together with the pPol-I L segment, and the two pPol-I S (S1 and S2) segments (*see* **Note 2**), where the NP ORF is replaced with a foreign gene (pPol-I S1 GPC/GOI 1), and the GPC ORF is replaced by another foreign gene in the second S segment (pPol-I S2 GOI 2/NP) (Fig. 3b) (*see* **Note 3**).

3.2 R3 Arenavirus Rescue Experimental Approach

Rescue of r3 arenaviruses is frequently done using the mouse Pol-I promoter and rodent BHK-21 cells, as this cell line is highly efficient with respect to transfection and easy to maintain, and is able to produce high viral titers [32, 37, 38, 41]. However, BHK-21 cells do not meet guidelines set forth by the FDA for human vaccine generation due to the presence of tumorigenic agents that may affect the purity of the vaccine seed [37]. Vero cells, on the other hand, have received approval from the FDA for the generation of vaccine seeds [37, 38, 59]. While Vero cells are easy to maintain and produce high viral titers, the transfection efficiencies in Vero cells are generally lower and thus may lead to difficulties in rescuing r3 arenaviruses [37]. Alternatively, human HEK293T cells can be used to generate r3 arenaviruses [37] (*see* **Note 2**). Unlike the Pol-II promoter, the transcriptional activity of the Pol-I promoter exhibits stringent species-specificity [37, 60] (*see* **Note 2**). For the generation of recombinant trisegmented (r3) arenavirus (Fig. 4), two pCAGGS protein expression plasmid encoding the

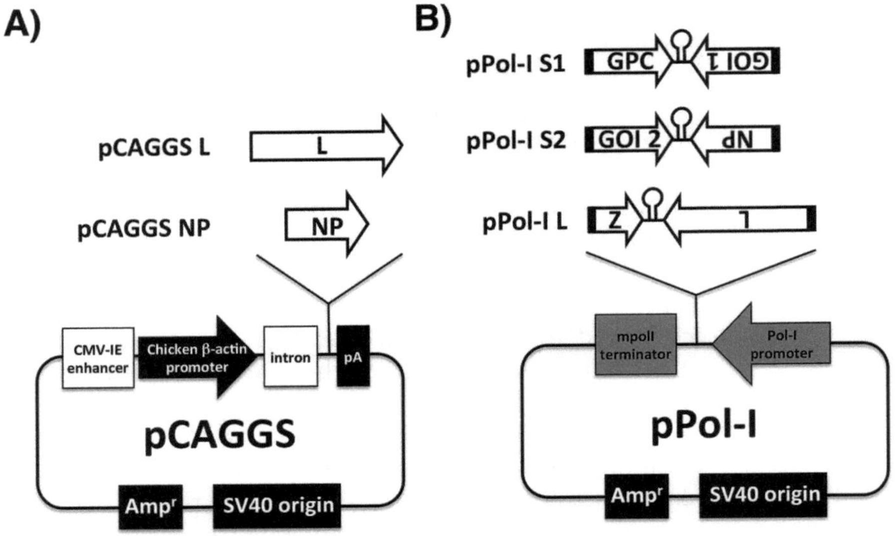

Fig. 3 Recombinant trisegmented (r3) arenavirus reverse genetics plasmids: The plasmids used for the generation of r3 arenaviruses can be transformed and amplified in DH5alpha competent cells and grown in LB media at 37 °C for 16–18 h, with the exception of the pPol-I L plasmid that we recommend growing at 30 °C for 24 h. Plasmids can be prepared using commercially available kits following the manufacturer's recommendations. Plasmids can be stored at −20 °C until use (*see* **Note 3**). (**a**) Schematic representation of the mammalian protein pCAGGS expression plasmid: Protein expression pCAGGS plasmids use the chicken beta-actin promoter (*black arrow*) and the rabbit beta-globin polyadenylation (pA) signal (*black box*) sequences [62] to direct the synthesis of the viral L (*top*) and NP (*bottom*) arenavirus proteins, which are the minimal viral *trans*-acting factors required for viral gene transcription and genome replication. These plasmids are required to provide the arenavirus minimal proteins required to initiate viral gene transcription and genome replication (*see* **Note 1**). (**b**) Schematic representation of the polymerase I-driven vRNA expression plasmid: vRNA expression plasmid under the control of the polymerase I (Pol-I) promoter (*gray arrow*) and terminator (*gray box*) sequences direct the synthesis of the arenavirus vRNA S (*top*) and L (*bottom*) segments. For the generation of recombinant arenavirus from murine or human cells, these plasmids contain the murine or human Pol-I promoters, respectively (*see* **Note 2**). For the generation of r3 arenaviruses, the pPol-I plasmid expressing the S vRNA segment is separated into two plasmids. In the pPol-I S1 plasmid, the viral NP is replaced by the gene of interest 1 (*top*) and in the pPol-I S2 plasmid, the viral GPC is replaced by the gene of interest 2 (*bottom*). Alternatively, gene of interest 1 can be expressed instead of the viral GPC in the pPol-I S2 plasmid and the gene of interest 2 from the pPol-I S1 plasmid (*see* **Note 4**)

arenavirus NP and L polymerase, which are the minimal viral *trans*-acting factors required for viral gene transcription and genome replication [2, 10, 11, 32, 33, 37–39, 43] (Fig. 3a) (*see* **Note 1**); and three pPol-I plasmids expressing the split S1 (pPol-I S1) and S2 (pPol-I S2), and L (pPol-I L) viral genomic or antigenomic RNAs are used (Fig. 3b) [32, 37, 38, 41]. In the pPol-I S1 plasmid, the viral NP is replaced by a foreign gene of interest 1 (GOI 1) and in the pPol-I S2 plasmid, the viral GPC is replaced by a foreign gene of interest 2 (GOI 2) (Fig. 3c) [32, 37, 38]. Instead, GOI 1 can be expressed instead of the viral GPC in the pPol-I S2 plasmid and GOI 2 from the pPol-I S1 plasmid (*see* **Note 4**).

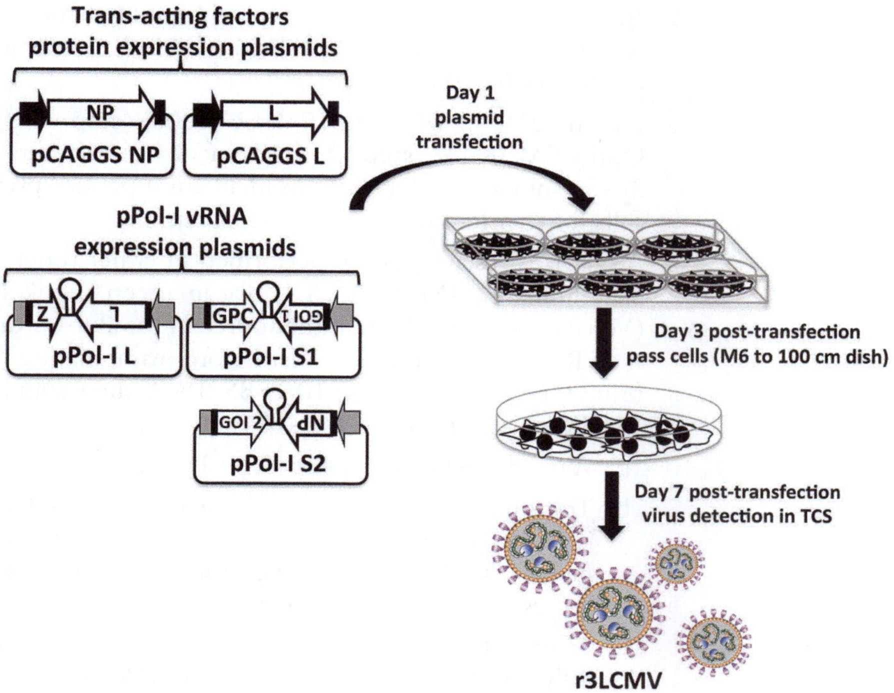

Fig. 4 Generation of r3 arenavirus: Recombinant r3 arenavirus rescues are performed in rodent BHK-21 (using the mouse Pol-I promoter) or in human (using the human Pol-I promoter) cells in 6-well plate format (triplicates) (*see* **Notes 2** and **5**). Cells are transiently co-transfected, using LPF2000, with the pCAGGS protein expression plasmids encoding the viral NP and polymerase L (required to initiate viral gene transcription and genome replication) (*see* **Note 1**) together with the pPol-I vRNA expression plasmids for the viral S1 and S2, and L segments (required to provide the arenavirus vRNAs to initiate viral gene transcription and genome replication). In the pPol-I S1 plasmid the viral NP is replaced by the gene of interest 1 (GOI 1), and in the pPol-I S2 plasmid the gene of interest 2 (GOI 2) replaces the viral GPC. Alternatively, the viral NP can be replaced by the GOI 2 and the viral GPC by the GOI 1 (*see* **Note 4**). Recommended mounts of plasmids, LPF2000, and cells for LCMV WT virus rescues are indicated in Table 1. At 72 h post-transfection, cells are trypsinized and scaled up into 10 cm dishes. After an additional 72 h incubation period, tissue culture supernatants are collected and the presence of virus is determined by immunofluorescence using arenavirus-specific antibodies (*see* **Note 7**). The chicken beta-actin promoter (*black arrow*) and the rabbit beta-globin polyadenylation (pA) signal are indicated in the pCAGGS protein expression plasmids. Viral untranslated regions (UTR, *black boxes*) and intergenic region (IGR) in the pPol-I vRNA expression plasmid are indicated. The Pol-I promoter and terminator sequences in the pPol-I plasmids are indicated by *gray arrows* and *boxes*, respectively. For more details see the text

1. Prepare 250 μl of OptiMEM media with 12 μg of LPF2000 (2.5 μg LPF2000/μg plasmid DNA) per transfection (Table 1). Virus rescues are performed in 6-well plates (*see* **Note 5**). Incubate the OptiMEM-LPF2000 mixture for 5–10 min at RT. During this incubation time, prepare the OptiMEM-DNA plasmid mixture.

2. In a separate tube, prepare the DNA plasmid mix using the recommended amounts provided in Table 1 in a total volume of 50 μl of OptiMEM media.
3. Pipette 250 μl of OptiMEM-LPF2000 (**step 1**) into the OptiMEM-DNA (**step 2**) and incubate this mixture for 20–30 min at RT. During this incubation period, prepare the cells for transient transfection in suspension.
4. Arenavirus rescues can be performed in either rodent (BHK-21), human (HEK293T), or African green monkey kidney (Vero) cells, depending on the source of the Pol-I promoter in the vRNA expression plasmids. Before manipulating the cells, bring the 1× PBS, DMEM 10% FBS, 1% PS media, and trypsin-EDTA mixture to 37 °C for ~10 min.
   (a) Wash the cells, twice, with 5 ml 1× PBS.
   (b) Trypsinize cells using 1 ml trypsin-EDTA. Cell detachment is usually accomplished by incubating the cells in a humidified 37 °C, 5% CO_2 chamber, for ~5 min. Gently tapping the tissue culture plate will uniformly detach the cells.
   (c) After cells are completely detached from the plate, carefully resuspend the cells with 9 ml of DMEM 10% FBS, 1% PS. Place the total media/cell mixture in a 15-ml centrifuge tube and centrifuge the cells for 5 min at 1000 × *g*.
   (d) Remove the media and resuspend the cells in 10 ml of fresh DMEM 10% FBS, 1% PS and count the cells using a hemocytometer. Adjust the cell concentration to ~1.0–1.2 × 10^6 cells/ml (Table 1).
5. After 20–30 min incubation, pipette into each LPF2000/DNA mixture tube (**step 3**) ~1.0–1.2 × 10^6 cells/well (**step 4**). Let the LPF2000/DNA and cell mixture incubate for ~5 min at RT.
6. Transfer the LPF2000/DNA/cells mixture into individual wells of a 6-well tissue culture plate. Gently tap the plate to distribute the cells uniformly and incubate the cells in a 5% CO_2 humidified 37 °C incubator for ~6–12 h.
7. After ~6–12 h incubation, replace the tissue culture supernatants from the transfection with 2 ml of infectious media and return the cells to the incubator and incubate for 48 h.
8. After 2-days incubation, transfected cells should reach ~100% confluence.
   (a) Remove the tissue culture supernatant and gently wash the cells, twice, with 1× PBS.
   (b) Trypsinize cells by adding 500 μl of trypsin-EDTA/well. Return the cells to the incubator and let them incubate for

~5 min. Gently tap the cells to complete detachment them from the plate.

(c) Carefully resuspend the cells with 1 ml of DMEM 10% FBS, 1% PS and transfer to a 1.5 ml microcentrifuge tube.

(d) Centrifuge the cells for 5 min at 5000 × *g*, 4 °C in a microcentrifuge.

(e) Remove the tissue culture supernatant and resuspend the cells in 1 ml of infectious media and transfer to a 10 cm tissue culture dish. Bring up the volume in the plate to 10 ml with infectious media. Gently shake the 10 cm tissue culture dish to allow uniform distribution of the cells and incubate the cells at 37 °C, 5% CO_2 for 72 h.

9. After 3–4 days of incubation, collect the tissue culture supernatant from the 10 cm tissue culture plates (**step 8**) into a 15-ml centrifuge tube and centrifuge at 2500 × *g*, 4 °C for 5 min. Collect the tissue culture supernatant containing the virus and discard the cell pellet.

10. Aliquot the virus into cryotubes and store them at −80 °C (*see* **Note 6**). Virus can be stored at −80 °C until confirmation of the presence of virus.

3.3 Confirmation of Successful r3 Arenavirus Rescue by Immunofluorescence

Arenaviruses do not display cytopathic effect (CPE) characteristically observed with other NS RNA viruses [1]. If the r3 arenavirus does not encode a reporter gene, presence and quantification of the rescued r3 arenavirus can be evaluated by immunofluorescence using an antibody specific for arenavirus NP [10, 11, 32, 33, 37–39, 43] (*see* **Note 7**), as described below. If r3 arenaviruses encode reporter genes, such as fluorescent or luminescent reporter genes [32, 37, 38, 41, 42], successful viral rescue and viral titers can be evaluated using the described protocol without the need for primary or secondary antibodies, under a fluorescence microscope (e.g., to detect GFP expression) [32, 37, 38, 41, 42]. Alternatively, a luciferase assay can be used to evaluate the presence of virus from the tissue culture supernatant [32, 37, 38, 41, 42].

1. A day before confirming viral rescue or titration, trypsinize Vero cells from 10 cm dishes as above. In this case, adjust the cell density to 2×10^5 cells/ml. Seed the cells in 96-well plates (100 μl/well) and gently tap the plate so that an uniform cell monolayer of 80–90% confluence (~4×10^4 cells/well) is reached the next day upon culturing the cells at 37 °C, 5% CO_2 (*see* **Note 8**).

2. On the day of virus titration, serially dilute (tenfold dilutions) viral tissue culture supernatants recovered from transfected cells in OptiMEM.

3. Remove the media and wash Vero cells twice with 50 μl of 1× PBS. Infect the cells with 50 μl of the serially diluted virus. Allow virus adsorption at 37 °C, 5% CO_2, for 90 min, rocking the plates every 15 min to allow uniform virus infection of the cell monolayer.
4. After 90 min post-infection, remove the viral inoculum and add 100 μl of infectious media. Allow the cells to incubate for 16–18 h (*see* **Note 9**).
5. Remove the tissue culture supernatants, fix and permeabilize the cells with 4% formaldehyde, 0.1% triton X-100 diluted in 1× PBS for 15 min at RT (*see* **Note 10**).
6. Remove the fixation/permeabilization solution and wash the cells, three times, with 1× PBS.
7. Block the cells with 2.5% BSA in 1× PBS for 1 h at RT (*see* **Note 11**).
8. During cell blocking, prepare the primary antibody. Antibodies specific to viral antigen should be diluted in blocking solution (2.5% BSA), and centrifuge for 15 min at 3500 × *g* before use (*see* **Note 7**).
9. After blocking the cells, remove the blocking solution and incubate the cells with 50 μl of the primary antibody and incubate at 37 °C, 5% CO_2 for 1 h.
10. After 1 h incubation with the primary antibody, wash the cells three times with 1× PBS and incubate with 50 μl of the fluorescein-conjugated secondary antibody diluted (following manufacturer's recommendations) in blocking solution (2.5% BSA) at 37 °C for 30 min (*see* **Note 12**).
11. Following the 30 min incubation remove the secondary antibody and wash the cells three times with 1× PBS.
12. r3 arenavirus rescue or titers can be determined under a fluorescence microscope. Viral titration is calculated by counting the fluorescent focus forming units (FFU) and the respective dilutions.

3.4 Amplification of Viral Rescue

Successful r3 arenavirus rescue depends on multiple factors including the proper maintenance of cells used for the generation of recombinant viruses, the quality of the plasmid preparations to generate recombinant arenaviruses, and the transfection efficiency of the cell line used for the generation of recombinant viruses, among others. Thus, we recommend performing the r3 arenavirus rescues in triplicate to increase the likelihood of a successful rescue (*see* **Note 5**). It is possible that r3 arenavirus titers in tissue culture supernatants from initial virus rescue are low and, therefore, the viruses need to be amplified to generate a stock. To that end, we recommend infecting fresh Vero or BHK-21 cells at low multiplicity of infection,

MOI (e.g., 0.01) and allow virus amplification for 48–72 h before collecting the new tissue culture supernatants for viral titration, as described above.

4 Notes

1. Other polymerase II (Pol-II) driven expression plasmids expressing arenavirus NP and L can be used instead of pCAGGS for r3 arenavirus rescue approaches.
2. It is important to choose the proper cell line to successfully generate r3 arenaviruses using plasmid-based reverse genetics techniques [37]. If r3 arenavirus rescue attempts are going to be performed in murine cells, the pPol-I vRNA expression plasmids should contain the murine Pol-I promoter [37, 61]. Alternatively, if human HEK293T or monkey Vero cells are used to assess viral replication and gene transcription (MG assay) or generation of recombinant viruses, the pPol-I plasmids should be used to drive the expression of the arenavirus vRNAs under the human Pol-I promoter [32, 37–39, 43].
3. All plasmids can be generated using standard cloning techniques and sequenced using standard protocols. Plasmid concentrations can be determined using spectrophotometry at 260 nm, with DNA purity being estimated using the 260:280 nm ratio (it is best to reach a 1.8–2.0 ratio for optimal arenavirus rescue).
4. It is important to state that reporter gene expression will depend on their location in the vRNA plasmid since it has been shown that arenavirus NP expression levels are higher than those of the viral GPC [32] during viral infection and therefore, foreign GOI expression will depend on their location in the viral S1 or S2 segments [32].
5. To increase the likelihood of successful r3 arenavirus rescue, virus rescues are attempted in triplicate. Therefore, prepare enough OptiMEM-LPF2000 based on the number of virus rescues planned.
6. Make small volume aliquots to prevent multiple thaw cycles, which may reduce virus titers.
7. An antibody specific to arenavirus NP is recommended, as NP is the most abundantly produced viral protein in infected cells and will assist in easy detection of the virus [1]. The species (e.g., mouse, rabbit, etc.), nature (e.g., monoclonal or polyclonal), and proper dilution of the antibody used for viral detection and/or titration must be determined. For LCMV, we use the mouse monoclonal antibody 1.1.3 from hybridoma tissue culture supernatants diluted in 2.5% BSA. In addition, it

is recommended to perform immunofluorescence with primary antibodies against the two foreign proteins encoded by the inserted GOI to demonstrate their efficient expression during r3 arenavirus infection.

8. Viral titers are usually evaluated in triplicate, using 96-well plates.
9. Viral infection lasting over 18 h post-infection may lead to secondary infections and, therefore, result in over-estimation of viral titers.
10. Alternatively, cells can be fixed with 4% formaldehyde diluted in 1× PBS for 15 min at RT, before permeabilizing the cells with 0.1% triton X-100 for 15 min at RT.
11. Alternatively, cells can be blocked overnight at 4 °C.
12. For LCMV NP, we use a secondary FITC-conjugated α-mouse antibody from Dako at 1:100 dilution [10, 11, 32, 33, 37–39, 43].

Acknowledgments

Current arenavirus research in LM-S laboratory is funded by the NIH grants R21 AI119775-01, R43 AI119775-01, and R21AI121550-01A1. Research in J.C.T. laboratory is supported by grants RO1 AI047140, RO1 AI077719, and RO1 AI079665.

References

1. Buchmeier MJ, Peter CJ, de la Torre JC (2007) Arenaviridae: the viruses and their replication, vol 2. Fields virology. Lippincott William and Wilkins, Philadelphia, PA
2. Lee KJ, Novella IS, Teng MN, Oldstone MB, de La Torre JC (2000) NP and L proteins of lymphocytic choriomeningitis virus (LCMV) are sufficient for efficient transcription and replication of LCMV genomic RNA analogs. J Virol 74(8):3470–3477
3. Strecker T, Eichler R, Meulen J, Weissenhorn W, Dieter Klenk H, Garten W, Lenz O (2003) Lassa virus Z protein is a matrix protein and sufficient for the release of virus-like particles (corrected). J Virol 77(19):10700–10705
4. Perez M, Craven RC, de la Torre JC (2003) The small RING finger protein Z drives arenavirus budding: implications for antiviral strategies. Proc Natl Acad Sci U S A 100(22): 12978–12983. doi:10.1073/pnas.2133782100
5. Urata S, Noda T, Kawaoka Y, Yokosawa H, Yasuda J (2006) Cellular factors required for Lassa virus budding. J Virol 80(8):4191–4195. doi:10.1128/JVI.80.8.4191-4195.2006
6. Pinschewer DD, Perez M, Sanchez AB, de la Torre JC (2003) Recombinant lymphocytic choriomeningitis virus expressing vesicular stomatitis virus glycoprotein. Proc Natl Acad Sci U S A 100(13):7895–7900. doi:10.1073/pnas.1332709100
7. Beyer WR, Popplau D, Garten W, von Laer D, Lenz O (2003) Endoproteolytic processing of the lymphocytic choriomeningitis virus glycoprotein by the subtilase SKI-1/S1P. J Virol 77(5):2866–2872
8. Rojek JM, Sanchez AB, Nguyen NT, de la Torre JC, Kunz S (2008) Different mechanisms of cell entry by human-pathogenic Old World and New World arenaviruses. J Virol 82(15):7677–7687. doi:10.1128/JVI.00560-08
9. Lee KJ, Perez M, Pinschewer DD, de la Torre JC (2002) Identification of the lymphocytic choriomeningitis virus (LCMV) proteins required to rescue LCMV RNA analogs into LCMV-like particles. J Virol 76(12):6393–6397
10. Ortiz-Riano E, Cheng BY, de la Torre JC, Martinez-Sobrido L (2012) Self-association of lymphocytic choriomeningitis virus nucleoprotein is mediated by its N-terminal region and is

not required for its anti-interferon function. J Virol 86(6):3307–3317. doi:10.1128/JVI.05503-11
11. Ortiz-Riano E, Cheng BY, de la Torre JC, Martinez-Sobrido L (2011) The C-terminal region of lymphocytic choriomeningitis virus nucleoprotein contains distinct and segregable functional domains involved in NP-Z interaction and counteraction of the type I interferon response. J Virol 85(24):13038–13048. doi:10.1128/JVI.05834-11
12. Pythoud C, Rodrigo WW, Pasqual G, Rothenberger S, Martinez-Sobrido L, de la Torre JC, Kunz S (2012) Arenavirus nucleoprotein targets interferon regulatory factor-activating kinase IKKepsilon. J Virol 86(15):7728–7738. doi:10.1128/JVI.00187-12
13. Martinez-Sobrido L, Emonet S, Giannakas P, Cubitt B, Garcia-Sastre A, de la Torre JC (2009) Identification of amino acid residues critical for the anti-interferon activity of the nucleoprotein of the prototypic arenavirus lymphocytic choriomeningitis virus. J Virol 83(21):11330–11340. doi:10.1128/JVI.00763-09
14. Martinez-Sobrido L, Giannakas P, Cubitt B, Garcia-Sastre A, de la Torre JC (2007) Differential inhibition of type I interferon induction by arenavirus nucleoproteins. J Virol 81(22):12696–12703. doi:10.1128/JVI.00882-07
15. Martinez-Sobrido L, Zuniga EI, Rosario D, Garcia-Sastre A, de la Torre JC (2006) Inhibition of the type I interferon response by the nucleoprotein of the prototypic arenavirus lymphocytic choriomeningitis virus. J Virol 80(18):9192–9199. doi:10.1128/JVI.00555-06
16. Borrow P, Martinez-Sobrido L, de la Torre JC (2010) Inhibition of the type I interferon antiviral response during arenavirus infection. Viruses 2(11):2443–2480. doi:10.3390/v2112443
17. Pythoud C, Rothenberger S, Martinez-Sobrido L, de la Torre JC, Kunz S (2015) Lymphocytic choriomeningitis virus differentially affects the virus-induced type I interferon response and mitochondrial apoptosis mediated by RIG-I/MAVS. J Virol 89(12):6240–6250. doi:10.1128/JVI.00610-15
18. Rodrigo WW, Ortiz-Riano E, Pythoud C, Kunz S, de la Torre JC, Martinez-Sobrido L (2012) Arenavirus nucleoproteins prevent activation of nuclear factor kappa B. J Virol 86(15):8185–8197. doi:10.1128/JVI.07240-11
19. Igonet S, Vaney MC, Vonrhein C, Bricogne G, Stura EA, Hengartner H, Eschli B, Rey FA (2011) X-ray structure of the arenavirus glycoprotein GP2 in its postfusion hairpin conformation. Proc Natl Acad Sci U S A 108(50):19967–19972. doi:10.1073/pnas.1108910108
20. Burri DJ, da Palma JR, Kunz S, Pasquato A (2012) Envelope glycoprotein of arenaviruses. Viruses 4(10):2162–2181. doi:10.3390/v4102162
21. Cao W, Henry MD, Borrow P, Yamada H, Elder JH, Ravkov EV, Nichol ST, Compans RW, Campbell KP, Oldstone MB (1998) Identification of alpha-dystroglycan as a receptor for lymphocytic choriomeningitis virus and Lassa fever virus. Science 282(5396):2079–2081
22. Kunz S, Borrow P, Oldstone MB (2002) Receptor structure, binding, and cell entry of arenaviruses. Curr Top Microbiol Immunol 262:111–137
23. Kunz S, Sevilla N, McGavern DB, Campbell KP, Oldstone MB (2001) Molecular analysis of the interaction of LCMV with its cellular receptor (alpha)-dystroglycan. J Cell Biol 155(2):301–310. doi:10.1083/jcb.200104103
24. Radoshitzky SR, Abraham J, Spiropoulou CF, Kuhn JH, Nguyen D, Li W, Nagel J, Schmidt PJ, Nunberg JH, Andrews NC, Farzan M, Choe H (2007) Transferrin receptor 1 is a cellular receptor for New World haemorrhagic fever arenaviruses. Nature 446(7131):92–96. doi:10.1038/nature05539
25. Pasqual G, Rojek JM, Masin M, Chatton JY, Kunz S (2011) Old world arenaviruses enter the host cell via the multivesicular body and depend on the endosomal sorting complex required for transport. PLoS Pathog 7(9):e1002232. doi:10.1371/journal.ppat.1002232
26. Capul AA, Perez M, Burke E, Kunz S, Buchmeier MJ, de la Torre JC (2007) Arenavirus Z-glycoprotein association requires Z myristoylation but not functional RING or late domains. J Virol 81(17):9451–9460. doi:10.1128/JVI.00499-07
27. Perez M, Greenwald DL, de la Torre JC (2004) Myristoylation of the RING finger Z protein is essential for arenavirus budding. J Virol 78(20):11443–11448. doi:10.1128/JVI.78.20.11443-11448.2004
28. Strecker T, Maisa A, Daffis S, Eichler R, Lenz O, Garten W (2006) The role of myristoylation in the membrane association of the Lassa virus matrix protein Z. Virol J 3:93. doi:10.1186/1743-422X-3-93
29. Loureiro ME, D'Antuono A, Levingston Macleod JM, Lopez N (2012) Uncovering viral protein-protein interactions and their role in arenavirus life cycle. Viruses 4(9):1651–1667. doi:10.3390/v4091651
30. de la Torre JC (2008) Reverse genetics approaches to combat pathogenic arenaviruses. Antiviral Res 80(3):239–250. doi:10.1016/j.antiviral.2008.08.002
31. Emonet SE, Urata S, de la Torre JC (2011) Arenavirus reverse genetics: new approaches

for the investigation of arenavirus biology and development of antiviral strategies. Virology 411(2):416–425. doi:10.1016/j.virol.2011.01.013

32. Cheng BY, Ortiz-Riano E, de la Torre JC, Martinez-Sobrido L (2015) Arenavirus genome rearrangement for the development of live-attenuated vaccines. J Virol. doi:10.1128/JVI.00307-15
33. Ortiz-Riano E, Cheng BY, de la Torre JC, Martinez-Sobrido L (2012) D471G mutation in LCMV-NP affects its ability to self-associate and results in a dominant negative effect in viral RNA synthesis. Viruses 4(10):2137–2161. doi:10.3390/v4102137
34. Russier M, Reynard S, Carnec X, Baize S (2014) The exonuclease domain of Lassa virus nucleoprotein is involved in antigen-presenting-cell-mediated NK cell responses. J Virol 88(23):13811–13820. doi:10.1128/JVI.01908-14
35. Reynard S, Russier M, Fizet A, Carnec X, Baize S (2014) Exonuclease domain of the Lassa virus nucleoprotein is critical to avoid RIG-I signaling and to inhibit the innate immune response. J Virol 88(23):13923–13927. doi:10.1128/JVI.01923-14
36. Seregin AV, Yun NE, Miller M, Aronson J, Smith JK, Walker AG, Smith JN, Huang C, Manning JT, de la Torre JC, Paessler S (2015) The glycoprotein precursor gene of Junin virus determines the virulence of Romero strain and attenuation of Candid #1 strain in a representative animal model of Argentine Hemorrhagic Fever. J Virol. doi:10.1128/JVI.00104-15
37. Ortiz-Riano E, Cheng BY, Carlos de la Torre J, Martinez-Sobrido L (2013) Arenavirus reverse genetics for vaccine development. J Gen Virol 94(Pt 6):1175–1188. doi:10.1099/vir.0.051102-0
38. Cheng BY, Ortiz-Riano E, de la Torre JC, Martinez-Sobrido L (2013) Generation of recombinant arenavirus for vaccine development in FDA-approved Vero cells. J Vis Exp 78. doi:10.3791/50662
39. Cheng BY, Ortiz-Riano E, Nogales A, de la Torre JC, Martinez-Sobrido L (2015) Development of live-attenuated arenavirus vaccines based on codon deoptimization. J Virol. doi:10.1128/JVI.03401-14
40. Rodrigo WW, de la Torre JC, Martinez-Sobrido L (2011) Use of single-cycle infectious lymphocytic choriomeningitis virus to study hemorrhagic fever arenaviruses. J Virol 85(4):1684–1695. doi:10.1128/JVI.02229-10
41. Emonet SF, Garidou L, McGavern DB, de la Torre JC (2009) Generation of recombinant lymphocytic choriomeningitis viruses with trisegmented genomes stably expressing two additional genes of interest. Proc Natl Acad Sci U S A 106(9):3473–3478. doi:10.1073/pnas.0900088106
42. Popkin DL, Teijaro JR, Lee AM, Lewicki H, Emonet S, de la Torre JC, Oldstone M (2011) Expanded potential for recombinant trisegmented lymphocytic choriomeningitis viruses: protein production, antibody production, and in vivo assessment of biological function of genes of interest. J Virol 85(15):7928–7932. doi:10.1128/JVI.00486-11
43. Ortiz-Riano E, Ngo N, Devito S, Eggink D, Munger J, Shaw ML, de la Torre JC, Martinez-Sobrido L (2014) Inhibition of arenavirus by A3, a pyrimidine biosynthesis inhibitor. J Virol 88(2):878–889. doi:10.1128/JVI.02275-13
44. Salvato M, Borrow P, Shimomaye E, Oldstone MB (1991) Molecular basis of viral persistence: a single amino acid change in the glycoprotein of lymphocytic choriomeningitis virus is associated with suppression of the antiviral cytotoxic T-lymphocyte response and establishment of persistence. J Virol 65(4):1863–1869
45. Nisii C, Castilletti C, Raoul H, Hewson R, Brown D, Gopal R, Eickmann M, Gunther S, Mirazimi A, Koivula T, Feldmann H, Di Caro A, Capobianchi MR, Ippolito G (2013) Biosafety Level-4 laboratories in Europe: opportunities for public health, diagnostics, and research. PLoS Pathog 9(1):e1003105. doi:10.1371/journal.ppat.1003105
46. Nogales A, Baker SF, Martinez-Sobrido L (2015) Replication-competent influenza A viruses expressing a red fluorescent protein. Virology 476:206–216. doi:10.1016/j.virol.2014.12.006
47. Flick R, Hobom G (1999) Transient bicistronic vRNA segments for indirect selection of recombinant influenza viruses. Virology 262(1):93–103. doi:10.1006/viro.1999.9895
48. Vieira Machado A, Naffakh N, Gerbaud S, van der Werf S, Escriou N (2006) Recombinant influenza A viruses harboring optimized dicistronic NA segment with an extended native 5′ terminal sequence: induction of heterospecific B and T cell responses in mice. Virology 345(1):73–87. doi:10.1016/j.virol.2005.09.050
49. Marschalek A, Finke S, Schwemmle M, Mayer D, Heimrich B, Stitz L, Conzelmann KK (2009) Attenuation of rabies virus replication and virulence by picornavirus internal ribosome entry site elements. J Virol 83(4):1911–1919. doi:10.1128/JVI.02055-08
50. Garcia-Sastre A, Muster T, Barclay WS, Percy N, Palese P (1994) Use of a mammalian internal ribosomal entry site element for expression of a foreign protein by a transfectant influenza virus. J Virol 68(10):6254–6261
51. Goto H, Muramoto Y, Noda T, Kawaoka Y (2013) The genome-packaging signal of the

influenza A virus genome comprises a genome incorporation signal and a genome-bundling signal. J Virol 87(21):11316–11322. doi:10.1128/JVI.01301-13
52. Liang Y, Hong Y, Parslow TG (2005) cis-Acting packaging signals in the influenza virus PB1, PB2, and PA genomic RNA segments. J Virol 79(16):10348–10355. doi:10.1128/JVI.79.16.10348-10355.2005
53. Ngo N, Cubitt B, Iwasaki M, de la Torre JC (2015) Identification and mechanism of action of a novel small-molecule inhibitor of arenavirus multiplication. J Virol 89(21):10924–10933. doi:10.1128/JVI.01587-15
54. Meyer BJ, de la Torre JC, Southern PJ (2002) Arenaviruses: genomic RNAs, transcription, and replication. Curr Top Microbiol Immunol 262:139–157
55. Buchmeier MJ (2002) Arenaviruses: protein structure and function. Curr Top Microbiol Immunol 262:159–173
56. Young PR, Howard CR (1983) Fine structure analysis of Pichinde virus nucleocapsids. J Gen Virol 64(Pt 4):833–842
57. Marsh GA, Rabadan R, Levine AJ, Palese P (2008) Highly conserved regions of influenza a virus polymerase gene segments are critical for efficient viral RNA packaging. J Virol 82(5):2295–2304. doi:10.1128/JVI.02267-07
58. Kohl A, Lowen AC, Leonard VH, Elliott RM (2006) Genetic elements regulating packaging of the Bunyamwera orthobunyavirus genome. J Gen Virol 87(Pt 1):177–187. doi:10.1099/vir.0.81227-0
59. Hess RD, Weber F, Watson K, Schmitt S (2012) Regulatory, biosafety and safety challenges for novel cells as substrates for human vaccines. Vaccine 30(17):2715–2727. doi:10.1016/j.vaccine.2012.02.015
60. Heix J, Grummt I (1995) Species specificity of transcription by RNA polymerase I. Curr Opin Genet Dev 5(5):652–656
61. Flatz L, Bergthaler A, de la Torre JC, Pinschewer DD (2006) Recovery of an arenavirus entirely from RNA polymerase I/II-driven cDNA. Proc Natl Acad Sci U S A 103(12):4663–4668. doi:10.1073/pnas.0600652103
62. Niwa H, Yamamura K, Miyazaki J (1991) Efficient selection for high-expression transfectants with a novel eukaryotic vector. Gene 108(2):193–199

Chapter 9

Development of Recombinant Measles Virus-Based Vaccines

Michael D. Mühlebach and Stefan Hutzler

Abstract

This chapter describes the development of recombinant measles virus (MV)-based vaccines starting from plasmid DNA. Live-attenuated measles vaccines are very efficient and safe. Since the availability of a reverse genetic system to manipulate MV genomes and to generate respective recombinant viruses, a considerable number of recombinant viruses has been generated that present antigens of foreign pathogens during MV replication. Thereby, robust humoral and cellular immune responses can be induced, which have shown protective capacity in a substantial number of experiments.

For this purpose, the foreign antigen-encoding genes are cloned into additional transcription units of plasmid based full-length MV vaccine strain genomes, which in turn are used to rescue recombinant MV by providing both full-length viral RNA genomes respective anti-genomes together with all protein components of the viral ribonucleoprotein complex after transient transfection of the so-called rescue cells. Infectious centers form among these transfected cells, which allow clonal isolation of single recombinant viruses that are subsequently amplified, characterized in vitro, and then evaluated for their immunogenicity in appropriate preclinical animal models.

Key words Recombinant measles virus, Rescue of *Morbillivirus*, Vaccine platform, *Paramyxoviridae*

1 Introduction

1.1 Background

Vaccines are the most effective way to prevent infectious disease in terms of safety and cost–benefit ratio. However, at present, the development of vaccines to the point of licensing for human use takes decades and sometimes has proven hardly possible as exemplified by the HIV pandemic. To minimize the time for vaccine development and to be safe, it is necessary to develop strategies that allow for the immediate initiation of standardized vaccine development, leading to successful and safe candidate vaccines in a minimal amount of time. One strategy is to use well-known, already authorized vaccines with exceptional safety and efficacy records as a platform to present critical antigens of the pathogen which is the focus of vaccine development. Thereby, efficacious immune responses are triggered in immunized animals and patients

Maureen C. Ferran and Gary R. Skuse (eds.), *Recombinant Virus Vaccines: Methods and Protocols*, Methods in Molecular Biology, vol. 1581, DOI 10.1007/978-1-4939-6869-5_9, © Springer Science+Business Media LLC 2017

not only against the vaccine vector, but also against the additionally present extra antigen. One of these potential vaccine platforms currently under development are recombinant vaccine strain-derived measles viruses.

1.2 Advantages of Measles Virus-Based Vaccines

Unmodified live-attenuated measles virus (MV) vaccine strains are efficient replicating vaccines. Besides revealing an excellent safety record, both humoral and cellular immune responses are elicited, which are responsible for long-lasting protection [1–3]. Therefore, the WHO targets eradication of measles by using these vaccines [4]. The vaccine's manufacturing process is extremely well established [5] and millions of doses can be generated quite easily and quickly. Generation of recombinant MV from DNA via reverse genetics became feasible [5] and allows for the robust expression of different antigens, as outlined below, during replication of the modified recombinant MV vaccine viruses.

Thereby, generally robust immune responses against vector and foreign antigens are induced after vaccination of transgenic MV-susceptible IFNAR$^{-/-}$-CD46Ge mice [6], nonhuman primates, or human patients (*see* Table 1) indicating the high efficiency of the system. Interestingly, pre-vaccinated animals with protective immunity against measles were still amendable to vaccination with the recombinant MV, since significant immune responses against the foreign antigen(s) are still induced [7, 8]. Also in human probands, levels of antibodies against chikungunya virus (CHIKV) Env antigens did not display a negative correlation with preexisting antibody levels against the MV vector backbone [9].

1.3 Potential Applications (i.e., Potential Deliverable Antigens/Disease Targets)

A plethora of different antigens of various viruses and of one bacterium have been cloned into recombinant MV genomes, and the respective recombinant viruses have already been rescued. These projects are summarized in the following table (Table 1).

As depicted, mainly structural proteins, especially viral envelope glycoproteins have been expressed as antigens by the yet generated recombinant MV-derived vaccines, simply due to the expectation that especially humoral immunity against these antigens may result in neutralizing antibodies with protective capacity. However, the vector system proved also capable to induce robust cellular immune responses. Moreover, also secreted, cytoplasmic, or membrane bound markers, such as different luciferases, GFP, lacZ [13], or cellular proteins such as carcinoembryonic antigen (CEA) [41] can be expressed by recombinant MV as demonstrated during its characterization and application as a potential oncolytic virus. Even membrane pore proteins such as the sodium iodide symporter (NIS) [42] and up to three different transgene cassettes with a size potentially exceeding 5 kb [13] have been successfully expressed by recombinant MV, demonstrating the general versatility of this vector system.

Table 1
Recombinant vaccines derived from measles virus

Pathogen	Antigen	Position[a]	Immunity[b]	Protection[c]	Reference
HBV	sHBsAg	P, H, L	ELISA, nAbs	n.t. (MV)	[10–12]
SIVmac	Env (+ Gag)	P	ELISA	n.t.	[13, 14]
MuV	HN, F	P	n.t.	n.t.	[14, 15]
WNV	E	P	nAbs, ELISpot	Yes	[16, 17]
HIV-1	Env	P	nAbs, ELISA, IFNγ-ICS	n.t.	[7, 18–24]
DENV	E, M; EDIII	P	ELISA, Cytokines	n.t.	[25–28]
SARS-CoV	S, N	P	ELISA, nAbs, ELISpot	Yes	[24, 29]
HPV	L1	P	ELISA, nAbs	n.t.	[30, 31]
HCV	C, E1, E2; E1/Ft, E2/Ft	P	ELISA, nAbs	n.t.	[32, 33]
Helicobacter pylori	NAP	N	ELISA, ELISpot	n.t.	[34]
RSV	F, G, M2-1, NP	N, P	ELISpot	Yes	[15, 35–37]
EBV	gB350	N, P	ELISpot	n.t.	[37]
MERS-CoV	S	H	ELISA, nAbs, ELISpot	Yes	[38]
NiV	G	N	ELISA	Yes	[39]
CHIKV	C-E3-E2-6k-E1	P	ELISA, nAbs, ELISpot	Yes	[8, 9]
JEV	prM-E	P	ELISA, nAbs	n.t.	[40]
FluV	HA	P	n.t.	n.t.	[15]

[a]Relative genomic position of the ATU; N indicates first position in the genom, P and H indicate position of the ATU directly following P and H gene cassettes, respectively
[b]Triggered antigen-specific immune responses after immunization determined by measuring total antibodies (ELISA), neutralizing antibodies (nAbs), or reactive T cells determined by ELISpot or intracellular cytokine staining (ICS)
[c]Protective capacity of vaccine-induced immune responses after challenge of the appropriate animal model determined by reduction of pathogen load or attenuation of etiopathology

The targeted viruses span a couple of genera and families. Also the developmental stage of the different vaccines is quite diverse, ranging from the demonstration of successful antigen expression by the recombinant MV, spanning the demonstration of humoral or cellular immunogenicity against the encoded antigen up to demonstration of the vaccine's protective efficacy in appropriate pre-clinical animal models. Of note, recombinant MV encoding the glycoprotein antigens of Chikungunya Virus, MV-CHIKV, has already been tested in a clinical phase I study in human volunteers [9]. After demonstrating efficacy in appropriate mouse and primate animal models [8], this recombinant vaccine delivered proof of principle for safety and immunogenicity in human patients, irrespective of preformed anti-measles immunity [9].

Thus, the route for clinical development of such recombinant, MV-derived vaccines is open. On the one hand, these recombinant vaccines may be valuable to be used during primary measles vaccination to immunize children simultaneously against measles and a secondary pathogen of concern for the respective pediatric population without the need to vaccinate these children with two different vaccines. As an example, MV expressing hepatitis B virus small antigen (HBsAG) may be used in regions with high HBV prevalence to protect children early on from this potentially chronic infection ("buy one, get one free" strategy).

On the other hand, recombinant MV is one of the potential vaccine platforms that can be used for the (fast track) development of vaccines against emerging pathogens, for which fast availability of a vaccine may be critical. In this respect, our MV-derived vaccine against the corona virus responsible for the Middle East Respiratory Syndrome (MERS-CoV) expressing the MERS-CoV glycoprotein S [38] has been among the first and most progressed vaccine candidates, which were evaluated by the Saudi Arabia Ministry of Health [43] and the WHO [44].

2 Materials

2.1 Plasmid DNA and cDNA

1. Full-length MV genome plasmids such as pBR-MV_{vac2}-GFP(H) [10] or p(+)PolII-MV_{vac2}-ATU(P) [38] (*see* **Note 1**).
2. The MV genomes encoded on these plasmids contain the so-called additional transcription units (ATUs). To facilitate insertion of foreign ORFs, usually single-cutter restriction endonuclease recognition sites are placed between the start and stop signals of the ATU, in the above mentioned examples 5′ *MluI* and 3′ *AatII* (*see* **Note 2**).
3. T7-promoter driven expression plasmids for MV proteins being components of the viral RNP complex (i.e., nucleocapsid protein N, phosphoprotein P, viral RNA-dependent RNA-Polymerase L), such as pEMC-Na, pEMC-Pa, or pEMC-La [5, 45], respectively.
4. PolII-Promoter driven expression plasmids for MV RNP complex proteins, such as pCA-MV-N, pCA-MV-L, and pCA-MV-P [46].
5. cDNA of the foreign antigen to be expressed by the recombinant vaccine. The ORF has to be flanked 5′ by *MluI* and 3′ by *AatII* restriction sites (or alternative sites being part of the ATU) such that the genome length of the putative recombinant vaccines obeys to the "rule-of-six" [47] (*see* **Note 3**).

2.2 PCR Components

1. Expand High-Fidelity PCR System (Roche) or standard PCR protocol.
2. Primers to generate antigen cDNA to be cloned into an ATU of MV genomes.
3. Sense primers have to encompass the 5′ restriction site being part of the ATU directly followed by the START-ATG codon and the approx. 20–25 following nucleotides of the antigen ORF.
4. Antisense primers have to encompass the 3′ restriction site being part of the ATU followed by a STOP codon and the approx. 20–25 preceding nucleotides of the antigen ORF. It may be necessary to include extra nucleotides between restriction site and STOP codon to obey the rule-of-six (*see* **Note 3**).

2.3 Enzymatic Restriction Reaction Components

1. Restriction endonucleases and respective buffers (e.g., purchased by New England Biolabs (NEB)).
2. Nuclease-free H_2O.
3. DNA to be digested.

2.4 Ligation Reaction Components

1. Standard ligation kit such as Rapid Ligation Kit (Roche).
2. Purified DNA fragments with compatible ends after restriction digest.

2.5 Bacteria Culture Components

1. Bacteria: *E. coli*, e.g., Top10 F′ (F′{*lac*I^q Tn10 (Tet^R)}, mcrA, Δ(*mrr-hsd*RMS-*mcr*BC), Φ 80 *lac*ZΔM15, Δ*lac*X74, *deo*R, *rec*A1, *ara*D139, Δ(*ara-leu*)7697, *gal*U, *gal*K, *rps*L (Str^R), *end*A1, *nup*G).
2. Luria–Bertani (LB) medium: Bacto tryptone 1% (v/w), yeast extract 0.5% (w/v), NaCl 1% (w/v), pH 7.0.
3. S.O.C. medium (Invitrogen): tryptone 2% (w/v), yeast extract 0.5% (w/v), NaCl 10 mM, KCl 2.5 mM, $MgCl_2$ 10 mM, $MgSO_4$ 10 mM, glucose 20 mM.
4. DNA isolation kits suited for DNA isolation from small (5 mL) or medium sized (200 mL) culture volumes.

2.6 Plasmid Transfection Components

1. $CaPO_4$-transfection: commercial Kit, e.g., ProFection Mammalian Transfection System.
2. 5 mL polystyrene roundbottom tube.
3. Lipofection: Lipofectamine® 2000 Transfection Reagent (Invitrogen).

2.7 Eukaryotic Cell Culture Components

1. Vero cells (African green monkey kidney): ATCC CCL-81.
2. 293T cells (human embryonal kidney): ATCC CRL-3216.
3. 293-3-46 (transgenic HEK cells) [5].
4. Geneticin (G418) solution, 100 mg/mL.

5. Cell are cultivated in DMEM supplemented with 10% fetal bovine serum and 2 mM L-Gln with additional 1.2 mg/mL of geneticin, when used for rescue as described in [5].
6. All cells were cultured at 37 °C in a humidified atmosphere containing 6% CO_2 for no longer than 6 months after thawing of the original stock.

2.8 Western Blot

1. RIPA lysis buffer (50 mM Tris-HCl, 150 mM NaCl, 1% (w/v) NP-40, 0.5% (w/v) sodium-desoxycholat, 0.1% (w/v) sodium dodecylsulfate (SDS), pH 8.0) supplemented with Protease Inhibitor Cocktail Complete (Roche Diagnostics, Mannheim, Germany).
2. Antibody/serum recognizing MV protein, e.g., nucleocapsid protein N.
3. Antibody/serum recognizing foreign antigen.
4. Standard SDS-PAGE and Western blot equipment and material.

2.9 Animal Experiments

1. IFNAR$^{-/-}$-CD46Ge: Mice deficient in (*knockout* insertion) α/β-interferon receptor (IFNAR) receptor gene, expressing human CD46 gene with human-like tissue specificity for human CD46 locus, derived from C57Bl/6 [6].
2. 30 G needles, one for each vaccine to be injected.
3. 2 mL syringes with fine scale, one for each vaccine to be injected.

3 Methods

3.1 Cloning of Full-Length Measles Virus Genomes Encoding Foreign Antigens

1. Generation of gene segments encoding the desired foreign antigen of the target pathogen may be generated by gene synthesis. The (codon-optimized) ORF encompassing START and STOP codons is flanked by the respective restriction sites, which allow direct cloning of the gene segment into the ATU of a full-length MV genome plasmid. It may be necessary to include a specific number of extra nucleotides between STOP codon and 3′restriction site to obey the rule-of-six (*see* **Note 3**).

   Alternatively, the desired ORF is amplified on the basis of (plasmid) cDNA or cDNA directly isolated (eventually after reverse transcription) from the target pathogens' genomes using (RT-)PCR. For this purpose, specific primers have to be designed as outlined above, depending on the exact structure of the ATU and the ORF to be amplified.
2. The resulting cDNA segments as well as the MV genome plasmids are then treated by the respective restriction endonucleases using the following standard reaction mix:

1–10 μg DNA.

5–10 U per restriction enzyme.

5 μl 10× NEB buffer (depending on the enzyme used).

5 μl 10× BSA (if required by the applied enzyme).

Fill up to 50 μl with nuclease-free H_2O.

DNA digestions proceeds at the temperature required by the respective enzymes to allow thorough digestion of the DNA, optimally overnight.

3. The desired segments are purified after restriction digestion by standard agarose gel electrophoresis (*see* **Note 4**). The purified genome-containing plasmid backbone and the antigen-ORF containing insert are ligated using standard ligation conditions with at least tenfold molar excess of the insert:

   50 ng vector DNA.

   150 ng insert DNA.

   2 μl 5× DNA dilution buffer.

   Fill up to 10 μl with nuclease-free water and mix.

   10 μl 2× T4 DNA ligation buffer.

   1 μl (5 U) T4 DNA ligase.

   Incubate for 10–15 min at room temperature.

4. Ligated DNA should be directly transformed into chemically competent *E. coli* strains such as Top10F′ being able to amplify large plasmids and cultured on LB-agar plates containing the selection antibiotic at the appropriate temperature (*see* **Note 1**).
5. After overnight or 48 h of cultivation, single bacterial colonies can be picked into 5 mL LB medium, each, containing the respective selection antibiotic.
6. After culture at the appropriate temperature (*see* **Note 1**) employing permanent shaking, a 500 μl probe of each sample is drawn the next morning or 48 h after picking the colonies, and stored for few hours at 4 °C during isolation of plasmid DNA using standard procedures for DNA preparation from small culture volumes.
7. The isolated DNA is analyzed by treatment with appropriate restriction enzymes (e.g., *HindIII* for Edmonston B-derived MV).
8. Probes of clones displaying the expected DNA pattern after agarose gel electrophoresis are used to inoculate 200 mL LB medium, each containing the respective selection antibiotic. 24 or 48 h after inoculation (the bacteria optimally being still in the logarithmic growth phase), bacteria are pelleted and

plasmid DNA is isolated using standard procedures for DNA isolation from medium sized bacterial cultures.

9. After checking the integrity and identity of the isolated plasmid DNA by enzymatic restriction nuclease treatment and agarose gel electrophoresis, the genome plasmids now containing the modified MV genomes are ready for the rescue of recombinant viruses.

3.2 Introduction to Rescue of Recombinant Measles Viruses

At least three protocols for the rescue of recombinant measles virus are available [5, 45, 46] (*see* **Note 5**), which differ mainly in the cell lines, plasmids, as well as the transfection protocol used for the transfection of recombinant MV DNA into the rescue cell line.

Carry out all procedures aseptically under laminar flow and at room temperature unless otherwise specified. Eukaryotic cells are generally cultured at 37 °C, 5% CO_2, and 95% humidity in an incubator.

3.3 Rescue by Transfection of the 293-3-46 Helper Cell Line [5]

1. Seed 8 × 10^5 293-3-46 cells/well in 2 mL complete DMEM + 1.2 mg/mL G418 into six-well plates and incubate overnight (*see* **Note 6**).
2. The next day, cells should be approximately 80% confluent bevor starting with transfection and the medium of the cells was replaced by medium without G418 approx. 3 h before transfection.
3. Transfection of 293-3-46 helper cells (calcium phosphate transfection): The ProFection Mammalian Transfection System is used for transfection. In detail, 5 μg of MV genome plasmid and 25 ng pEMC.La are added to 25 μl $CaCl_2$ [2 M] in a 1.5 mL reaction tube. The reaction volume is filled up to 200 μl with nuclease-free H_2O. 200 μl 2× HBS buffer are filled into a 5 mL polystyrene round bottom tube and strongly vortexed, while the DNA containing solution is carefully added dropwise to the 2× HBS buffer. The transfection mix is then incubated for 30 min at RT, added dropwise to the medium of the cells, and cells with transfection mix are incubated for 24 h. After incubation, a heat shock of the transfected 293-3-46 cells is done for 3 h at 42 °C in a water bath (*see* **Note 7**).
4. In parallel, overlay cell cultures are prepared by seeding 8 × 10^5 Vero cells/10 cm cell culture dish in 10 mL complete DMEM. After the heat shock, 293-3-46 cells are cultivated for further 48 h, before 293-3-46 cells are overlaid onto prepared overlay cells. During the incubation period examine for syncytia formation, daily (*see* **Note 8**).

3.4 Transfection Protocol Using a PolII Polymerase-Based Rescue System [46]

1. Seed 8 × 10^5 293T cells/well in 2 mL complete DMEM into six-well plates and incubate overnight (*see* **Note 6**).
2. The next day, cells should be approx. 80% confluent bevor starting transfection.
3. Transfection: 4 μg of the respective MV genomic cDNA plasmid are mixed with 0.4 μg pCA-MV-N, 0.4 μg pCA-MV-L, and 0.1 μg pCA-MV-P (helper-plasmids); add 250 μl Opti-MEM to this mixture (*see* **Note 9**). In parallel mix 12.5 μl Lipofectamine 2000 and fill up to 250 μl with Opti-MEM. Incubate both mixtures for 5 min. Mix both solutions and gently mix by vortexing at level 4. Incubate for 20 min to build lipid–DNA complexes. During the incubation period change medium on the prepared six-well plates to 1.5 mL Opti-MEM. After incubation add the total of the lipid–DNA complex solution (500 μl) dropwise to the six-well. Incubate for 4 h. Then, change medium again to complete DMEM and incubate for 2 days.
4. Seed 3 × 10^6 Vero cells/10 cm cell culture dish in 10 mL complete DMEM and incubate for 4 h. Completely suspend transfected 293T cells by pipetting up and down and spread 1 mL of the solution evenly onto the prepared 10 cm cell culture dish (overlay; *see* isolation of single MV clones). Incubate for 3 days. During the incubation period examine for syncytia formation, daily (*see* **Note 8**).

3.5 Transfection Protocol Using T7 Polymerase Based Rescue System and a T7 Pol Expressing Vaccinia Virus [45]

1. Seed 5 × 10^5 Vero cells/well in 2 mL complete DMEM into six-well plates and incubate overnight (*see* **Note 6**).
2. The next day, cells should be approx. 80% confluent bevor starting transfection.
3. Infection: Cells are infected with a T7-encoding vaccinia virus such as MVA-T7 at an MOI of 1–5 (*see* **Note 10**). 45 min after infection, the medium is replaced and cells are transfected.
4. Transfection: 1.5 μg of the respective MV genomic cDNA plasmid are mixed with 1.5 μg pEMC-Na, 1.5 μg pEMC-Pa, and 0.5 μg EMC.La (helper plasmids) and transfected using a commercially available lipofection method as described above in the protocol using the PolII-based rescue system. Transfected cells are cultured and examined for syncytia formation, daily (*see* **Note 8**).

3.6 Isolation of Single Infectious MV Clones

1. If you find syncytia, pick them as outlined below (*see* Subheading 3.6, **step 4**).
2. If no syncytia are visible on day 4 post overlay, split the overlay culture by passaging the culture 1:4. For that purpose, seed 8 × 10^5 Vero cells/10 cm cell culture dish in 10 mL complete DMEM and incubate for 4 h. Aspirate the medium from the 10 cm cell culture dish of the overlay and wash once with 5 mL

PBS. Detach the cells by incubating with 1.5 mL trypsin–EDTA for 5 min. After complete detaching (check by microscope) stop trypsin incubation by adding 2.5 mL complete DMEM and suspend the cells by pipetting up and down. Seed 25% of the cell suspension to the prepared 10 cm cell culture dish. The remaining 75% of the cell suspension are transferred into a 15 mL tube and snap-frozen in liquid nitrogen for 5 min. The frozen cell suspension is thawed at 37 °C in a water bath and the resulting cell debris is pelleted by centrifugation at 3000 × *g* for 5 min at 4 °C. Transfer the supernatant to the 10 cm cell culture dish dropwise and incubate overnight (*see* **Note 11**).

3. Again check for syncytia formation (*see* **Note 8**). If there is no syncytia formation wait for one additional day and if there is still no syncytia formation, repeat the rescue.
4. If there is syncytia formation, seed one six-well plate/virus with 3×10^5 Vero cells/well in 2 mL complete DMEM per well and incubate for 4 h. Identify six different syncytia (*see* **Note 8**) and mark them by surrounding the syncytia at the bottom side of the 10 cm cell culture dish. Harvest one syncytium by scratching the marked area with a 200 μl pipette tip and aspirating in parallel 60 μl. Transfer the aspirated 60 μl to one of the prepared six wells. Repeat the procedure to obtain six different virus clones (one six-well plate/virus).
5. Incubate the six-well plate and check regularly for the level of infection (at least twice a day). If a well is near complete infection, aspirate 1 mL medium and detach the infected cells by scratching with a cell scraper. Transfer the remaining 1 mL including the virus to a 15 mL tube and snap-freeze in liquid nitrogen for 5 min (*see* **Note 12**). Thaw the frozen virus solution at 37 °C in a water bath (*see* **Note 13**) and pellet the remaining cell debris by centrifugation at 3000 × *g* for 5 min at 4 °C. Aliquot the so-called "passage 0" (P0) virus supernatant at 300 μl each and store at −80 °C.
6. For infection of virus in passage 1 (P1), seed 5×10^6 Vero cells/15 cm cell culture dish in 20 mL complete DMEM and incubate for 4 h. Thaw one of the P0 virus aliquots at room temperature and distribute the virus suspension across the 15 cm cell culture dish. Slew the 15 cm cell culture dish immediately for a few seconds (*see* **Note 14**). Incubate the 15 cm cell culture dish and check regularly for the level of infection (*see* **Note 15**).
7. When the 15 cm cell culture dish is completely infected, aspirate the medium completely and add 1 mL Opti-MEM. Detach the infected cells by scratching with a cell scraper. Transfer the medium including all cell debris by a 1 mL pipette (*see* **Note 16**)

to a 15 mL falcon and snap-freeze in liquid nitrogen for 5 min (*see* **Note 12**). Thaw the frozen virus solution at 37 °C in a water bath (*see* **Note 13**) and pellet the remaining cell debris by centrifugation at 3000 × *g* for 5 min at 4 °C. Distribute the P0 virus supernatant into 300 μl aliquots and store at −80 °C. To obtain the virus titer measured as 50% tissue culture infective dose ($TCID_{50}$), perform an endpoint dilution assay with one aliquot according to Spearman–Karber [48].

3.7 Amplification of Recombinant Measles Viruses (See Note 17)

1. For generation of P1 virus stocks 5 × 10^6 Vero are seeded in quadruplicates into 15 cm dishes and cultivated for around 4 h at 37 °C.
2. The cells were infected with 300 μl of P0 stock. Vero cells infected with MV vaccine strains are cultivated at 32 °C.
3. When almost all cells are infected (*see* **Notes 8** and **15**), the P1 culture is harvested by freezing and thawing of cells. The medium of the infected cells is completely removed (*see* **Note 18**) and 1 mL Opti-MEM is added to the infected cells. The cells were carefully detached using a cell scraper and the cell suspension is transferred into a 15 mL tube, which is snap-frozen in liquid nitrogen (*see* **Note 12**). The suspension is then thawed at 37 °C (*see* **Note 13**) and subsequently centrifuged at approx. 3000 × *g*, 5 min, 4 °C. The supernatant is aliquoted into 300 μl aliquots in cryotubes and stored at −80 °C (*see* **Note 19**). The P1 virus stocks are titrated on Vero cells according to Kaerber and Spaerman [48].
4. To generate P2 and subsequent MV cultures (*see* **Note 20**), 5 × 10^6 Vero cells are seeded in quadruplicates in 15 cm dishes and cultivated for around 4 h at 37 °C. Then, the cells are infected with a multiplicity of infection (MOI) of 0.03 of the titrated parental virus stock and cultivated at 32 °C. When almost all cells are infected, the P2 culture is harvested as described above and titrated on Vero cells [48].

3.8 Characterization of Recombinant Measles Virus-Based Vaccines by Western Blot Analysis

1. For the preparation of cell lysates 3 × 10^5 Vero cells/well in 2 mL complete DMEM per well are incubated for around 4 h.
2. The cells are infected with an MOI of 0.03 of the respective virus.
3. When almost all cells are infected, medium is removed and the cells are washed with 1 mL PBS at 4 °C for 5 min (*see* **Note 21**).
4. The cells are then incubated with 500 μl RIPA buffer for 10 min on ice (*see* **Note 22**).
5. The cell suspension is transferred into precooled 1.5 mL reaction tubes and centrifuged at 17,000 × *g* for 15 min at 4 °C to remove the cell debris.

6. The protein containing supernatant is transferred into a fresh pre-cooled 1.5 mL reaction tube and stored at −80 °C. Frozen cell lysates are thawed on ice for further Western blot applications according to standard conditions using antibodies recognizing an MV protein, e.g., the nucleocapsid protein, to standardize for infection, and another antibody recognizing the foreign antigen to allow assessment of proper antigen expression by the recombinant vaccine.

3.9 Vaccine Characterization by Determining Viral Growth Kinetics in Vitro

1. For the generation of growth curves, 1×10^5 Vero are seeded per well of a 12-well plate. After 24 h, the cells are infected with the virus of interest with an MOI of 0.03 in six replicates.
2. Released virus in the supernatant and cell-associated virus is sampled 24, 48, 72, 96, 120, and 144 h post infection.
3. To harvest the supernatant, 500 μl medium are removed in duplicates and transferred into pre-cooled 1.5 mL reaction tubes and quick-frozen.
4. To harvest the cell-associated virus 1 mL Opti-MEM is added to one well of infected cells, which are detached from the well using a cell scraper and transferred into a pre-cooled 1.5 mL reaction tube and quick-frozen.
5. The cell suspension is thawed at 37 °C (*see* **Note 13**) and subsequently centrifuged at 855 × *g*, 5 min, and 4 °C. The virus containing supernatant was also stored 2× 500 μl aliquots at −80 °C.
6. Both the released virus and the cell-associated virus are titrated on Vero cells in 8 two-fold dilutions with two replicates per time point and virus.

3.10 In Vivo Characterization of Recombinant Vaccine Viruses

1. IFNAR$^{-/-}$-CD46Ge mice (*see* **Note 23**) aged 6–12 weeks receive 1×10^5 $TCID_{50}$ MV diluted in Opti-MEM in a final volume of 200 μl.
2. Mice are injected i.p. into the left, caudal abdomen using a 30 G needle.
3. After 4 weeks, mice receive a booster immunization of 1×10^5 $TCID_{50}$ MV diluted in Opti-MEM to a final volume of 200 μl, which are injected as before (*see* **Note 24**).
4. Four to 7 days after booster immunization, splenozytes are harvested from immunized mice to assess abundance of antigen- or vector-specific T cells by ELISpot or intracellular cytokine staining after stimulation with respective antigens or peptides, either following standard protocols or using commercially available kits according to the manufacturer's instructions.

5. Before immunization ("pre-bleed"), directly before the booster vaccination ("post-prime") or 21 days after booster vaccination ("post-boost"), 200 μl blood are taken from each mouse, and sera are separated to assess abundance of vector- or target-specific antibodies by titrating neutralizing titers or total antibody titers by ELISA.
6. If the IFNAR$^{-/-}$-CD46Ge mouse strain is susceptible to the pathogen to which the vaccine is directed against, vaccinated mice can be challenged subsequent to immunization. The challenge relies on an established infection protocol of (unvaccinated) animals, which results in symptomatic infections or even death, thereby allowing to test the protective capacity of the vaccine. Parameters such as course of disease or pathogen load in specific organs are assed (*see* **Note 25**).

4 Notes

1. Both examples pBR-MV$_{vac2}$-GFP(H) and p(+)PolII-MV$_{vac2}$-ATU(P) contain, as all genome plasmids for the rescue of recombinant MV, a full-length MV vaccine strain genome. pBR-MV$_{vac2}$-GFP(H) is derived from the plasmid backbone pBR322 (low copy) and expresses the viral RNA antigenome under the control of a T7-promoter, whereas p(+)PolII-MV$_{vac2}$-ATU(P) has a pBluescript (high copy) backbone and is PolII-driven. Plasmids containing full-length MV genomes tend to be a bit delicate to handling procedures. Therefore, plasmids with a high-copy plasmid backbone should be amplified in *E. coli* at 30 °C, whereas low-copy plasmids can be amplified at 37 °C. In addition, it pays to directly pick clones or isolate plasmids from growing cultures instead of storing liquid bacteria cultures or colony plates with MV genome-containing plasmids at 4 °C for more than few hours (≪ over-night!). As an alternative, bacteria pellets can be stored frozen at −20 °C before plasmid isolation.
2. Each MV gene cassette is flanked by conserved genetic elements representing start and stop signals for the viral polymerase complex. By duplicating these highly conserved intergenic sequences, a new transcription unit can be inserted in virtually any position of the virus genome, allowing insertion and expression of foreign genes such as antigen ORFs. The relative genomic position of the ATU allows regulation of the inserted gene's expression due to the transcriptional gradient found in *Mononegavirales*. The further upstream the ATU cassette is located, the higher the amount of mRNA being transcribed in infected cells and the higher protein expression. However, if the encoded gene product interferes with MV replication, too

high expression levels of the encoded antigen may be detrimental.

3. The number of nucleotides in MV genomes can be exactly divided by 6, presumably due to one N protein binding to six nucleotides. Also recombinant genomes have to obey this rule; otherwise no recombinant virus can be rescued. Therefore, it has to be considered that the length of the inserted gene segment can be divided with the same rest by 6 as the length of the segment removed from the genome during cloning, if gene cassettes are inserted into genome plasmids. Thereby, one makes sure that the length of the resulting full-length genome is multiple of 6, again.
4. Due to the size of the genome-containing plasmid (approx. 20 kDa), voltage during agarose gel electrophoresis should be restricted to max. 70 V.
5. While T7-based rescue of MV, especially using the helper cell line 293-3-46, is the standard rescue system guaranteeing precise start and stop of the transcribed anti-genomic viral RNA due to the precise start of T7-driven transcription and stop due to specific termination signals in conjunction with the ribozyme flanking the viral genome sequences [5], efficiency of the rescue is quite variable and depends considerably on the status of the rescue cells. Moreover, syncytia formation using 293-3-46 cells after overlay is not too efficient [5], further limiting rescue efficiency especially of virus variants with limited fusion activity (unpublished own observation). Vaccinia Virus driven rescue allows usage of cell lines other than 293, which may be better suited for propagation of one specific MV variant, but depends on the quality of the used plasmids. PolII-driven virus rescue is very efficient and usually results in recombinant MV with precise genomes, but the lower precision of start and stop of Poll II transcription may allow completion of virus from genomes not being in line with the rule of six [46].
6. Prepare one more six-well plate than required for the rescue of the different MV. This additional well is used as transfection control.
7. Seal six-well plate properly to avoid contamination of the cells.
8. If the recombinant MV will additionally express GFP or other fluorescent marker proteins, check for GFP-expression with the help of a fluorescence microscope to identify syncytia. If no easy marker protein for easy evaluation is encoded, check for syncytia formation via light microscope in phase contrast.
9. For transfection control, use 4 μg of for example EGFP expression plasmids such as pEGFP-N1 without any MV cDNA or helper-plasmids and transfect as described for MV cDNA.

10. If using another Vaccinia Virus than MVA for T7 Pol expression, one has to make sure that the rescued recombinant MV can be separated from (co-) replicating Vaccinia Virus, which may be a tedious process due to the laborious methods needed to physically separate the different virus populations.
11. **Step 2** seems to be slightly more efficient in our hands, but it includes one additional freeze–thaw cycle.
12. After quick-freezing in liquid nitrogen, the tube containing the virus suspension can be stored at −80 °C for several days.
13. Check thawing of the virus regularly, the virus is heat sensitive and incubating the virus at 37 °C will lead to significantly reduced virus titers.
14. It is essential to slew the cell culture dish immediately as well as properly to avoid erratic infection of Vero cells, which will lead to lower virus titers.
15. The growth rate is depending on the virus strain and might be modulated by the additional genetic information. Therefore, check the virus growth regularly to develop a feeling for the growth rate.
16. Scratch the cells to on edge of the cell culture dish and hold the plate inclined while aspirating the medium including all cell debris.
17. While MV vaccine strains authorized to be used as human vaccines are usually regarded as safe and accordingly being handled under BSL-1 conditions, recombinant viruses—even those bearing identical vaccine strain genomes—may be handled under BSL-1 or BSL-2 conditions depending on the locally responsible national or regional regulatory authorities. Under very rare circumstances, single recombinant MV may be placed into BSL-3, depending on the nature of the expressed foreign antigen.
18. Try to remove the medium completely while following **Note 16**. This will increase virus titers.
19. The number of aliquots can be modified, depending on freezer-space and experimental plans.
20. For passages >P5 it is sufficient to infect only one 15 cm dish and store around five aliquots, because those viruses are not used for experiments, normally.
21. Slew the plate gently a few times during incubation.
22. Slew the plate vigorously a few times during incubation.
23. Experimental mouse work has to be carried out in compliance with the regulations of the respective animal protection law.
24. Mice are sacrificed or used for further studies dependent on the respective experimental schedule.

25. Efficacy of the recombinant vaccines can be most directly assessed using a challenge experiment directly revealing protection by abolishing or attenuating the etiopathology. In absence of an appropriate challenge, quantitative abundance of antigen-specific (neutralizing) antibodies or T cell reactivity can indicate the protective efficacy of the recombinant vaccine.

Acknowledgment

The authors are indebted to R. Cattaneo for introduction into the exciting field of recombinant MV and thank U. Schneider for providing the PolII Rescue System. The project was supported by Federal ministry for Education and Research of Germany (BMBF) grant 031A010B (M.D. Mühlebach).

References

1. Griffin DE (2002) Measles virus. In: Wiley encyclopedia of molecular medicine. John Wiley & Sons, Inc., Hoboken, NJ, USA
2. Davidkin I, Jokinen S, Broman M et al (2008) Persistence of measles, mumps, and rubella antibodies in an MMR-vaccinated cohort: a 20-year follow-up. J Infect Dis 197(7):950–956. doi:10.1086/528993
3. Hilleman MR (2001) Current overview of the pathogenesis and prophylaxis of measles with focus on practical implications. Vaccine 20(5–6):651–665
4. WHO Global eradication of measles. Sixty-Third World Health Assembly
5. Radecke F, Spielhofer P, Schneider H et al (1995) Rescue of measles viruses from cloned DNA. EMBO J 14(23):5773–5784
6. Mrkic B, Pavlovic J, Rulicke T et al (1998) Measles virus spread and pathogenesis in genetically modified mice. J Virol 72(9):7420–7427
7. Lorin C, Mollet L, Delebecque F et al (2004) A single injection of recombinant measles virus vaccines expressing human immunodeficiency virus (HIV) type 1 clade B envelope glycoproteins induces neutralizing antibodies and cellular immune responses to HIV. J Virol 78(1):146–157
8. Brandler S, Ruffie C, Combredet C et al (2013) A recombinant measles vaccine expressing chikungunya virus-like particles is strongly immunogenic and protects mice from lethal challenge with chikungunya virus. Vaccine 31(36):3718–3725. doi:10.1016/j.vaccine.2013.05.086
9. Ramsauer K, Schwameis M, Firbas C et al (2015) Immunogenicity, safety, and tolerability of a recombinant measles-virus-based chikungunya vaccine: a randomised, double-blind, placebo-controlled, active-comparator, first-in-man trial. Lancet Infect Dis 15(5):519–527. doi:10.1016/S1473-3099(15)70043-5
10. del Valle JR, Devaux P, Hodge G et al (2007) A vectored measles virus induces hepatitis B surface antigen antibodies while protecting macaques against measles virus challenge. J Virol 81(19):10597–10605. doi:10.1128/JVI.00923-07
11. Reyes-del Valle J, Hodge G, McChesney MB et al (2009) Protective anti-hepatitis B virus responses in rhesus monkeys primed with a vectored measles virus and boosted with a single dose of hepatitis B surface antigen. J Virol 83(17):9013–9017. doi:10.1128/JVI.00906-09
12. Singh M, Cattaneo R, Billeter MA (1999) A recombinant measles virus expressing hepatitis B virus surface antigen induces humoral immune responses in genetically modified mice. J Virol 73(6):4823–4828
13. Zuniga A, Wang Z, Liniger M et al (2007) Attenuated measles virus as a vaccine vector. Vaccine 25(16):2974–2983. doi:10.1016/j.vaccine.2007.01.064
14. Wang Z, Hangartner L, Cornu TI et al (2001) Recombinant measles viruses expressing heterologous antigens of mumps and simian immunodeficiency viruses. Vaccine 19(17–19):2329–2336
15. Swett-Tapia C, Bogaert L, de Jong P et al (2016) Recombinant measles virus incorporat-

ing heterologous viral membrane proteins for use as vaccines. J Gen Virol. doi:10.1099/jgv.0.000523
16. Brandler S, Marianneau P, Loth P et al (2012) Measles vaccine expressing the secreted form of West Nile virus envelope glycoprotein induces protective immunity in squirrel monkeys, a new model of West Nile virus infection. J Infect Dis 206(2):212–219. doi:10.1093/infdis/jis328
17. Despres P, Combredet C, Frenkiel M-P et al (2005) Live measles vaccine expressing the secreted form of the West Nile virus envelope glycoprotein protects against West Nile virus encephalitis. J Infect Dis 191(2):207–214. doi:10.1086/426824
18. Guerbois M, Moris A, Combredet C et al (2009) Live attenuated measles vaccine expressing HIV-1 Gag virus like particles covered with gp160DeltaV1V2 is strongly immunogenic. Virology 388(1):191–203. doi:10.1016/j.virol.2009.02.047
19. Stebbings R, Fevrier M, Li B et al (2012) Immunogenicity of a recombinant measles-HIV-1 clade B candidate vaccine. PLoS One 7(11):e50397. doi:10.1371/journal.pone.0050397
20. Stebbings R, Li B, Lorin C et al (2013) Immunogenicity of a recombinant measles HIV-1 subtype C vaccine. Vaccine 31(51):6079–6086. doi:10.1016/j.vaccine.2013.09.072
21. Lorin C, Segal L, Mols J et al (2012) Toxicology, biodistribution and shedding profile of a recombinant measles vaccine vector expressing HIV-1 antigens, in cynomolgus macaques. Naunyn Schmiedebergs Arch Pharmacol 385(12):1211–1225. doi:10.1007/s00210-012-0793-4
22. Lorin C, Delebecque F, Labrousse V et al (2005) A recombinant live attenuated measles vaccine vector primes effective HLA-A0201-restricted cytotoxic T lymphocytes and broadly neutralizing antibodies against HIV-1 conserved epitopes. Vaccine 23(36):4463–4472. doi:10.1016/j.vaccine.2005.04.024
23. Liniger M, Zuniga A, Tamin A et al (2008) Induction of neutralising antibodies and cellular immune responses against SARS coronavirus by recombinant measles viruses. Vaccine 26(17):2164–2174. doi:10.1016/j.vaccine.2008.01.057
24. Hu H-M, Chen H-W, Hsiao Y-J et al (2016) The successful induction of T-cell and antibody responses by a recombinant measles virus-vectored tetravalent dengue vaccine provides partial protection against dengue-2 infection. Hum Vaccin Immunother 12(7):1678–1689. doi:10.1080/21645515.2016.1143576
25. Harahap-Carrillo IS, Ceballos-Olvera I, Valle JR-D (2015) Immunogenic subviral particles displaying domain III of dengue 2 envelope protein vectored by measles virus. Vaccines (Basel) 3(3):503–518. doi:10.3390/vaccines3030503
26. Brandler S, Lucas-Hourani M, Moris A et al (2007) Pediatric measles vaccine expressing a dengue antigen induces durable serotype-specific neutralizing antibodies to dengue virus. PLoS Negl Trop Dis 1(3):e96. doi:10.1371/journal.pntd.0000096
27. Brandler S, Ruffie C, Najburg V et al (2010) Pediatric measles vaccine expressing a dengue tetravalent antigen elicits neutralizing antibodies against all four dengue viruses. Vaccine 28(41):6730–6739. doi:10.1016/j.vaccine.2010.07.073
28. Escriou N, Callendret B, Lorin V et al (2014) Protection from SARS coronavirus conferred by live measles vaccine expressing the spike glycoprotein. Virology 452–453:32–41. doi:10.1016/j.virol.2014.01.002
29. Lininger M, Zuniga A, Morin TNA et al. (2009) Recombinant measles virus exp ressing single or multiple antigens of human immunodeficiency virus (HIV-1) in duce cellular and humoral immune responses. Vaccine 27(25–26):3299–3305. doi:10.1016/j.vaccine.2009.01.057
30. Gupta G, Giannino V, Rishi N et al (2016) Immunogenicity of next-generation HPV vaccines in non-human primates: measles-vectored HPV vaccine versus Pichia pastoris recombinant protein vaccine. Vaccine. doi:10.1016/j.vaccine.2016.07.051
31. Cantarella G, Liniger M, Zuniga A et al (2009) Recombinant measles virus-HPV vaccine candidates for prevention of cervical carcinoma. Vaccine 27(25–26):3385–3390. doi:10.1016/j.vaccine.2009.01.061
32. Satoh M, Saito M, Tanaka K et al (2010) Evaluation of a recombinant measles virus expressing hepatitis C virus envelope proteins by infection of human PBL-NOD/Scid/Jak3null mouse. Comp Immunol Microbiol Infect Dis 33(6):e81–e88. doi:10.1016/j.cimid.2010.02.006
33. Reyes-del Valle J, de La Fuente C, Turner MA et al (2012) Broadly neutralizing immune responses against hepatitis C virus induced by vectored measles viruses and a recombinant envelope protein booster. J Virol 86(21):11558–11566. doi:10.1128/JVI.01776-12
34. Iankov ID, Haralambieva IH, Galanis E (2011) Immunogenicity of attenuated measles virus engineered to express Helicobacter pylori neutrophil-activating protein. Vaccine 29(8):1710–1720. doi:10.1016/j.vaccine.2010.12.020
35. Sawada A, Komase K, Nakayama T (2011) AIK-C measles vaccine expressing fusion protein of respiratory syncytial virus induces protective antibodies in cotton rats. Vaccine

29(7):1481–1490. doi:10.1016/j.vaccine.2010.12.028
36. Yamaji Y, Nakayama T (2014) Recombinant measles viruses expressing respiratory syncytial virus proteins induced virus-specific CTL responses in cotton rats. Vaccine 32(35):4529–4536. doi:10.1016/j.vaccine.2014.06.024
37. Mok H, Cheng X, Xu Q et al (2012) Evaluation of measles vaccine virus as a vector to deliver respiratory syncytial virus fusion protein or Epstein-Barr virus glycoprotein gp350. Open Virol J 6:12–22. doi:10.2174/1874357901206010012
38. Malczyk AH, Kupke A, Prufer S et al (2015) A highly immunogenic and protective middle east respiratory syndrome coronavirus vaccine based on a recombinant measles virus vaccine platform. J Virol 89(22):11654–11667. doi:10.1128/JVI.01815-15
39. Yoneda M (2014) Study of pathogenicity of Nipah virus and its vaccine development. Uirusu 64(1):105–112. doi:10.2222/jsv.64.105
40. Higuchi A, Toriniwa H, Komiya T et al (2016) Recombinant measles AIK-C vaccine strain expressing the prM-E antigen of Japanese encephalitis virus. PLoS One 11(3):e0150213. doi:10.1371/journal.pone.0150213
41. Peng K-W, Facteau S, Wegman T et al (2002) Non-invasive in vivo monitoring of trackable viruses expressing soluble marker peptides. Nat Med 8(5):527–531. doi:10.1038/nm0502-527
42. Dingli D, Peng K-W, Harvey ME et al (2004) Image-guided radiovirotherapy for multiple myeloma using a recombinant measles virus expressing the thyroidal sodium iodide symporter. Blood 103(5):1641–1646. doi:10.1182/blood-2003-07-2233
43. Excler J-L, Delvecchio CJ, Wiley RE et al (2016) Toward developing a preventive MERS-CoV vaccine-report from a workshop organized by the Saudi Arabia Ministry of Health and the International Vaccine Institute, Riyadh, Saudi Arabia, November 14–15, 2015. Emerg Infect Dis 22(8). doi:10.3201/eid2208.160229
44. Modjarrad K, Moorthy VS, Ben Embarek P et al (2016) A roadmap for MERS-CoV research and product development: report from a World Health Organization consultation. Nat Med 22(7):701–705. doi:10.1038/nm.4131
45. Schneider H, Spielhofer P, Kaelin K et al (1997) Rescue of measles virus using a replication-deficient vaccinia-T7 vector. J Virol Methods 64(1):57–64
46. Martin A, Staeheli P, Schneider U (2006) RNA polymerase II-controlled expression of antigenomic RNA enhances the rescue efficacies of two different members of the Mononegavirales independently of the site of viral genome replication. J Virol 80(12):5708–5715. doi:10.1128/JVI.02389-05
47. Calain P, Roux L (1993) The rule of six, a basic feature for efficient replication of Sendai virus defective interfering RNA. J Virol 67(8):4822–4830
48. Kärber G (1931) Beitrag zur kollektiven Behandlung pharmakologischer Reihenversuche. Arch Exp Pathol Pharmakol 162(4):480–483. doi:10.1007/BF01863914

Chapter 10

Recombinant Tri-Segmented Pichinde Virus as a Novel Live Viral Vaccine Platform

Rekha Dhanwani, Hinh Ly, and Yuying Liang

Abstract

Pichinde virus (PICV) is a nonpathogenic arenavirus with a bi-segmented RNA genome (L and S segments) that encodes four viral genes. We have developed a reverse genetics system to generate recombinant tri-segmented PICV (rP18tri) that packages three RNA segments (L, S1, and S2) and can encode up to two foreign genes. Using influenza virus HA and NP as model antigens, we show that the rP18tri vector can induce strong humoral and cell-mediated immunity, which further increases upon a booster dose. We propose that this novel rP18tri vector can be developed into a useful vaccine platform for other antigens, particularly when strong cellular immunity and prime-boost vaccination strategy are desired.

Key words Viral vaccine vector, Pichinde virus, Arenavirus, Vaccine

1 Introduction

Pichinde virus (PICV) is an enveloped RNA virus within the *Arenaviridae* family. PICV was first isolated from its natural hosts *Oryzomys albigularis* (rice rats) in the Pichinde valley of Colombia, South America [1], and is not known to cause disease in humans or animals. The sero-prevalence is very low even among humans living or working in close association with habitats of infected rodents [1]. Therefore, there is virtually no preexisting immunity against PICV in the general population. This is in contrast to another prototypic arenavirus, lymphocytic choriomeningitis virus (LCMV), which has a global distribution with up to 5% seroprevalence in human populations. The PICV genome consists of two RNA segments, the long (L) and short (S) segments. Each segment encodes two genes in the opposite orientation (Fig. 1a). The L segment encodes the small RING-domain containing matrix protein Z and a large L polymerase protein. The S segment encodes the glycoprotein GPC and the nucleoprotein NP. All four genes are essential for the basic life cycle of the virus. The 15-kDa Z protein mediates virus budding and regulates viral RNA synthesis. The L protein (~200 kDa) is the

Maureen C. Ferran and Gary R. Skuse (eds.), *Recombinant Virus Vaccines: Methods and Protocols*, Methods in Molecular Biology, vol. 1581, DOI 10.1007/978-1-4939-6869-5_10, © Springer Science+Business Media LLC 2017

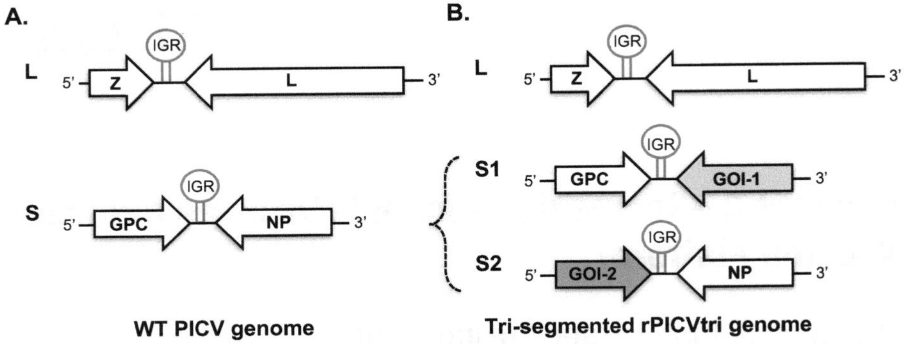

Fig. 1 Genomic organization of PICV and tri-segmented rPICVtri. (**a**) Wild-type (WT) PICV genome consists of two genomic RNA segments (L and S), each encoding two viral genes in opposite orientation. (**b**) Tri-segmented recombinant PICV (rPICVtri) genome consists of three RNA segments, L, S1, and S2. S1 encodes GPC and the gene of interest (GOI-1). S2 encodes GOI-2 and NP. *GOI* gene-of-interest, *IGR* intergenic region

RNA-dependent RNA polymerase (RdRp) that is required for viral RNA transcription and replication. The GPC glycoprotein precursor is posttranslationally cleaved into three subunits, stable signal peptide (SSP), GP1, and GP2, which together form a tripartite complex that mediates receptor binding and membrane fusion. The NP protein encapsidates the viral genomic RNAs and plays an essential role in viral RNA synthesis. In addition, the NP and Z proteins have been found to play important roles in suppressing the host innate immune responses [2].

Arenaviruses target dendritic cells (DCs) and macrophages early in the infection; therefore, these viruses are considered potential vaccine vectors [3–6]. Following a strategy first developed by de la Torre group for LCMV [4], we have recently generated a tri-segmented PICV (P18 strain) vaccine vector (rP18tri) that can simultaneously express dual foreign antigens in addition to its own genes (Fig. 1b). The rP18tri-based viruses are attenuated in vitro and in vivo, and can effectively induce strong T cell and humoral responses with limited anti-vector neutralizing antibodies [7]. Therefore, this novel rP18tri vector exhibits multiple features of an ideal live viral vector including safety, immunogenicity, robust antigen-encoding capacity, targeting antigen-presenting cells (APCs), and the lack of a strong anti-vector immunity.

2 Materials

2.1 Plasmids

1. pP18S1-GPC/MCS: This plasmid (Fig. 2a) expresses the antigenomic strand of the rP18 S1 segment under control of the T7 promoter. The rP18 S1 segment encodes the glycoprotein GPC and a multiple-cloning-site (MCS) that replaces the NP

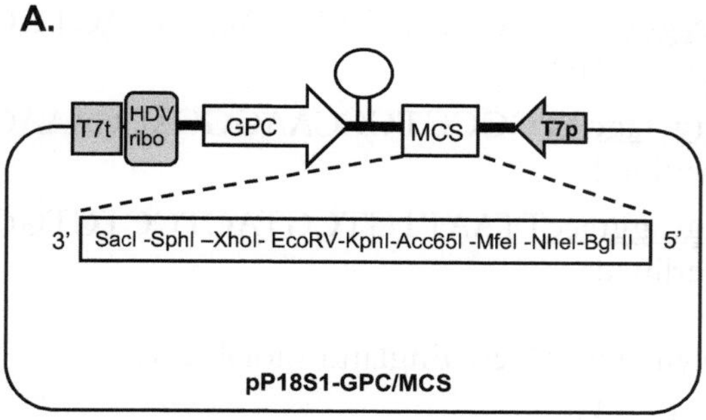

Fig. 2 Vector maps of plasmids encoding S1 and S2 RNA segments. Plasmids pP18S1-GPC/MCS (**a**) and pP18S2-MCS/NP (**b**) are based on the PICV P18 reverse genetics system plasmid pP18S, which encodes the full-length P18 S RNA segment, followed by hepatitis delta virus ribozyme sequence (HDVribo), under a T7 promoter. Genomic organization of the rP18tri vector expressing eGFP together with influenza virus A/PR8HA (rP18tri-G/H) or NP (rP18tri-G/P). *IAV* influenza virus, *IGR* intergenic region, *MCS* multiple cloning sites

gene and allows the convenient cloning of a gene of interest. The stem-loop structure represents the intergenic region (IGR) of viral RNA. The hepatitis delta virus ribozyme (HDVribo) sequence, which immediately follows the P18S1 RNA segment and precedes the T7 terminator sequence (T7t), is used to generate authentic PICV S RNA ends [8].

2. pP18S2-MCS/NP: This plasmid (Fig. 2b) expresses the antigenomic strand of the rP18 S2 segment under control of the T7 promoter. The rP18 S2 segment encodes the nucleoprotein NP and a multiple-cloning site (MCS) that replaces the GPC gene and allows the convenient cloning of a gene of interest. The stem-loop structure represents the intergenic region (IGR) of viral RNA. The hepatitis delta virus ribozyme (HDVribo) sequence, which immediately follows the P18S1 RNA segment and precedes the T7 terminator sequence (T7t), is used to generate authentic PICV S RNA ends [8].
3. pPolI-HA and pPolI-NP plasmids: These plasmids express the segment 4 (encoding Hemagglutinin HA) and the segment 5 (encoding nucleoprotein NP), respectively, of influenza A virus H1N1 laboratory strain A/PR8, and were obtained from Drs. Brownlee and Fodor (Oxford University, UK).
4. pP18L: This plasmid expresses the full-length antigenomic strand of the rP18 L segment under the control of the T7 promoter. The hepatitis delta virus ribozyme (HDVribo) sequence, which immediately follows the P18S1 RNA segment and precedes the T7 terminator sequence (T7t), is used to generate authentic PICV S RNA ends [8].

2.2 Primer Sequences

1. HA Forward: <u>ggtgctagc</u>ATGAAGGCAAACCTACTGGTCCTG (Nhe I site is underlined).

2. HA Reverse: gcaggtaccTCAGATGCATATACTGCACTGC (Kpn I site is underlined).
3. NP Forward: ggtgctagcATGGCGTCCCAAGGCACCAAAC (Nhe I site is underlined).
4. NP Reverse: gcaggtaccTTAATTGTCGTACTCCTCTGC (Kpn I site is underlined).

2.3 Molecular Cloning

1. Phusion DNA polymerase (New England Biolabs, MA).
2. Qiagen gel purification kit.
3. Restriction enzymes Nhe I and Kpn I.
4. Qiagen nucleotide removal kit.
5. Antarctic Phosphatase (New England Biolabs, MA).
6. T4 DNA ligase (New England Biolabs, MA).
7. Qiagen mini-prep kit.

2.4 Cell Lines

1. Baby hamster kidney (BHK-21) cells.
2. BSRT7-5 cells (obtained from Dr. K.-K. Conzelmann, Ludwig-Maximilians-Universität, Germany) are BHK-21 cells stably expressing the T7 RNA polymerase.
3. African green monkey kidney (Vero) cells.
4. Madin-Darby canine kidney (MDCK) cells.

2.5 Cell Culture Reagents

1. BHK-21 cells are grown in Dulbecco's modified Eagle medium (DMEM with high glucose) supplemented with 10% fetal bovine serum (FBS) and 50 μg/mL penicillin-streptomycin.
2. BSRT7-5 cells are grown in Minimal essential medium (MEM) supplemented with 10% FBS, 1 μg/mL Geneticin, and 50 μg/mL penicillin-streptomycin.
3. Vero cells are grown in MEM supplemented with 10% FBS and 50 μg/mL penicillin-streptomycin.
4. MDCK cells are grown in MEM supplemented with 10% FBS and 50 μg/mL penicillin-streptomycin.

2.6 Transfection Reagents

1. Opti-MEM.
2. Lipofectamine-2000.

2.7 Plaque Assay

1. First overlay: 0.6 mL of 2% agar and 2.4 mL of complete MEM medium supplemented with 10% FBS and 50 μg/mL penicillin-streptomycin.
2. Second overlay: 0.4 mL of 2% agar, 1.6 mL of complete MEM medium, 120 μl of neutral red dye stock solution (0.33% stock concentration).

2.8 Mouse Experiment

1. Six- to eight-week-old female C57BL/6 mice were obtained from Charles River Laboratories.
2. Influenza A virus A/PR8 is a laboratory mouse-adapted strain that causes lethal infection in mice [9] and was obtained from Dr. Richard W. Compans (Emory University, GA).
3. Isoflurane is used to sedate mice prior to intranasal (IN) inoculation.

3 Methods

3.1 Cloning of Antigen Genes into the PICV-Based rP18tri Vectors

1. PCR amplification of antigen genes: Influenza A virus HA and NP genes are used as model antigens to explain the construction and usage of the rP18tri-based vaccine candidates. HA and NP open-reading-frames (ORFs) were amplified from the pPolI-HA and pPolI-NP plasmids, respectively, with the 5′ primers containing the NheI site (HA Forward and NP Forward) and the 3′ primers containing the KpnI site (HA Reverse and NP Reverse), in a 50-μl reaction that contains 1× Phusion HF buffer, 50 ng of plasmid DNA, 25 pmol of each primer, 10 μM dNTPs, and 1 U of Phusion DNA polymerase. The PCR conditions were 98 °C for 30 s, and 30 cycles of 98 °C for 10 s, 55 °C for 15 s, and 72 °C for 30 s. The 1.7-kb and 1.5-kb PCR products for HA and NP, respectively, were purified from agarose gel slices using Qiagen gel purification kit and digested with NheI and KpnI in a 40-μl reaction that contains 1× CutSmart Buffer, 1 μl of NheI (10 U), and 1 μl of KpnI-HF (20 U), at 37 °C for 4 h (*see* **Note 1**). The digested PCR fragments were purified using Qiagen nucleotide removal kit.
2. Digestion of the viral vector plasmids. One microgram of each of the pP18S1-GPC/MCS and pP18S2-MCS/NP plasmids (Fig. 2) was digested with NheI and KpnI in a 30-μl reaction that contains 1× CutSmart Buffer, 1 μl of NheI (10 U) and 1 μl of KpnI-HF (20 U), at 37 °C for 4 h (*see* **Note 1**). At the end of the restriction enzyme reaction, 3 μl of 10× Antarctic Phosphatase Buffer and 1 μl of Antarctic Phosphatase were added and incubated at 37 °C for 1 h followed by a 5-min incubation at 70 °C to inactivate the enzyme.
3. Ligation and transformation. The NheI/KpnI-treated HA PCR fragment was ligated into the digested pP18S1-GPC/MCS vector, while the NheI/KpnI-treated NP PCR fragment was ligated with the digested pP18S2-MCS/NP vector, at an insert-to-vector ratio of 3 to 1. The 10-μl ligation reaction contains 1 μl of T4 ligase buffer, 1 μl of 10 mM dNTPs, and 1 μl of T4 DNA ligase (400 U) (*see* **Note 2**). After incubating at room temperature for 2 h (*see* **Note 3**), 5 μl of the ligation

reaction was used to transform 100 μl of *E. coli* competent Stbl2 cells that were plated on LB-Amp plate (*see* **Note 4**). Plasmid DNAs were extracted from the bacterial cultures using the Qiagen mini-prep kit and screened by restriction enzyme digestion using the NheI and KpnI-HF enzymes. The positive clones were verified by sequencing and named pP18S1-GPC/H and pP18S2-P/NP, respectively.

3.2 Generation of Recombinant Tri-Segmented PICVs from Plasmid Transfection

Recombinant tri-segmented PICVs are generated by simultaneously transfecting three plasmids encoding the L, S1, and S2 RNA segments (Fig. 3) into BSRT7-5 cells that constitutively express the T7 RNA polymerase. Supernatants were collected from the transfected cells and detected for infectious viruses by plaque assaying on Vero cells. Single plaques were picked from plates and amplified in BHK-21 cells to prepare viral vaccine stocks (Fig. 3).

1. Seed 4 × 10^5 BSRT7-5 cells (*see* **Note 5**) per well in a 6-well plate with antibiotics-free culture medium and incubate the cells overnight at 37 °C and 5% CO_2.
2. The following day, change to fresh medium 1 h prior to transfection.
3. Mix 250 μl of Opti-MEM (*see* **Note 6**) with three plasmids, pP18L, pP18S1-GPC/MCS containing gene of interest, and

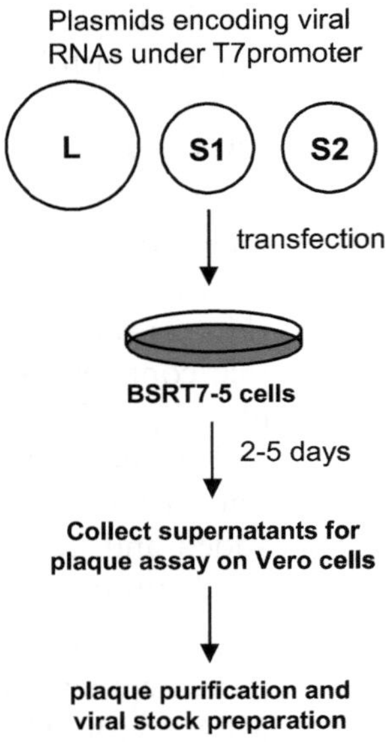

Fig. 3 Steps to generate the tri-segmented rP18tri-based vaccine stocks. BSR-T7 cells are transfected with three plasmids encoding the L, S1, and S2 RNA segments. Supernatants from the transfected cells are detected for infectious viruses by plaque assay. Virus stocks are prepared by growing up plaque-purified viruses in BHK-21 cells

pP18S2-MCS/NP containing gene of interest, each at 1 μg, and incubate for 5 min at room temperature.

4. Mix 250 μl of Opti-MEM with 7 μl of Lipofectamine-2000 and incubate for 5 min at room temperature.
5. Mix Opti-MEM/plasmids with Opti-MEM/lipofectamine and further incubate the mixture for 30 min at room temperature before adding dropwise to the cells.
6. After 4-h incubation at 37 °C, replace the transfection medium with antibiotics-free culture medium.
7. Incubate the cells at 37 °C and 5% CO_2. Collect 100 μl of supernatants daily from 2 to 5 days post-transfection for plaque assay to determine whether viable tri-segmented rP18tri-HA/NP virus has been generated (*see* **Note 7**).

3.3 Plaque Assay

1. Seed 3 × 10^5 Vero cells per well in 6-well plates and incubate overnight at 37 °C and 5% CO_2.
2. Conduct tenfold serial dilutions (normally from 10^1 to 10^6 dilutions) of the collected supernatants in MEM medium (*see* **Note 8**).
3. Aspirate medium from the cells and add 500 μl of the appropriate dilution to each well. Gently rock the plate to make sure that the cell monolayer is evenly covered with the viral dilution.
4. Incubate the infected cells for 1 h at 37 °C and 5% CO_2; rock the plate every 10 min.
5. Prepare the first overlay and keep in 55 °C water bath. Melt the 2% agar by microwave and equilibrate to 55 °C before adding to the complete MEM medium.
6. Remove the infection medium and immediately add 3 mL of the first overlay per well. After the agar has solidified, incubate cells at 37 °C and 5% CO_2 for 4 days.
7. Add 2 mL of the second overlay per well and, after agar has solidified, incubate cells at 37 °C and 5% CO_2 for 1 day.
8. Count plaques and calculate viral titers as plaque-forming unit (PFU)/mL.
9. Proceed to the plaque purification step.

3.4 Plaque Purification

1. Add 1 mL of MEM medium to 1.5-mL microtubes.
2. Choose an isolated plaque that is well separated from other plaques in the plaque assay plate (*see* **Note 9**).
3. Use a P1000 pipette to insert a 1-mL pipette tip into the agar straight down to the plaque and gently aspirate a small volume of materials.

4. Pipet up and down to dispense the collected agar into a 1-mL MEM in a microtube.
5. Vortex at high speed. In a microcentrifuge, spin at 200 × g for 5 min. Collect the 1-mL supernatants and store at −80 °C, or immediately infect BHK-21 cells for viral stock preparation.

3.5 Preparation of the rP18tri-Based Viral Vaccine Stocks

1. Seed 8 × 10^5 BHK-21 cells in a 10-cm culture dish and incubate overnight at 37 °C and 5% CO_2.
2. Aspirate the culture medium, add 1 mL of supernatants from a single plaque (*see* **Note 10**), incubate for 1 h at 37 °C and 5% CO_2, rock plate every 15 min.
3. Add another 7 mL of fresh culture medium to the infected cells, further incubate for 48 h at 37 °C and 5% CO_2.
4. Collect supernatants, centrifuge at 200 × *g* for 5 min to remove debris, filter supernatants through a 0.45 μm filter (Millipore, MA).
5. Aliquot and store viral stocks at −80 °C (*see* **Note 11**).
6. To make concentrated viral stocks, gently dispense 40 mL of viral sample on the top of 5 mL of 20% sucrose cushion and centrifuge the sample at 13,000 × *g* for 2 h in a SW28 rotor (Beckman Coulter, CA). Resuspend the pellet in 500 μl of PBS. Aliquot and store at −80 °C.
7. Quantify viral titer by plaque assaying as described in Subheading 3.3 (*see* **Note 12**).

3.6 Immunization of Mice with rP18tri-HA/NP in a Lethal Flu-Mouse Model

1. Inoculation of C57BL/6 mice with recombinant viruses is conducted in a biosafety cabinet (*see* **Note 13**).
2. For intraperitoneal (IP) inoculation, use a 25-gauge needle and 1-mL syringe to inject 1 × 10^5 pfu (*see* **Note 14**) of rP18tri-HA/NP in 60 μl volume into the peritoneum of the mouse. For intramuscular (IM) inoculation, restrain the mouse in a restrainer, use a 25-gauge needle and 1-mL syringe to inject 1 × 10^5 pfu of rP18tri-HA/NP in 50-μl volume into the thigh muscle. A booster dose can be given 21 days later.
3. Monitor the mouse body weight and other disease signs daily (*see* **Note 15**).
4. For blood collection, 100 μl of blood is taken from facial vein using a 21-gauge needle and 1-mL syringe (*see* **Note 16**). Blood cells were collected at 7 days after each dose in heparinized tubes and used immediately for analysis of T cell response [7]. Blood was collected at 14 days after each dose into 1.5-mL microtubes. After blood clotting at 37 °C for 1 h, collect the serum by centrifugation at 4000 × *g* for 10 min in a microfuge. Serum can be stored at −20 °C until being used for analysis of neutralizing antibodies [7].

5. For a challenge study, immunized mice were inoculated intranasally (IN) with 10× 50% mouse-lethal dose (MLD_{50}) of influenza A virus A/PR8 (*see* **Note 13**). Mice were anesthetized with 5% isoflurane in the anesthesia machine. Hold the anesthetized mouse (*see* **Note 17**) in one hand, tilt the mouse backward slightly, and use a P200 pipet to inoculate 50 μl of A/PR8 virus into the right and left nostrils [9]. Place the mouse back into the cage (*see* **Note 18**). Monitor mouse body weight and disease signs daily up to 14 dpi. Mice are euthanized when reaching the predetermined terminal points (*see* **Note 19**).

4 Notes

1. The restriction enzyme digestion reactions can be kept overnight in a 37 °C water bath.
2. A vector-alone ligation reaction should be conducted as a negative control.
3. The ligation reaction can be carried out at either ambient (room) temperature or 16 °C for variable lengths of time from 30 min to overnight.
4. We prefer to propagate PICV reverse genetics plasmids in Stbl2 cells at 30 °C, partly because arenavirus genome contains the high GC-rich intergenic region (IGR) that can be responsible for genomic instability if amplified in conventional competent cells (e.g., DH5α) and at higher temperature (e.g., 37 °C).
5. In order to increase transfection efficiency, use low passaged BSRT7-5 cells. Higher passaged cells may limit transfection efficiency and thereby reduce virus yield.
6. For plasmid transfection, use fresh aliquots of Opti-MEM. Avoid repeated opening of Opti-MEM bottle to avoid its oxidation.
7. All work with recombinant viruses should be performed in a biosafety cabinet. Centrifugation of recombinant viruses is conducted in a sealed rotor. Proper personal protection equipment (PPE) such as lab coats, gloves, and toe-covered shoes is required.
8. For serially diluting the virus, add 900 μl medium to each of six tubes. Transfer 100 μl of the PICV stock virus to the first tube containing 900 μl of medium. Vortex the mixture for 15 s and transfer 100 μl of the diluted virus to the next tube.
9. We normally pick single plaques from samples that were collected at the earliest time points after plasmid transfection.

Viruses collected at earlier times are less likely to contain spontaneous mutations.

10. High-titer viral stocks are generated from plaque-purified virus.
11. Store virus stocks in small aliquots to avoid repeated freeze-thaw cycles.
12. Titers of the rP18tri-based viral vaccines can vary from 10^5 to 10^7 pfu/mL.
13. Inoculation of mice with viruses should be conducted in a biosafety cabinet inside an ABSL-2 facility. Proper PPEs include disposable long-sleeved gown, surgical mask, hair cover, shoe cover, and gloves.
14. Lower dose of viral vaccines such as 1000 pfu was found to provide protective immunity in the lethal influenza-mouse model [7].
15. Mice immunized with the rP18tri-based vaccine vectors can be downgraded from ABSL-2 to ABSL-1 facility 3 days after inoculation, as these vaccine vectors are severely attenuated in vitro and in vivo [7].
16. Maximal volume of blood collected from one mouse per week is 0.5% of the mouse's body weight.
17. Anesthesia is confirmed by toe pinching.
18. Mice infected with influenza A virus A/PR8 were housed in an ABSL-2 facility.
19. Endpoints are determined using an established scoring system [9]. Hunched posture is 3 points, ruffled fur is 3 points, not eating or drinking 2 points, greater than 20% body weight loss 10 points, neurological symptoms (hind-limb paralysis) 10 points. When the total points exceed 16, the animal should be euthanized.

Acknowledgment

This work was supported by NIH grants R21AI094133 and R01AI083409 to Y.L., and R01AI093580 to H.L.

References

1. Trapido H, Sanmartin C (1971) Pichinde virus, a new virus of the Tacaribe group from Colombia. Am J Trop Med Hyg 20:631–641
2. Meyer B, Ly H (2016) Inhibition of innate immune responses is key to pathogenesis by arenaviruses. J Virol 90:3810–3818
3. Flatz L, Hegazy AN, Bergthaler A, Verschoor A, Claus C, Fernandez M et al (2010) Development of replication-defective lymphocytic choriomeningitis virus vectors for the induction of potent CD8+ T cell immunity. Nat Med 16:339–345

4. Emonet SF, Garidou L, McGavern DB, de la Torre JC (2009) Generation of recombinant lymphocytic choriomeningitis viruses with trisegmented genomes stably expressing two additional genes of interest. Proc Natl Acad Sci U S A 106:3473–3478
5. Popkin DL, Teijaro JR, Lee AM, Lewicki H, Emonet S, de la Torre JC et al (2011) Expanded potential for recombinant trisegmented lymphocytic choriomeningitis viruses: protein production, antibody production, and in vivo assessment of biological function of genes of interest. J Virol 85:7928–7932
6. Ortiz-Riano E, Cheng BY, Carlos de la Torre J, Martinez-Sobrido L (2013) Arenavirus reverse genetics for vaccine development. J Gen Virol 94:1175–1188
7. Dhanwani R, Zhou Y, Huang Q, Verma V, Dileepan M, Ly H et al (2015) A novel live Pichinde virus-based vaccine vector induces enhanced humoral and cellular immunity upon a booster dose. J Virol 90(5):2551–2560
8. Lan S, McLay SL, Wang J, Kumar N, Ly H, Liang Y (2009) Development of infectious clones for virulent and avirulent pichinde viruses: a model virus to study arenavirus-induced hemorrhagic fevers. J Virol 83:6357–6362
9. Matsuoka Y, Lamirande E W, and Subbarao K (2009) The mouse model for influenza. Curr Protoc Microbiol Chapter 15, Unit 15G 13

Chapter 11

Human Rhinovirus-A1 as an Expression Vector

Khamis Tomusange, Danushka Wijesundara, Eric James Gowans, and Branka Grubor-Bauk

Abstract

Expression vectors that are based on live human rhinoviruses (HRVs) are attractive, yet often overlooked in vaccine development due to their limited capacity for foreign gene inserts and poor genetic stability. This chapter describes a novel methodology to engineer a replication-competent genetically stable recombinant HRV (rHRV) without affecting viral replication capability. We have previously used these methods to generate live, genetically stable recombinant HRVs encoding HIV Gag and Tat proteins (rHRV-Gag-Tat), a potential mucosally targeted HIV vaccine.

Key words HRV-A1, Live vaccine vector, HIV-Gag and HIV-Tat

1 Introduction

1.1 Classification of Human Rhinoviruses (HRVs)

HRVs are single-stranded, positive-sense RNA viruses belonging to the genus Enteroviruses of the *Picornaviridae* family [1]. Other genera within this family are the Hepatoviruses [2], Kobu viruses [3], and Parechoviruses [4] all of which cause diseases in humans and other animals. Perhaps the most important species among the picornaviruses are the polioviruses and human rhinoviruses (HRVs) owing to their historical clinical associations. HRVs are closely similar to polioviruses, but differ by being acid labile with low temperature culture requirements [5]. Polioviruses cause poliomyelitis in humans, while HRVs are mainly isolated from individuals with acute and chronic respiratory illnesses [6]. Infections with polioviruses have been reduced and the viruses are nearing global eradication as a result of the global vaccination campaign. HRV infections tend to be seasonal, peaking during the winter months and are usually self-limiting.

1.2 Virion Structure and Genome Organization

HRVs are icosahedral viruses with a diameter of ~30 nm with a RNA genome of ~7.4 kb enclosed in a capsid [7]. The 5′-end of the genome contains a 5′ UTR encompassing an internal ribo-

Maureen C. Ferran and Gary R. Skuse (eds.), *Recombinant Virus Vaccines: Methods and Protocols*, Methods in Molecular Biology, vol. 1581, DOI 10.1007/978-1-4939-6869-5_11, © Springer Science+Business Media LLC 2017

somal entry site and the VPg protein which primes genome replication, followed by the P1 region that encodes the capsid (VP1–VP4) proteins, and the P2 and P3 regions that encode the non-structural proteins (2Apro to 2C and 3A to 3D, respectively). The genome is terminated by a 3′ UTR and a poly-A tail which are required for efficient genome replication.

The VP1 protein possesses a canyon required during cell entry to bind the cellular receptor, the VP2, VP3, and VP4 proteins contain the neutralizing antibody immunogenic regions (NIm-IB, NIm-II, and NIm-III) and VP4 also anchors the RNA into the capsid. The 2A protease ($2A^{pro}$) cleaves the viral polyprotein to separate the structural from the non-structural proteins. The 3C protease ($3C^{pro}$) cleaves the polyprotein into the individual mature VP1, VP3, 2B, 2C, 3A, 3B, and 3D proteins. Together with $2A^{pro}$, $3C^{pro}$ shuts-off 5′cap-dependent host cellular translation to ensure that the cellular machinery is directed towards viral translational and replication. The 2B, 2C, and 3A proteins are involved in cell membrane rearrangement and the formation of cytoplasmic vesicles, and also influence the host range for HRVs. The 3D protein acts as a RNA-dependent RNA polymerase ($3D^{Pol}$) and the 3B protein is the VPg protein.

1.3 HRV Genotypes and Serotypes

HRVs are classified as genotype A, B, or C (HRV87 is the only currently identified C strain) based on phylogenetic analysis of the 5′ UTR and capsid coding sequences [8, 9]. HRV genotypes A and B are further classified into the major and minor receptor groups based on receptor recognition [10]. The major receptor groups HRVs use for cell entry are the intracellular adhesion molecule (ICAM-CD5) or the heparin sulfate proteoglycans (HSPG) [11, 12]. These molecules constitute about 90% of all HRVs receptors (all genotype B and a few genotype A strains) [1]. The minor receptor group HRVs (genotype A only) use a family of low density lipoprotein receptors (LDLRs) including: LDLR, VLDLR, LDLR-related proteins and megalin [13], which are located on the surface of human and murine cells [7]. Therefore, most minor group HRVs can infect both human and murine cells [14, 15]. The receptor used by HRV-C remains poorly understood, but previous evidence shows that a sialoprotein is used [16]. HRVs have also been further divided into species A (74 serotypes) and B (25 serotypes) based on susceptibility to antiviral agents such as capsid-binding compounds, for example pleoconaril [7]. They have also been divided into M-strains which grow in human and monkey kidney cells, and H-strains that initially grew in human cell lines before they were adapted to grow in monkey cells [5].

1.4 Viral Replication

The actual mechanism of HRV replication is poorly understood. However, upon successful attachment to the membrane, viruses are either endocytosed or micropinocytosed into the cell. This is followed by conformational changes in the virion induced by the endosomal microenvironment, resulting in the formation of hydrophobic virus particles [5]. The viral RNA exits the endosome via membrane pores into the cytosol where it is translated in a cap-independent manner in association with cytoplasmic membranous vesicles into a polyprotein of ~250 kDa, which is auto-catalytically and co-translationally cleaved by the viral proteases into precursor and mature proteins. Generally, HRV RNA can be detected 5 h post infection. Viral replication is completed ~12 h post-infection and the peak viral load is reached 48 h post-infection in permissive cell lines.

1.5 Human Rhinoviruses Serotype A1 (HRV-A1) as Vaccine Vectors

Thanks to the global success of the poliovirus vaccines, (especially the live-attenuated oral polio vaccine) and the near eradication of poliovirus infections, interest in utilizing live polioviruses as effective recombinant expression vectors grew [17–19]. This interest is further supported by the mucosal transmission of polioviruses, which indicates that vectors based on these viruses could potentially be used to deliver mucosally targeted vaccines against diverse viral infections. Live poliovirus vectors have been mainly evaluated in animal models as candidate vaccines against human immunodeficiency virus (HIV) infections. These vaccines have been shown to induce simian immunodeficiency virus (SIV)-specific immune responses that protect vaccinated macaques against intravaginal challenge with a pathogenic SIVmac251 [19–21], a surrogate macaque HIV challenge model. However, the high level of prior immunity to polioviruses in humans has prevented further testing of vaccines delivered by live poliovirus vectors. Prior immunity to a vaccine vector resulted in poor responses in a large-scale clinical trial evaluating a potential HIV vaccine [22].

On the other hand, the close similarity between polioviruses and HRVs imply that vaccines delivered by live HRV vectors might be equally immunogenic relative to live poliovirus vaccines. Indeed, early evidence showed that HIV vaccines delivered by HRV vectors were highly immunogenic in animals [17, 18, 23–26] and this was further supported by data from a more recent study [27]. Unfortunately, the same reasons (i.e., preexisting immunity) that hampered testing vaccines delivered by a live poliovirus vector have affected the use of live HRV vectors in humans.

Nevertheless, HRV-A1 a member of the minor group HRVs has emerged as a potential suitable expression vector. This serotype is considered the rarest among all HRVs circulating in the human population [28, 29] which suggests that prior immunity to this serotype among humans is uncommon. Furthermore, HRV-A1 can infect mice and humans [14, 15], permitting experiments to evaluate the efficacy of recombinant HRV-A1 vaccines in a mouse model prior to human clinical trials. We have recently produced the first evidence that HRV-A1 can be engineered into a genetically stable, replication-competent expression vector [30]. We inserted the HIV *gag* or *tat* genes, as outlined in Subheading 3, to generate a live recombinant HRV vaccine encoding HIV Gag or Tat proteins (rHRV-Gag/Tat) as a potential mucosally targeted HIV vaccine.

2 Materials

2.1 Cells

1. H1-HeLa cells (only this cell strain is used in all experiments unless otherwise stated).
2. *E. coli* DH5α cells.

2.2 Enzymes

1. Restriction endonucleases: Apal, Mlul, and Xhol2.4DNA ligase.
2. Antarctic phosphatase.

2.3 Growth Media

1. LB-broth: 1% w/v tryptone, 0.5% w/v yeast extract, and 200 mM NaCl. Sterilize by autoclaving.
2. LB-Agar: 1% w/v tryptone, 0.5% w/v yeast extract, 1.5% w/v agar, and 200 mM NaCl. Sterilize by autoclaving.
3. SOC medium 1% w/v tryptone, 0.5% w/v yeast extract, 5 M NaCl, 1 M KCl, 1 M $MgCl_2$, 1 M $MgSO_4$ and 1 M glucose. Sterilize by autoclaving.
4. Cell culture media: 10% w/v FCS, 1% w/v Pen/Strep in 500 ml DMEM.
5. Virus growth media: 10% w/v FCS, 1% w/v penicillin/strepto mycin, 30 mM $MgCl_2$ in 500 ml DMEM.
6. Virus harvest media: PBS (1×), 30 mM $MgCl_2$, and 30 mM $CaCl_2$. (Filter to sterilize.)
7. Opti-MEM® I reduced serum media.

2.4 Preparative Kits

1. KAPA™HiFi PCR kit.
2. KAPA™Taq PCR kit.
3. PureLink® Quick Plasmid Miniprep Kit.
4. PureLink® Quick Gel Extraction Kit.
5. PureLink® PCR Purification Kit.
6. RNeasy Mini Kit.
7. TransIT®-mRNA Transfection Kit.
8. MEGAscript® T7 Transcription Kit.
9. MEGAclear™ Transcription Clean-Up Kit.
10. QIAGEN OneStep RT-PCR Kit.

2.5 Reagents, General Materials, and Instrumentation

1. RNase AWAY™ Decontamination Reagent.
2. 70% and 100% ethanol.

3. 10 and 50 ml Falcon tubes.
4. Corning® cell scrapers.
5. Nalgene™ 0.2 and 0.45 μm syringe filters.
6. Amicon Ultra-15 Centrifugal Filter Units, NMWL 100 kDa (Millipore, MA, USA).
7. Polyethylene glycol 6000.
8. 5 M sodium chloride. Filter to sterilize and store at room temperature.
9. Syringes (2–20 ml).
10. Dry ice.
11. Sterile, cotton plugged pipette tips.
12. Sterile single-wrapped transfer pipettes.
13. Sterile six-well tissue culture plates.
14. Sterile T75 and T175 tissue culture flasks.
15. DNA Engine PCR machine.
16. NanoDrop 2000c.
17. V5 mouse monoclonal antibody (Thermo Fisher Scientific).
18. Goat anti-mouse IgG (H+L) secondary antibody, Alexa Fluor 488 conjugate (Thermo Fisher Scientific).
19. 2% paraformaldehyde.

3 Methods

3.1 General Procedure to Generate Recombinant HRV (rHRV)

By analogy with the polioviruses, there are several potential sites within the HRV genome into which exogenous genes may be inserted without abrogating viral replication, including the P1/P2 junction, the VPg/VP1 junction, the 2C/3A junction and the VPg/3C^{pro} junction [17]. Exogenous HIV *gag* or *tat* genes are inserted into the P1/P2 junction of the HRV genome (Fig. 1a) to ensure that the resultant recombinant HRVs remained replication-competent by utilizing the autocatalytic activity of the HRV-2A^{pro} to cleave the Gag/Tat proteins from the recombinant viral polyprotein [30].

Several technical issues must be addressed when inserting exogenous genes into the HRV genome to ensure expression of the corresponding proteins in cells infected with the recombinant viruses:

1. Like all picornaviruses, HRVs have a limited capacity for the insertion of foreign genes to ensure that the final genome is ≤115% that of wild type HRV RNA. Thus, exogenous genes of around 1100 bases may be considered. Inserts which exceed

this limit will be naturally lost and the recombinant virus will probably revert to wild type upon serial passage.

2. The P1/P2 junction of the cDNA encoding the HRV-A1 genome contains a unique ApaI restriction endonuclease site. Therefore, this site can be used to insert exogenous genes. ApaI restriction enzyme sites in foreign genes must therefore be mutated or a linker containing a multiple cloning site (MCS) with various restriction endonuclease sites can be introduced into the P1/P2 junction.
3. To ensure that the protein encoded by the inserted gene is cleaved from the recombinant polyprotein, nucleic acid sequences which encode the $2A^{pro}$ cleavage sequence should be introduced at the 5′ and 3′ends of the exogenous gene insert.
4. To enhance the genetic stability of recombinant viruses, it is necessary to reduce the sequence homology of the two $2A^{pro}$ cleavage sites and thus inhibit detrimental homologous recombination.

These concerns are addressed as follows:

1. The full length *gag* gene (~1500 bp) must be divided into five discrete overlapping fragments (*gag-1* to *gag-5*) ranging from 393 to 513 bp, within the putative capacity of HRVs, and then individually clone each fragment into a separate HRV plasmid to generate five rHRVs each encoding an adjacent region of Gag (rHRV-Gag-1 to rHRV-Gag-5). Although up to 1100 bp of exogenous genes could theoretically be inserted into the HRV genome, it is best to insert *gag* fragments of up to 513 bp to closely mimic the previous construction of highly immunogenic recombinant Sabin poliovirus vectors [19]as shown in Table 1. Each of the *gag* fragments contains a unique ApaI site, thus an MCS containing a XhoI site can be inserted to aid the insertion of these gene fragments into the P1/P2 junction. However, the full length *tat* gene (303 bp) is within the insertion limit, and thus the full length gene can be cloned into HRV-A1 to generate a single rHRV encoding full length Tat protein (rHRV-Tat).
2. To ensure that the Gag and Tat proteins are cleaved from the recombinant viral polyprotein, PCR is employed to introduce a second $2A^{pro}$ cleavage site upstream of all the *gag* and *tat* inserts (Fig. 1b).
3. To enhance the genetic stability of the rHRV-Gag/Tat, several silent mutations can be introduced into the coding sequences of both flanking $2A^{pro}$ cleavage sites to reduce the homology between the $2A^{pro}$ cleavage sequences, of these sites from 100% to 77% (Fig. 1c).

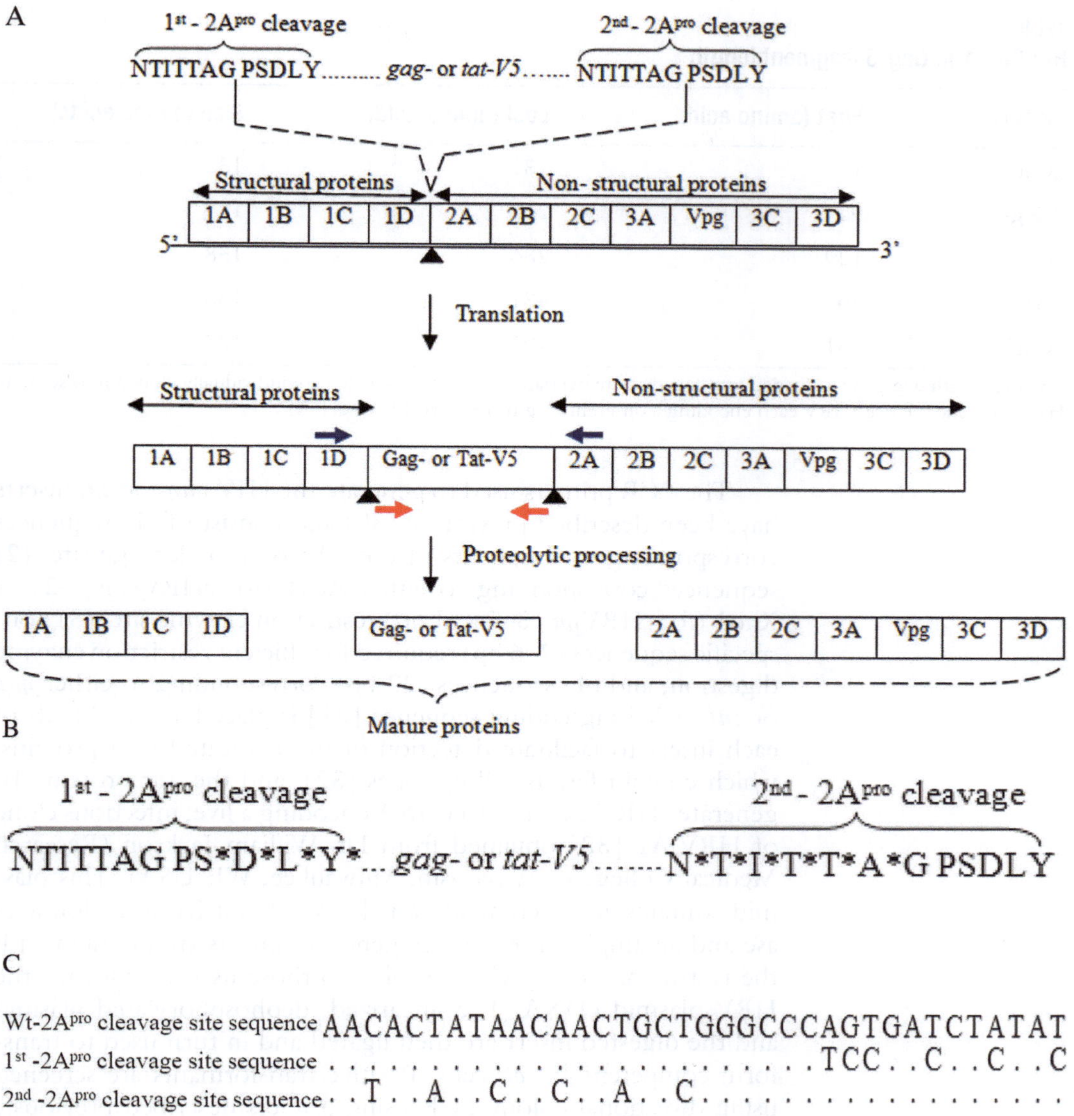

Fig. 1 Cloning strategy and production of replication-competent recombinant HRVs. (**a**) Schematic presentation of the construction of the replication-competent, recombinant HRV-A1 vector and the expression strategy for the recombinant viral proteins. HRV genes and proteins are presented in *boxes*. 2Apro cleavage at points indicated by *solid triangles* separates HRV structural from non-structural proteins and releases HIV proteins. *Solid red arrows* indicate the binding sites for insert-specific primers and *solid blue arrows* indicate binding sites for primers that anneal to HRV-A1 sequences flanking the inserts. (**b**) Amino acid sequence of the first and second 2Apro auto-cleavage sites. *Asterisk* indicates silently mutated codons for these amino acids. (**c**) RNA sequences encoding the 2Apro auto-cleavage site of wt-HRV-1A (*top line*) and the sequences of the mutated sites; the first-2Apro auto-cleavage site (*middle line*) and the second-2Apro auto-cleavage site (*bottom line*). *Dots* correspond to nucleotides in the first and second-2Apro auto-cleavage sites that are homologous to the wt-HRV-A1 2Apro auto-cleavage site sequence. This figure is reproduced from Virus Research, 2015 with permission from Elsevier Limited, License number 3841340715142, issued on 03/04/2016

Table 1
HIV Gag-1 to Gag-5 fragment length

Insert	First (amino acid)	Last (amino acid)	Size (amino acids)
Gag-1	1	131	132
Gag-2	92	262	171
Gag-3	129	286	158
Gag-4	264	431	168
Gag-5	361	497	137

The full length gag gene is divided into five discrete overlapping fragments which are individually cloned into separate HRVs to generate five rHRV each encoding a different Gag protein (rHRV-Gag-1–5)

The PCR primers used to generate the HIV *gag* and *tat* inserts have been described previously [30] and consist of (1) sequences corresponding to fragments of the 2Apro auto cleavage site, (2) sequences corresponding to either Apa1 (for rHRV*gag* 1–2) or Xho1 (for rHRV*gag* 3–5 and *tat*) restriction enzyme site, (3) non-specific sequences (2–6 bp) required for efficient restriction enzyme digestion, and (4) sequences (22 bp) corresponding to either *gag* or *tat*. A V5 tag coding sequence [31] is placed at the 3′ends of each insert to facilitate detection of the truncated Gag proteins, which contain few B cell epitopes [32], and the Tat protein. To generate rHRVs, we used a cDNA encoding a live, infectious clone of HRV-Al [33] obtained from Dr. William Jackson (Research Medical College of Wisconsin, Milwaukee, WI, USA). This plasmid contains an inherent site for the Mlu1 restriction endonuclease and an ampicillin resistance gene. All inserts are digested with the restriction endonuclease similar to those used to linearize the HRV plasmid cDNA. The linearized, dephosphorylated plasmid and the digested insert are then ligated and in turn used to transform competent *E. coli* cells. Positive transformants are screened using directional colony PCR using primers described previously [30]. Plasmid mini-preparations of positively transformed colonies are prepared and the authenticity of these plasmids confirmed by sequencing. This plasmid DNA is linearized using Mlu1 and then used in an in vitro transcription assay to generate rHRV mRNA. The purified mRNA is used to transfect H1-HeLa cells from which rHRVs are produced, harvested, and purified. The recombinant viruses are stored in small volume aliquots at −80 °C.

3.2 PCR Amplification of HIV Gag or Tat Inserts

All reactions to amplify HIV *gag* or *tat* inserts are carried out using the KAPA™HiFi PCR kit.

1. In a sterile PCR tube, mix 1× KAPA HiFi Buffer, 0.3 mM of each dNTP, 0.3 μM forward primer, 0.3 μM reverse primer,

Table 2
Generating gag/tat inserts

Number of cycles	1	30	30	30	1
Temperature (°C)	95	98	Tm[a]	72	72
Time (minutes)	2	0.5	0.5	60/Kb	5

Summary of PCR thermocycling conditions to amplify the required DNA for the different HIV gag or tat inserts
[a]Tm, the primer annealing temperature, depended on the length and guanine–cytosine (G-C) composition of the primer (>50–65 °C)

100 ng DNA template, and 0.5 U KAPA HiFi DNA polymerase. Include a negative control for the reaction (use sterile distilled water instead of the DNA template).

2. Run the reaction in the DNA Engine PCR machine using thermocycler conditions summarized in Table 2.
3. Load the PCR products on a 1% w/v agarose gel in TBE buffer (0.22 M trizma-base, 180 mM boric acid, 5 mM EDTA, pH 8.3, with 5% v/v Gel red™) in parallel with a suitable marker.
4. Run the PCR products on a 1% w/v agarose gel at 120 kVA for approximately 1.5 h.
5. Cut-out the band corresponding to the predicted product size from the gel using a sterile scalpel blade.
6. Extract and purify from the gel DNA using PureLink® Quick Gel Extraction Kit following the manufacturer's instruction.
7. Quantify the harvested DNA using the NanoDrop 2000c spectrophotometer at 280 nm absorbance.
8. Store DNA at +4–8 °C for short term only or use immediately.

3.3 Preparing the HRV Vector

It is important to completely linearize the plasmid backbone before ligating it with the insert as this improves the cloning efficiency and reduces the number of false positive bacterial colonies formed as a result of uncut plasmid backbone.

1. Cut ~2 μg of HRV-A1 plasmid cDNA with Apa1 or Xho1 in 1× enzyme buffer with 2 U enzyme for 3–4 h at 25 °C (for Apa1) or 37 °C (for Xho1).
2. Heat at 65 °C for 20 min to inactivate the enzyme.
3. Load on to a 1% w/v agarose gel and run as stated in Subheading 3.1, **steps 3** and **4**.
4. Cut out the desired band corresponding to the linearized plasmid.

5. Extract and purify DNA from the gel as stated in Subheading 3.2, **step 6**.

3.4 Dephosphorylating the Vector

Since restriction endonuclease digestion of plasmid DNA is performed with a single restriction endonuclease, the chances of plasmid re-ligation are high, thus dephosphorylating a digested plasmid minimizes this possibility.

1. Dephosphorylate ~500 ng of linearized plasmid DNA with 1 U of antarctic phosphatase in 1× enzyme buffer.
2. Incubated the reaction for 1 h at 37 °C.
3. Inactivate the enzyme by incubating the reaction at 65 °C for 10 min.
4. Purify the linearized, dephosphorylated plasmid DNA as stated in Subheading 3.2, **step 6**.

3.5 Preparing the HIV Inserts

1. A restriction enzyme site for ApaI endonuclease flanks the HIV *gag-1* and *gag-2* inserts, whereas a restriction enzyme site for XhoI flanks *gag 3–5* and *tat*, thus *gag-1* and *gag-2*are digested with ApaI while *gag 3–5* and *tat* are digested with XhoI. About 1 μg of gel-extracted PCR-amplified DNA was digested as stated in Subheading 3.3, **step 1**.
2. Load all products onto a 1% w/v agarose gel and run as stated in Subheading 3.2.
3. Extract and purify DNA as stated in Subheading 3.3.

3.6 Ligating the Vector and Insert

1. Ligation reactions are setup to ligate the HIV inserts with the HRV-A1 vector digested with the same restriction endonucleases. The relative amounts of insert and vector are calculated using the equation: *Insert [ng] = ((170[ng] vector* × *insert size [kb])/vector size [kb]))/insert [ng]* (*see* **Note 1**). In an Eppendorf tube, mix the appropriate volume of insert and vector in a reaction containing 1 U of DNA ligase enzyme and 1× enzyme buffer. A vector only control should be included, i.e., no insert in added to the ligation reaction.
2. Incubate the mixture at 4 °C overnight.

3.7 Transforming Bacterial Cells

The heat shock method is used to transform competent DH5α *E. coli* cells with the ligated *HRV-gag* or *tat* DNA.

1. Thaw a vial of competent DH5α cells (50 μl per vial) on ice for 3–5 min.
2. Pipette 5 μl of the ligation mixture (from a 10 μl reaction) and mix with thawed DH5α cells on ice.
3. Incubate the cells on ice for 30 min.
4. Incubate the cells at 42 °C for 45 s.

5. Place the cells back on ice for 2 min.
6. Add 500 μl of sterile SOC media to cells and close the vial tightly.
7. Rock the cells in the vial at 225 rpm for 1 h at 37 °C.
8. Centrifuge the vial at 15,000 × *g* to pellet cells.
9. Resuspend the pellet in ~50 μl LB broth.
10. Spread the cells on LB-agar plates containing 0.1% v/v ampicillin.
11. Incubate the plates at 37 °C for at least 16 h.
12. Count the number of colonies formed on each plate. Ideally, no colonies should appear on the vector control plate, but some colonies may appear if the vector was not completely dephosphorylated. However, this number should be 5- to 10-fold lower than that from plates inoculated with the ligated insert and vector.

3.8 Colony Screening

Screening for colonies transformed with the plasmid/insert is performed using the rapid colony PCR method (*see* **Note 2**).

1. Randomly select and pick up several colonies from each inoculated plate and emulsify each in 10 μl of sterile water in a separate sterile PCR tube. The number of colonies picked from each plate depends on the number of colonies present on the "vector only" plate. Fewer colonies on this plate indicate that fewer colonies need to be screened from the "insert plus vector" plates and vice versa.
2. Setup the PCR using the KAPA™Taq PCR kit in a reaction containing 0.25 U KAPA™ Taq polymerase (0.08 μl), 1× KAPA Taq buffer, 0.4 mM of each dNTP, 0.8 μM forward primer, 0.8 μM reverse primer, and 5 μl of emulsified bacteria colony.
3. Run the reaction under conditions summarized in Table 3.
4. Load the PCR products on to a 1% w/v agarose gel and run gel as stated in Subheading 3.2, **step 6**.
5. Select colonies which show the expected band sizes on the gel and use these to generate plasmid DNA by the mini-preparation method.

3.9 Preparing rHRV-Gag/Tat Plasmid DNA Mini-Preps

Generally, ~1 μg of plasmid DNA is required for transcription and transfection experiments, thus it is necessary to prepare plasmid DNA mini-preps from transformed bacterial cells to yield the required amount of DNA.

1. Into a clean, sterile 10 ml centrifuge tube and in a safety hood, dispense 5 ml of LB-broth supplemented with 0.1% v/v ampicillin.

2. Inoculate the LB-broth with ~5 μl of bacterial suspension.
3. Close the tube and place on a rack.
4. Incubate tube at 37 °C overnight in a rocking incubator at 220 rpm.
5. Take ~500 μl of the bacterial culture and add it to the same volume of sterile 100% glycerol to make a glycerol stock that can be used in the future to culture the same bacterial clone. Store this at −80 °C.
6. Pellet the remaining bacterial culture at 3000 × *g* for 5 min at room temperature.
7. Discard the supernatant and use the pellet to extract plasmid DNA.
8. Extract and purify plasmid DNA using the PureLink® Quick Plasmid Miniprep Kit following the manufacturer's instructions.
9. Quantify the harvested DNA as stated in Subheading 3.2, **step** 7.
10. Store DNA at +4 °C for short-term storage, at −80 °C for long-term storage or use immediately in subsequent experiments.
11. Validate the authenticity of plasmid constructs. It is important to authenticate plasmid DNA before using it in any experiments to ensure the validity of the experimental results. Only colonies with the correct plasmid and insert sequences should be selected for further use.

3.10 Linearizing Plasmid HRV-Gag/Tat Plasmid DNA

Since HRVs are positive sense RNA viruses, to cultivate these viruses in vitro requires transfection of susceptible cell lines with in vitro transcribed mRNA generated from a linearized plasmid DNA template (*see* **Note 3**).

1. Linearize the recombinant HRV plasmid DNAs using Mlu1 in a reaction consisting of 1× enzyme buffer, 3 μg plasmid DNA, and 10 U of Mlu1.
2. Incubate the mixture at 37 °C for at least 10 h to ensure total digestion of the template. Inactivate the enzyme by incubating the mixture at 65 °C for 20 min.

Table 3
Colony PCR

Number of cycles	1	30	30	30	1
Temperature (°C)	95	95	55 °C	72	72
Time (min)	2	0.5	0.5	1 min/Kb	2

Summary of thermocycling conditions used to screen correctly transformed *E. coli* colonies

3. Analyse the reaction products on agarose gel as stated in Subheading 3.2, **steps 3** and **4**.
4. Cut-out the band corresponding to linearized plasmid from the gel.
5. Extract and purify DNA as stated in Subheading 3.2, **step 6**.
6. Determine the DNA yield as stated in Subheading 3.2, **step 7**.
7. Use the harvested plasmid DNA immediately in a transcription reaction. Do not keep this DNA for future use as the probability of re-annealing and therefore re-circularizing are extremely high.

3.11 Transcription of rHRV-Gag/Tat mRNA

All experiments should be setup in a clean RNA preparation room. It is always a good habit to wipe down all apparatus and workspace with RNase AWAY™ to remove any RNases that might compromise RNA yield. Always wear fresh gloves.

1. Use the MEGAscript™ transcription kit and follow the manufacturer's recommendation.
2. In a clean, sterile PCR tube, add ~200 ng of linear plasmid DNA, 1× recommended buffer, 150 mM of each dNTPs, and 2 U of the enzyme mix.
3. Incubate the reaction at 37 °C for at least 6 h.
4. Terminate the reaction by adding 2 U of DNase and incubate the reaction at 37 °C for 15 min to remove any traces of template DNA.
5. Purify the RNA transcripts using the MEGAclear™ Kit following the manufacturer's instructions.
6. Quantify the RNA yield using the Nanodrop 2000c spectrophotometer at 260 nm absorbance.
7. As RNA is very unstable, store the harvested mRNA at −80 °C or use immediately in a transfection experiment.

3.12 Transfecting H1-HeLa Cells with HRV-Gag/Tat mRNA

All experiments are to be performed in a clean, sterile cell culture hood using aseptic techniques. Wipe down the hood and all other apparatus with RNase AWAY™ to remove any RNases that might compromise RNA quality.

1. One day prior to transfection, seed ~1×10^5 H1-HeLa cells per well of a six-well plate in 500 μl of cell culture media ensuring that the cells reach ~80% confluence before transfection.
2. On the day of transfection, replace the cell culture media with ~500 μl of fresh virus growth media ~3 h prior to transfection.
3. Setup the transfection solution using the TransIT®-mRNA Transfection Kit following the manufacturer's instructions in a reaction containing 3 μg of transcribed RNA, 6 μl of mRNA

boost reagent, 6 μl of TransIT-mRNA reagent, and 250 μl of Opti-MEM per well. Include a transfection control, i.e., containing all reagents except in vitro transcribed RNA and a cell only control (no transfection mixture added).

4. Incubate the transfection mixture at room temperature for not more than 5 min.
5. Add the mixture dropwise to the cells.
6. Incubate the cells between 32 and 33 °C rather than 37 °C (*see* **Note 4**) in 5% CO_2 and monitor daily for evidence of virus-induced cytopathic effect (CPE).

3.13 Harvesting rHRVs

1. Using a sterile cell scrapper, scrap the cell monolayer infected with rHRV into the culture media when 70–80% of cells show evidence of infection. Avoid extended incubation as this can result in low virus yields, due to the release of rHRV into the cell culture supernatant.
2. Transfer the cells and supernatant to a sterile 50 ml falcon tube.
3. Pellet the cells by centrifuging at 500 × *g* for 10 min at 4 °C.
4. Discard the supernatant and keep the cell pellet.
5. Resuspend the pellet in ~500 μl of virus harvest media.
6. Lyse the cells and release the virus by freeze-thawing three times. Freeze in a dry ice–ethanol bath and thaw in a 37 °C water bath.
7. Centrifuge at 3000 × *g* for 15 min at 4 °C to remove cell debris.
8. Harvest the virus-rich supernatant into a sterile 1.5 ml sterile Eppendorf tube. This represents passage zero (P_o virus).
9. Store viruses at −80 °C until required or subsequently passage it in fresh cells.

3.14 Large Scale Preparation of rHRVs

Reserve an aliquot (~200 μl) of the P_o virus as a backup and for future reference (*see* **Note 5**) or to confirm the presence of *gag* or *tat* inserts (*see* Subheading 3.15) and the expression of Gag or Tat proteins (*see* Subheading 3.16). An appropriate volume of virus should be reserved after each virus passage for the same purposes. Store these at −80 °C.

1. Seed ~1 × 10^6 H1-HeLa cells in one T75 flask with 15 ml of cell culture media to ensure 80% confluent at the time of infection.
2. Dilute ~250 μl of P_o virus in 10–15 ml of fresh virus growth media.
3. Prior to infection, wash the cells with sterile PBS and replace the culture media with virus growth media prepared in **step 2**.

Ensure that the whole H1-HeLa monolayer is covered with medium by gently rocking the flask side-to-side.

4. Incubate the flask as stated in Subheading 3.12, **step 6** until 70–80% CPE is observed.
5. Harvest the virus (P_1 virus) in ~1 ml of virus harvest media as stated in Subheading 3.13.
6. Passage ~300–500 μl of P_1 rHRV in one T175 flask with cells at 80% confluence and maintained in ~20–25 ml of fresh virus growth media.
7. Continue harvesting and passaging virus using a 1:4 ratio, i.e., from 1× T175 flask to 4× T175 flasks until the desired virus volume is reached. This process can also be referred to as scaling-up virus volume and titer (*see* **Note 6**). Assuming 35× T175 flasks are infected, harvest infected H1-HeLa cells as stated in Subheading 3.13. Pool the pellets from 3× T175 flasks to facilitate freeze-thawing. Resuspend the cell pellet in 10 ml of medium. This yields ~100 ml of crude virus preparation that needs to be concentrated and titrated (*see* Subheading 3.17).

3.15 RT-PCR

RT-PCR is performed to confirm the retention of the exogenous HIV gag/tat inserts upon serial passage of rHRVs as an indication of the genetic stability of the rHRVs.

1. Plate H1-HeLa cells at 3×10^5 per well of a six-well cell culture plate and incubate as stated in Subheading 3.12, **step 6**.
2. Wash the cells with sterile 1× PBS and then inoculate with virus at a multiplicity of infection (M.O.I) of 5 at a particular passage number in virus growth media. *See* Subheading 3.17 for virus titration and determining M.O.I. Include a cell only (no virus) control.
3. Incubate the cells at 32–33 °C in 5% CO_2 until 70–80% of cells show evidence of infection.
4. Using a sterile cell scraper, scrape the cells into the culture media and pellet at 800 × *g* for 10 min at 4 °C.
5. Discard the supernatant and wash the cells twice with ice-cold 1× PBS.
6. Extract rHRV RNA from the cell pellet using the RNeasy kit following the manufacturer's instructions.
7. Quantify harvested RNA as stated in Subheading 3.11, **step 6**.
8. Use ~1 μg of this RNA in a reverse transcription reaction using the QIAGEN OneStep RT-PCR Kit as per manufacturer's protocol to generate rHRV cDNA.
9. Prepare two separate PCR mixtures using the KAPA HiFi kit as stated in Subheading 3.2 with 1 μl of rHRV cDNA generated

in **step 8** and using either insert-specific primers (in PCR-1) or primers flanking the insert (in PCR-2).

10. Load the PCR products in two separate 1% w/v agarose gels and run gels as stated in Subheading 3.2.
11. Analyse the banding patterns on each gels for the presence of exogenous gene inserts, i.e., in PCR-1, only a band corresponding to the exogenous gene insert is observed (Fig. 2a), whereas in PCR-2 a larger band corresponding to the inserted exogenous gene along with HRV gene sequences flanking the insert is observed (Fig. 2b). PCR-1 yields no band, if the exogenous gene insert is deleted.

3.16 Immunofluorescence

Immunofluorescence is performed to confirm the expression of Gag and Tat proteins in cells infected with rHRVs at a particular passage number.

1. Plate cells at 1 × 10^5 per well of a 24-well cell culture plate and incubate as stated in Subheading 3.12.
2. Wash the cells with sterile 1× PBS and then refeed with fresh virus culture media containing virus at a M.O.I = 5 for a particular passage number. Remember to include a cell only (no virus) control.
3. Incubate cells as stated in Subheading 3.12 until 70–80% of cells show evidence of infection.
4. Carefully remove virus culture media, wash the cells with ice-cold 1× PBS and then add 100 μl of 2% paraformaldehyde to each well.
5. Cover the plate and incubate at 4 °C for 10 min to fix cells.
6. Wash the plate 2× with ice-cold 1× PBS while taking extra care not to lift the cells off the surface.
7. Block the wells with ice-cold 1% w/v BSA at room temperature for 30–45 min.
8. Wash the plates 2× with ice-cold 1× PBS.
9. Add 100 μl per well of primary antibody diluted in 1% w/v BSA (V5 mouse monoclonal antibody diluted at 1:5000).
10. Incubate the plate for 1 h at 37 °C.
11. Wash 2× with 1× PBS.
12. Add 100 μl per well of fluorescently labelled secondary antibody diluted in 1% w/v BSA (Alexa 488 conjugated anti-mouse, use at 1:10,000).
13. Incubate at 37 °C for 1 h.
14. Wash 2× with 1× PBS.

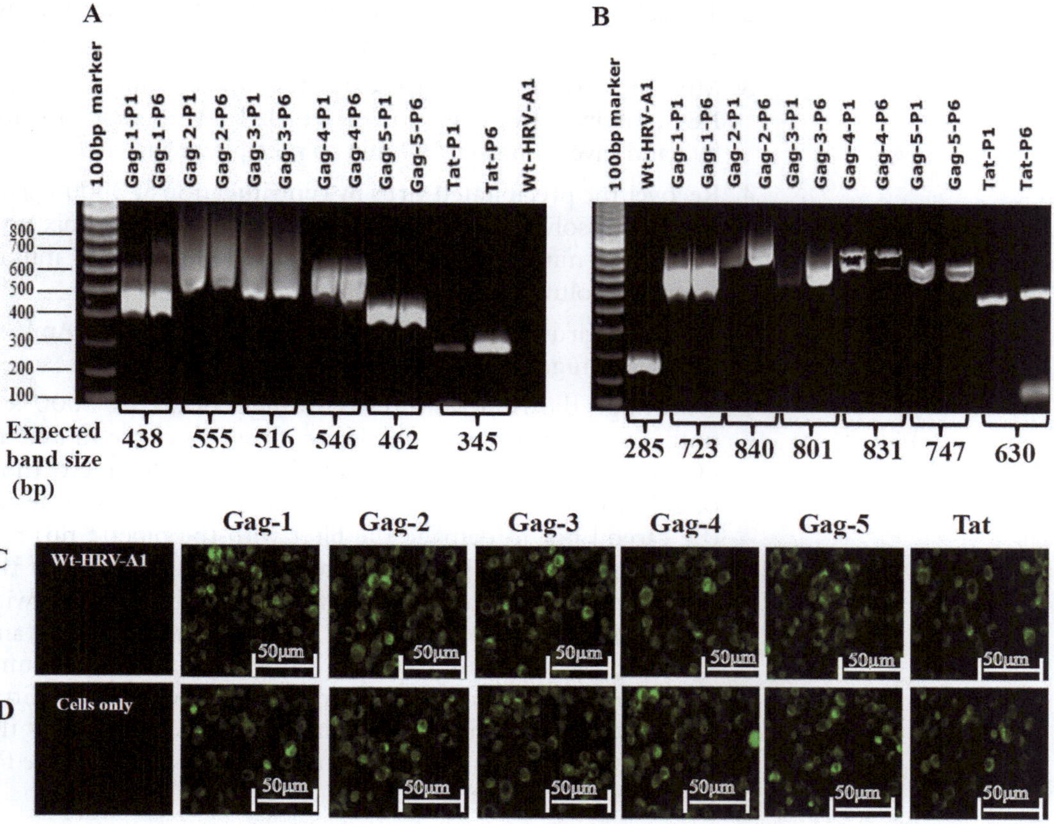

Fig. 2 Agarose gel electrophoresis of RT-PCR products to examine the genetic stability of rHRVs and immunofluorescence to detect expression of Gag-1 to Gag-5 and Tat. (**a**) gel electrophoresis of PCR products generated using insert-specific primers and (**b**), using primers which anneal to HRV sequences flanking the HIV inserts. In (**a**), fragments of 438, 555, 516, 546, 462, and 345 bp corresponding to Gag-1, Gag-2, Gag-3, Gag-4, Gag-5, and Tat, respectively were amplified. No band was amplified corresponding to wt-HRV-A1. In (**b**), fragments of 285, 723, 840, 801, 831, 747, and 630 bp corresponding to wt-HRV-A1, rHRV-Gag-1, rHRV-Gag-2, rHRV-Gag-3, rHRV-Gag-4, rHRV-Gag-5, and rHRV-Tat, respectively were amplified. Expression of Gag and Tat proteins in H1-HeLa cells infected with (**c**), P1 viruses (M.O.I = 5) and (**d**), cells infected with P6 viruses (M.O.I = 5) at 48 h post-infection. This figure is reproduced from Virus Research, 2015 with permission from Elsevier Limited, License number 3841340715142, issued on 03/04/2016

15. View the plates under a fluorescence microscope to detect the expression of exogenous V5-tagged HIV Gag or Tat proteins. *See* Fig. 2c and d for the expected fluorescence.

3.17 Concentrating, Titrating and Storing rHRVs

The rHRVs intended for animal vaccinations to evaluate vaccine immunogenicity should be concentrated and titrated before use (*see* **Note 7**).

1. Filter the virus-containing supernatant through a 0.2 μm syringe filter.

2. To each 10 ml of clarified virus, add 2.8 g of polyethylene glycol (PEG)-6000 and 4 ml of 5 M NaCl.
3. Mix on a roller at room temperature for 5 min to dissolve PEG, followed by incubation on ice for 1 h with gentle mixing by hand inversion every 20 min to precipitate the virus.
4. Recover the precipitated virus by centrifugation at 3000 × *g* for 1 h and dissolve the virus pellet in 15 ml of 1× PBS, mix on a roller for 5 min and then centrifuge at 3000 × *g* for 15 min to remove insoluble debris.
5. Filter the virus using a 0.2 μm syringe filter into an Amicon ultra centrifugal device.
6. Centrifuge the Amicon ultra centrifugal device at 3000 × *g* until the supernatant (containing virus) is concentrated to ~0.5 ml in the Amicon device. Add 10 ml of PBS, pipette thoroughly to mix the concentrated virus in the filtration device (be careful not to damage the filter with the pipette tip) and repeat the process. Harvest the concentrate and wash out the device with additional 2× 1 ml of PBS. Combine washes with 0.5 ml virus to yield 2.5 ml total. Aliquot into 2× 250 μl and 4× 500 μl or as required and store at −80 °C. A small volume (~50–100 μl) of concentrated virus should be saved for titration. Avoid freeze-thawing the virus stocks as this reduces the titer. Titrated viruses should be thawed and used only once for vaccination experiments.
7. Measure the infectious titer of rHRVs using H1-HeLa cells. Serially dilute purified rHRV stock to yield dilutions from 10^{-1} to 10^{-8} and add 50 μl of each dilution to eight replicate wells of HeLa cells in a 96-well plate. Include a "no virus" or cell only control.
8. Incubate the plate at 32–33 °C in 5% CO_2 for 4 days.
9. On day 4 post-infection, determine the highest dilution where CPE is still visible using a light microscope.
10. Determine the tissue culture infective dose 50% ($TCID_{50}$)/ml value by scoring the sum of positive wells. The highest dilution where CPE is still visible is determined by counting the number of wells showing CPE. A Spearman–Karber formula can be used to estimate the TCID50. Alternatively, the Reed and Muench end point assay can be used with the formula: *TCID50 = log10 dilution factor (% of infection at next above 50%) − 50%/(% of infection at next above 50%) − (% of infection at next below 50%).*

4 Notes

1. The volume (μl) of insert or vector used in the ligation reaction depends on the corresponding DNA concentration. A "no insert" or "vector only" control must be included as this control accounts for any colonies resulting from vector re-ligation.
2. Directional colony PCR is used to screen inoculated agar plates for correctly transformed *E. coli* colonies. This method allows rapid screening of multiple transformants (within 2 h) and simultaneously determines the orientation of the inserts. The forward primers used in this PCR anneal to sequences in the plasmid upstream of the insert, whereas the reverse primers anneal to sequences at the 3′end of the insert. Alternatively, digestion of plasmid DNA prepared from selected colonies with restriction endonucleases can also be used. In this case, the banding pattern obtained after resolving the digested DNA can provide information to select positive colonies. However, this method is labour intensive, uses more reagents and results are normally obtained after 2 days.
3. Plasmid DNA must be completely linearized with Mlu1 before it is used in an in vitro transcription assay because the presence of circular plasmid templates will generate long, heterogeneous RNA transcripts. It is extremely important to confirm complete linearization of the plasmid by agarose gel electrophoresis as the presence of even small traces of uncut circular plasmid will generate a large proportion of transcripts.
4. For efficient in vitro cultivation of HRV-A1, it is desirable that the cultures are maintained between 32–33 °C because HRV-A1 is particularly sensitive to high temperatures, and thus its growth is affected when cultures are incubated at temperatures >33 °C. Efficient packaging of HRV-A1 requires Mg^{2+} and Ca^{2+}; therefore, the virus will not grow in cell culture unless these salts are added to the growth media.
5. After every passage, it is important to demonstrate the presence of the gene inserts by RT-PCR and protein expression from these genes by immunofluorescence as stated in Subheadings 3.15 and 3.16. This is absolutely vital as it confirms the genetic stability of the rHRVs before they are passaged or used for animal vaccination experiments. Note the passage number to ensure that viruses from the same stock are always used in any experiment, and in the event of any change in growth characteristics or stability of the rHRV at a given passage, then trouble shooting is easier.
6. Normally, considerable virus is lost during purification and concentration, which necessitates starting with a high volume

of high titer virus. In this case, it may be necessary to scale up the virus to 25–35× T175 flasks.

7. For mouse vaccination experiments, it is important that the viruses are purified to remove cellular debris that might elicit undesired immunological responses. These nonspecific immune responses might obscure the desired antigen-specific immune response which impacts vaccine efficacy. Furthermore, a small volume of virus (<100 μl) with a high titer is desired for vaccination as this is more likely to be well tolerated.

References

1. Palmenberg AC, Spiro D, Kuzmickas R, Wang S, Djikeng A, Rathe JA, Fraser-Liggett CM, Liggett SB (2009) Sequencing and analyses of all known human rhinovirus genomes reveal structure and evolution. Science 324:55–59
2. Cuthbert JA (2001) Hepatitis A: old and new. Clin Microbiol Rev 14:38–58
3. Reuter G, Boros A, Pankovics P (2011) Kobuviruses—a comprehensive review. Rev Med Virol 21:32–41
4. Li L, Victoria J, Kapoor A, Naeem A, Shaukat S, Sharif S, Alam MM, Angez M, Zaidi SZ, Delwart E (2009) Genomic characterization of novel human parechovirus type. Emerg Infect Dis 15:288–291
5. Jacobs SE, Lamson DM, St George K, Walsh TJ (2013) Human Rhinoviruses. Clin Microbiol Rev 26:135–162
6. Jackson DJ, Gangnon RE, Evans MD, Roberg KA, Anderson EL, Pappas TE, Printz MC, Lee WM, Shult PA, Reisdorf E, Carlson-Dakes KT, Salazar LP, DF DS, Tisler CJ, Gern JE, Lemanske RF Jr (2008) Wheezing rhinovirus illnesses in early life predict asthma development in high-risk children. Am J Respir Crit Care Med 178:667–672
7. Mackay IM (2008) Human rhinoviruses: the cold wars resume. J Clin Virol 42:297–320
8. Arden KE, Mackay IM (2010) Newly identified human rhinoviruses: molecular methods heat up the cold viruses. Rev Med Virol 20:156–176
9. Ledford RM, Patel NR, Demenczuk TM, Watanyar A, Herbertz T, Collett MS, Pevear DC (2004) VP1 sequencing of all human rhinovirus serotypes: insights into genus phylogeny and susceptibility to antiviral capsid-binding compounds. J Virol 78:3663–3674
10. Hayden FG (2004) Rhinovirus and the lower respiratory tract. Rev Med Virol 14:17–31
11. Winther B, Arruda E, Witek TJ, Marlin SD, Tsianco MM, Innes DJ, Hayden FG (2002) Expression of ICAM-1 in nasal epithelium and levels of soluble ICAM-1 in nasal lavage fluid during human experimental rhinovirus infection. Arch Otolaryngol Head Neck Surg 128:131–136
12. Khan AG, Pickl-Herk A, Gajdzik L, Marlovits TC, Fuchs R, Blaas D (2011) Entry of a heparan sulphate-binding HRV8 variant strictly depends on dynamin but not on clathrin, caveolin, and flotillin. Virology 412:55–67
13. Savolainen C, Blomqvist S, Hovi T (2003) Human rhinoviruses. Paediatr Respir Rev 4:91–98
14. Reithmayer M, Reischl A, Snyers L, Blaas D (2002) Species-specific receptor recognition by a minor-group human rhinovirus (HRV): HRV serotype 1A distinguishes between the murine and the human low-density lipoprotein receptor. J Virol 76:6957–6965
15. Tuthill TJ, Papadopoulos NG, Jourdan P, Challinor LJ, Sharp NA, Plumpton C, Shah K, Barnard S, Dash L, Burnet J, Killington RA, Rowlands DJ, Clarke NJ, Blair ED, Johnston SL (2003) Mouse respiratory epithelial cells support efficient replication of human rhinovirus. J Gen Virol 84:2829–2836
16. Bochkov YA, Palmenberg AC, Lee WM, Rathe JA, Amineva SP, Sun X, Pasic TR, Jarjour NN, Liggett SB, Gern JE (2011) Molecular modeling, organ culture and reverse genetics for a newly identified human rhinovirus C. Nat Med 17:627–632
17. Andino R, Silvera D, Suggett SD, Achacoso PL, Miller CJ, Baltimore D, Feinberg MB (1994) Engineering poliovirus as a vaccine vector for the expression of diverse antigens. Science 265:1448–1451
18. Mandl S, Sigal LJ, Rock KL, Andino R (1998) Poliovirus vaccine vectors elicit antigen-specific cytotoxic T cells and protect mice against lethal challenge with malignant melanoma cells expressing a model antigen. Proc Natl Acad Sci U S A 95:8216–8221
19. Crotty S, Miller CJ, Lohman BL, Neagu MR, Compton L, Lu D, Lu FXS, Fritts L, Lifson

JD, Andino R (2001) Protection against simian immunodeficiency virus vaginal challenge by using Sabin poliovirus vectors. J Virol 75:7435–7452

20. Crotty S, Andino R (2004) Poliovirus vaccine strains as mucosal vaccine vectors and their potential use to develop an AIDS vaccine. Adv Drug Deliv Rev 56:835–852
21. Crotty S, Lohman BL, Lu FX, Tang S, Miller CJ, Andino R (1999) Mucosal immunization of cynomolgus macaques with two serotypes of live poliovirus vectors expressing simian immunodeficiency virus antigens: stimulation of humoral, mucosal, and cellular immunity. J Virol 73:9485–9495
22. Buchbinder SP, Mehrotra DV, Duerr A, Fitzgerald DW, Mogg R, Li D, Gilbert PB, Lama JR, Marmor M, del Rio C, McElrath MJ, Casimiro DR, Gottesdiener KM, Chodakewitz JA, Corey L, Robertson MN, Team SSP (2008) Efficacy assessment of a cell-mediated immunity HIV-1 vaccine (the Step Study): a double-blind, randomised, placebo-controlled, test-of-concept trial. Lancet 372:1881–1893
23. Arnold GF, Resnick DA, Smith AD, Geisler SC, Holmes AK, Arnold E (1996) Chimeric rhinoviruses as tools for vaccine development and characterization of protein epitopes. Intervirology 39:72–78
24. Resnick DA, Smith AD, Gesiler SC, Zhang A, Arnold E, Arnold GF (1995) Chimeras from a human rhinovirus 14-human immunodeficiency virus type 1 (HIV-1) V3 loop seroprevalence library induce neutralizing responses against HIV-1. J Virol 69:2406–2411
25. Smith AD, Geisler SC, Chen AA, Resnick DA, Roy BM, Lewi PJ, Arnold E, Arnold GF (1998) Human rhinovirus type 14: human immunodeficiency virus type 1 (HIV-1) V3 loop chimeras from a combinatorial library induce potent neutralizing antibody responses against HIV-1. J Virol 72:651–659
26. Dollenmaier G, Mosier SM, Scholle F, Sharma N, McKnight KL, Lemon SM (2001) Membrane-associated respiratory syncytial virus F protein expressed from a human rhinovirus type 14 vector is immunogenic. Virology 281:216–230
27. Arnold GF, Velasco PK, Holmes AK, Wrin T, Geisler SC, Phung P, Tian Y, Resnick DA, Ma X, Mariano TM, Petropoulos CJ, Taylor JW, Katinger H, Arnold E (2009) Broad neutralization of human immunodeficiency virus type 1 (HIV-1) elicited from human rhinoviruses that display the HIV-1 gp41 ELDKWA epitope. J Virol 83:5087–5100
28. Monto AS, Fendrick AM, Sarnes MW (2001) Respiratory illness caused by picornavirus infection: a review of clinical outcomes. Clin Ther 23:1615–1627
29. Martin EK, Kuypers J, Chu HY, Lacombe K, Qin X, Strelitz B, Bradford M, Jones C, Klein EJ, Englund JA (2015) Molecular epidemiology of human rhinovirus infections in the pediatric emergency department. J Clin Virol 62:25–31
30. Tomusange K, Yu W, Suhrbier A, Wijesundara D, Grubor-Bauk B, Gowans EJ (2015) Engineering human rhinovirus serotype-A1 as a vaccine vector. Virus Res 203:72–76
31. Garrod TJ, Grubor-Bauk B, Gargett T, Li Y, Miller DS, Yu W, Major L, Burrell CJ, Wesselingh S, Suhrbier A, Gowans EJ (2014) DNA vaccines encoding membrane-bound or secreted forms of heat shock protein 70 exhibit improved potency. Eur J Immunol 44:1992–2002
32. French MA, Center RJ, Wilson KM, Fleyfel I, Fernandez S, Schorcht A, Stratov I, Kramski M, Kent SJ, Kelleher AD (2013) Isotype-switched immunoglobulin G antibodies to HIV Gag proteins may provide alternative or additional immune responses to 'protective' human leukocyte antigen-B alleles in HIV controllers. AIDS 27:519–528
33. Quiner CA, Jackson WT (2010) Fragmentation of the Golgi apparatus provides replication membranes for human rhinovirus 1A. Virology 407:185–195

Chapter 12

Generating Recombinant Vesicular Stomatitis Viruses for Use as Vaccine Platforms

John B. Ruedas and John H. Connor

Abstract

The unique properties of vesicular stomatitis virus (VSV) make it a promising vaccine platform. With the advent of plasmid-based approaches to generate recombinant VSV viruses that express glycoproteins of other viruses, researchers now have the means to generate vaccine candidates targeting a variety of human pathogens. This chapter gives a general overview of the workings of VSV as a vaccine platform and provides a detailed protocol for the generation of recombinant VSV from plasmids.

Key words Vesicular stomatitis virus, Vaccine platform, Reverse genetics, Vaccinia virus, T7 RNA polymerase

1 Introduction

Vesicular stomatitis virus (VSV) is a veterinary pathogen associated with sporadic outbreaks in North and South America. VSV is not known to be a significant human pathogen, but it has proven to be highly tractable for laboratory investigation. VSV is also notable for being easily pseudotyped; meaning a glycoprotein gene from a different virus can be cloned into its genome and expressed on the virus surface. Since viral glycoproteins are typically major antigens that induce immune responses, infection with a pseudotyped VSV can generate an immune response against the glycoprotein, thereby generating an immune response to the virus from which the glycoprotein originated. For this reason VSV has been extensively investigated as a vaccine platform to target specific viral agents, and has been used to develop candidate vaccines for several human pathogens. Experimental studies in animals report that VSV-based candidate vaccines provide protection against virus challenge for influenza, HIV, Lassa, Marburg, and Ebola [1–3]. Most notably, VSV-based candidate vaccines for HIV and Ebola have advanced

Maureen C. Ferran and Gary R. Skuse (eds.), *Recombinant Virus Vaccines: Methods and Protocols*, Methods in Molecular Biology, vol. 1581, DOI 10.1007/978-1-4939-6869-5_12,

to human testing where studies indicate these vaccines are effective in mounting protective responses without major side effects [4–6]. Moreover, the VSV vaccine platform can be multivalent, with a single injection of a vaccine candidate engineered to express protective epitopes against multiple diseases as shown by Mire et al. [7]. The results seen with the VSV vaccine platform has encouraged interest for developing additional VSV-based vaccines that target other viruses. As a result, generation of recombinant VSV (rVSV) encoding foreign glycoproteins is becoming an increasingly important tool for therapeutic development in the fields of virology and vaccinology.

As the prototypic member of the Rhabdoviruses, replication of VSV has been extensively characterized. The virus genome is composed of a single negative-sense RNA molecule that is fully encapsidated by the virus nucleoprotein (N) to form the ribonucleoprotein (RNP) core. The virally encoded RNA polymerase complex, comprising the large (L) protein and phosphoprotein (P) cofactor, utilizes the RNP as a template to synthesize virus transcripts. Monocistronic transcripts made for each VSV protein are initiated at a defined transcription start sequence and terminated at a consensus termination sequence. These sequences can be appended to any ORF to confer transcription from the VSV genome. The genome also includes a gene for the transmembrane glycoprotein that protrudes from the virus surface and functions in virus attachment and entry into the cell.

Generation of rVSV begins with cloning a gene of interest into the genome plasmid by recombinant DNA techniques. In the VSV vaccine platform, this is accomplished by replacing the VSV glycoprotein gene with a glycoprotein gene from the desired vaccine target. As mentioned above, more than one glycoprotein can be expressed in an individual rVSV. Upon completion of the cDNA construction of a VSV genome containing the desired glycoprotein insert(s), replicating virus can be generated from this cDNA by transfecting the genome plasmid as well as support plasmids individually encoding VSV N, P, and L proteins into eukaryotic cells. Generally, each plasmid is under the control of a T7 promoter and as such can be transfected into eukaryotic cells infected with a recombinant vaccinia virus encoding the T7-RNA polymerase (T7-RNAP). However, due to concerns that low-level vaccinia contamination could conceivably be present in rVSV stocks intended for human use, cell lines stably expressing T7 RNAP, such as BSR-T7/5, can be used as a vaccinia-free alternative. This chapter details vaccinia-dependent and vaccinia-independent approaches for rVSV development.

2 Materials

2.1 Preparation of Plasmid Encoding VSV Genome Containing Gene of Interest

1. pVSV-FL(+): plasmid containing cDNA encoding the VSV genome [8]. Available through Kerafast (Boston, MA, cat. no. EH1001).
2. *Alternative plasmid* pVSV-ΔG-GFP: plasmid containing cDNA encoding the VSV genome with VSV G gene substituted by the GFP gene [9]. Available through Kerafast (cat. no. EH1003).
3. cDNA encoding gene to be cloned into VSV genome.

2.2 Cell Culture and Transfection

1. Class II biological safety cabinet.
2. Six-well tissue culture plates.
3. Conical tubes: 15 ml.
4. Dulbecco's modified Eagle's medium (DMEM) containing 10% fetal bovine serum.
5. Phosphate-buffered saline (PBS): 10 mM Na_2HPO_4, 1.8 mM KH_2PO_4, 137 mM NaCl, 2.7 mM KCl, pH 7.4
6. 0.25% trypsin–EDTA (1×): Gibco, cat. no. 25200-056.
7. Water: sterile and nuclease-free.
8. Polyethyleneimine "Max" (Polysciences, Inc., cat. no. 24765), or commercial source of PEI-based transfection reagent.
9. Fluorescence microscope.
10. Transfection control plasmid (*optional*). *See* **Note 1**.

2.3 Vaccinia-Dependent Method

1. Baby Hamster Kidney cells (BHK): ATCC (CCL-10) *or* Kerafast (cat. no. EH1011).
2. Recombinant vaccinia virus expressing the bacteriophage T7 RNA polymerase gene, vTF7-3 [10].
3. Syringe-filters: EMD Millipore Millex-GS 0.22 μm (cat. no. SLGS025NB). *See* **Note 2**.
4. 5 ml syringe.
5. Cytosine D-arabinofuranoside (Ara-C), *optional*.
6. pBS-N-ϕT: support plasmid encoding VSV N gene [8]. Available through Kerafast (cat. no. EH1013).
7. pBS-P-ϕT: support plasmid encoding VSV P gene [8]. Available through Kerafast (cat. no. EH1014).
8. pBS-L-ϕT: support plasmid encoding VSV L gene [8]. Available through Kerafast (cat. no. EH1015).

2.4 Vaccinia-Free Method

1. BSR-T7/5 cells: BHK-derived cell line stably expressing T7 RNA polymerase gene [11].
2. pTM1-N: IRES-containing plasmid encoding VSV N gene [12].

3. pTM1-P: IRES-containing plasmid encoding VSV P gene [12].
4. pTM1-L: IRES-containing plasmid encoding VSV L gene [12].

2.5 Growing rVSV Stocks

1. Agarose (high-purity and low-melting): Invitrogen, cat. no. 16520-050.
2. Pasteur pipettes.
3. Conical tubes: 15 and 50 ml.
4. Six-well tissue culture flask.
5. T-75 tissue culture flask.
6. T-150 tissue culture flask.
7. 1.5 ml microcentrifuge tubes.

3 Methods

3.1 General Overview of the Procedure

Generating rVSV first involves the preparation of a plasmid containing cDNA that encodes the desired recombinant virus. It also requires the preparation of appropriate support plasmids (pN, pP, and pL) and an appropriate source of T7 polymerase to drive transcription from these plasmids. The preparation of these support reagents enables a transfection-based virus recovery approach that begins with the seeding of cells in six-well plates, infecting the cells with Vaccinia-T7 (VV-T7) if the vaccinia method is used, and transfecting the cells with the three support plasmids and genome plasmid. rVSV virions produced by the transfected cells will be amplified on fresh cell monolayers for visual confirmation of their recovery. Upon recovery of the desired rVSV, virus stocks will be grown. Figure 1 provides a flowchart summarizing the key steps for generating rVSV. Note that because VSV infection in cattle resembles foot-and-mouth disease, the USDA lists VSV as a select agent. Therefore, production and handling of rVSV should first be approved by an Institutional Biosafety Committee and all work conducted in a BSL-2 certified laboratory. Accordingly, all steps in this protocol should be done in a Class II biosafety cabinet.

3.2 Preparation of Plasmids

The VSV genome is composed of negative-sense single-stranded RNA that is entirely encapsidated by the virus nucleocapsid (N) protein. The genome is flanked at its 3′ and 5′ ends by noncoding sequences known as the leader and trailer regions, respectively, where critical promoter sequences are found. Five genes are positioned between the leader and trailer in the order 3′-le-N-P-M-G--L-tr-5′. Genes are separated from each other by an intergenic dinucleotide sequence (C/GA) and all genes are flanked by VSV-specific transcription start and stop sequences that are common for each gene. Transcription of the genome by the virus polymerase complex (P and L proteins) yields monocistronic transcripts in a decreasing gradient from the 3′ to 5′ direction [13]. Thus, the

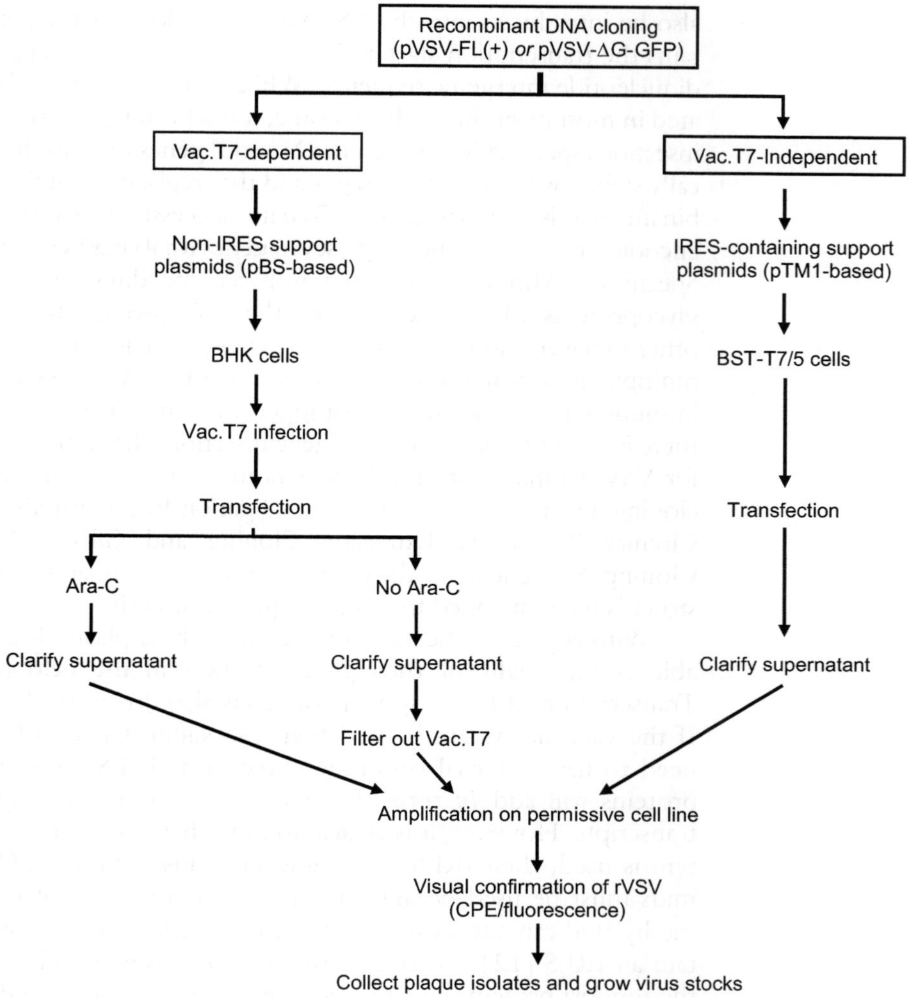

Fig. 1 Flowchart showing key steps in generating rVSV

expression level of a given gene is dependent on its proximity to the 3′ end. Cloning a heterologous glycoprotein gene into VSV is done by using a plasmid containing cDNA that encodes the VSV genome. Importantly, the plasmid is driven by T7 RNAP to generate a positive-sense transcript of the VSV genome (e.g., antigenome strand). It is important to remember that the positive-sense sequence of the gene to be cloned be on the same strand as the positive-sense genome strand. Also, care should be taken during cloning to preserve all important regulatory elements in the plasmid. Lawson et al. detail the construction of the genome-encoding plasmid [8].

Generating rVSV to serve as a vaccine platform involves replacing the VSV glycoprotein ORF with a foreign glycoprotein from a targeted virus while preserving the transcription start and stop sequences. Barr et al. provide an excellent review on sequence requirements for VSV transcription [14]. An additional gene can also be introduced into the VSV genome as long as the gene contains the transcription start and stop sequences and the appropriate dinucleotide intergenic sequence. While an extra gene can be tolerated in most positions in the genome, it has been reported that gene insertions specifically between the N and P genes may not be genetically stable over multiple passages and that replication of the recombinant virus is attenuated [14]. To date, successful recovery of rVSV encoding two extra genes (e.g., seven genes total) has been reported. Specifically, Mire et al. reported an rVSV encoding three different glycoproteins where one replaced the VSV glycoprotein and the other two were cloned as additional genes [7]. The ability to express multiple glycoproteins increases the value of rVSV as a prophylactic immunogen for a number of pathogens. It is not currently known if there is a limit to the number of gene insertions that can be tolerated for VSV. Cloning into the VSV genome can be done by standard cloning techniques as well as with ligation-free methods such as Circular Polymerase Extension Cloning and Gibson Assembly Cloning. Sequencing of the cloned regions in the final plasmid construct is recommended to ensure sequence integrity.

With regard to the support plasmids, these plasmids are available commercially or through researchers in the field [8, 12]. Transcription of the support plasmids is also driven by T7 RNAP. If the vaccinia system is used then the support plasmids do not need to have internal ribosome entry sites (IRES) since vaccinia proteins will add *in trans* the essential 5′-methylated cap to T7 transcripts. However, it is critical to note that if a vaccinia-free system is used, then IRES-containing plasmids such as pTM1 plasmids must be used because the T7 transcripts will not have a 5′ methylated cap and as such will not be translated unless they contain an IRES [12]. Therefore, the type of plasmids to be used for the support proteins needs to be taken into account when deciding whether to use a vaccinia-dependent or vaccinia-independent system to generate rVSV. Note that the genome plasmid should not have an IRES element regardless of the method used.

3.3 Preparing Cells for Transfection

1. Trypsinize and dilute BHK cells so that they can be seeded into two 6-well plates. Choose a density so that the monolayers will be 75–90% confluent on the following day (*see* **Note 3**). If the vaccinia-free method is used, seed BSR-T7 cells instead.
2. Shake cells constantly in a side-to side and forward-reverse (X–Y) motion for the first 2 min after seeding to allow consistent distribution of the cells.
3. Incubate the cells at 37 °C, 5% CO_2 overnight in a tissue culture incubator, shaking again briefly at 10 and 20 min after seeding to ensure even cell spreading which will lead to uniform monolayers.
4. On the next day, examine the cells using an inverted brightfield microscope to confirm cell monolayers are evenly distributed

and 75–90% confluent. Infection and transfection conditions will be suboptimal if the confluency conditions are incorrect.

5. If using the Vaccinia-independent method, proceed to Subheading 3.5 for transfection.

3.4 Infecting the Cells with Vaccinia-T7

The volume of VV-T7 virus needed to infect each cell at an MOI of 5 will need to be calculated. The starting VV-T7 stock concentration should be 10^8 PFU/ml or greater. *See Methods in Molecular Biology: volume 269*, for a review on growing vaccinia stocks [15]. A master mix for 14 wells (12 samples + 2 extra) should be prepared.

1. Calculate the volume of VV-T7 needed to infect each cell at an MOI of 5 in one well of a six-well dish. There are approximately 10^6 cells per well at 90% confluence. If, for example, the VV-T7 stock is 10^8 PFU/ml, then 0.05 ml will be needed per well.
2. Multiply the calculated volume by 14 (12 wells plus 2 extra to allow for error).
3. Add this amount of VV-T7 stock to a polystyrene 15 ml conical tube.
4. Add DMEM to reach a final total volume of 2.8 ml. Some researchers opt to include a DNA synthesis inhibitor to prevent vaccinia replication (*see* **Note 4**).
5. Mix the master mix thoroughly by vortex or inverting multiple times.
6. Remove the media from each well by aspiration.
7. Infect each well by adding 0.2 ml of the VV-T7 master mix. Work quickly to prevent cells from drying.
8. Shake plates constantly in an X–Y motion during the first 5 min of infection (virus absorption) to allow for even infection of the cell monolayer.
9. Incubate at 37 °C, 5% CO_2 for 60–90 min, shaking the plates briefly every 5–10 min to prevent monolayers from drying.
10. During the virus absorption period, proceed to preparing the transfection mixes as described below.

3.5 Transfection

3.5.1 Preparation of 10× PEI Transfection Reagent Stock

A concentrated 10× stock of PEI should be prepared and frozen in advance. Polyethyleneimine "Max" (cat. no. 24765) from Polysciences, Inc. is a readily soluble PEI powder that is recommended for this procedure (*see* **Note 5**). Note that a commercial source of ready-to-use PEI transfection reagent is also available through Polyplus (JetPEI).

1. Make a 10× PEI stock by adding 51.7 mg of PEI "Max" to 10 ml of sterile nuclease-free water.
2. Mix or vortex well. The powder should readily dissolve in water and the solution should look clear.

3. Filter-sterilize the solution with a 0.22 μm syringe filter.
4. Freeze the 10× stock at −20 °C in 0.5 ml aliquots.

3.5.2 Preparing the Plasmid Transfection Mixes

Most transfection methods, including the method described here, have a time-sensitive step of pre-mixing plasmids with the transfection reagent just prior to adding to the cells. Hence, careful timing should be taken such that the reagent–plasmid mix is ready to add to the cells just after the VV-T7 absorption period has concluded (*see* below).

1. Thaw an aliquot of 10× PEI and make a 1× working stock by diluting 1:10 in sterile nuclease-free water.
2. Thaw the pTM1-GFP transfection control plasmid (*optional*) and the four VSV plasmids, referred to here as pN, pP, pL, and pGenome (*see* **Note 6**).
3. In ten separate microcentrifuge tubes, add the following amounts of plasmid to each tube for a total of 4 μg of plasmid per tube: 0.6 μg of pN, 1.4 μg of pP, 0.9 μg of pL, and 1.1 μg of pGenome (*see* **Notes 7** and **8**). This will be used to create ten separate recovery trials within the experiment.
4. The total volume of the plasmid mix should not exceed 30 μl for each tube. If needed, adjust the plasmid stock concentrations accordingly.
5. Prepare a "No L" negative control by adding the amount of each plasmid indicated above into a microcentrifuge tube *except* that no pL plasmid is to be added. This control will serve as a useful indicator to determine if VV-T7 is efficiently filtered out during the amplification step. *See* Subheading 3.9 for more information. To maintain a constant amount of overall DNA per sample, 1.1 μg of empty vector or salmon sperm DNA should be added in place of the pL plasmid in the "No L" control.
6. Prepare a transfection control by adding 4 μg of pTM1-GFP (or fluorescent maker of choice) into a microcentrifuge tube.
7. Add 0.3 ml of serum-free media to each tube.
8. When there is 10 min remaining for the VV-T7 virus absorption period, add 32 μl of 1× PEI transfection reagent to each tube containing plasmid. If the amount of plasmid DNA is varied, maintain a ratio of 8 μl of 1× PEI per μg of DNA.
9. Mix the plasmid-PEI solutions well and spin-down by *brief* centrifugation (~1000 × *g* for 30 s).
10. Incubate plasmid-PEI solution at room-temperature for 15 min.
11. Proceed to removing the VV-T7 inoculum from the cells (*see* below).

3.5.3 Removing the VV-T7 Inoculum

1. At the end of the VV-T7 absorption period, remove the virus inoculum by aspirating.
2. Wash each well with 2 ml of PBS that has been pre-warmed at 37 °C.
3. Remove the PBS wash by aspirating.
4. Add 3 ml of fresh DMEM with serum to the each well. Include Ara-C (40 μg/ml) *if desired* to inhibit VV-T7 production (*see* **Note 4**).

3.5.4 Adding Transfection Mixes to Cells

1. At the end of the plasmid-PEI incubation period, add the transfection mixes to their respective wells in a dropwise fashion. Drops should be dispersed evenly on top of the media. Wells 1–10 receive the ten replicates, well #11 receives the 'No L' control, and well #12 receives the transfection control. Work swiftly so as to not prolong the plasmid-PEI incubation time.
2. Shake cells constantly in an X–Y motion for 5 min. Shake carefully to avoid spilling media.
3. Incubate at 37 °C for 48 h, shaking the plates briefly at 15 and 30 min after addition of the transfection mix to ensure evenly dispersed transfection.
4. Clear signs of VV-T7-mediated cytopathic effect (CPE) should appear by 48 h post-infection. *See* Fig. 2a.

3.6 Preparing Cells for Virus Amplification

Recombinant VSV that has been produced and budded from the transfected cells is likely to be present at a low concentration in the supernatant (<10^3 PFU/ml). Moreover, because the transfected cells were infected with a high MOI of VV-T7, it is not possible to detect the presence of rVSV by CPE or fluorescence in the transfected cells. Therefore, a second set of cells is needed to amplify the rVSV to confirm that it has been successfully generated. The cell type to be used for virus amplification depends on the heterologous glycoprotein that was engineered into the rVSV genome plasmid. A cell line that is permissive for the target virus should be used (e.g., Vero E6 cells for Ebola). If the rVSV being recovered encodes the endogenous VSV glycoprotein then BHK cells are recommended to obtain the highest virus titer.

1. On the day after transfection, seed the appropriate cell line on two 6-well plates so that the monolayers will be nearly confluent on the following day (*see* **Note 9**).
2. Shake cells constantly in an X–Y motion for the first 2 min after seeding to ensure evenly spread monolayers.
3. Incubate overnight at 37 °C, 5% CO_2, shaking cells again briefly in an X–Y motion at 10 and 20 min after seeding.

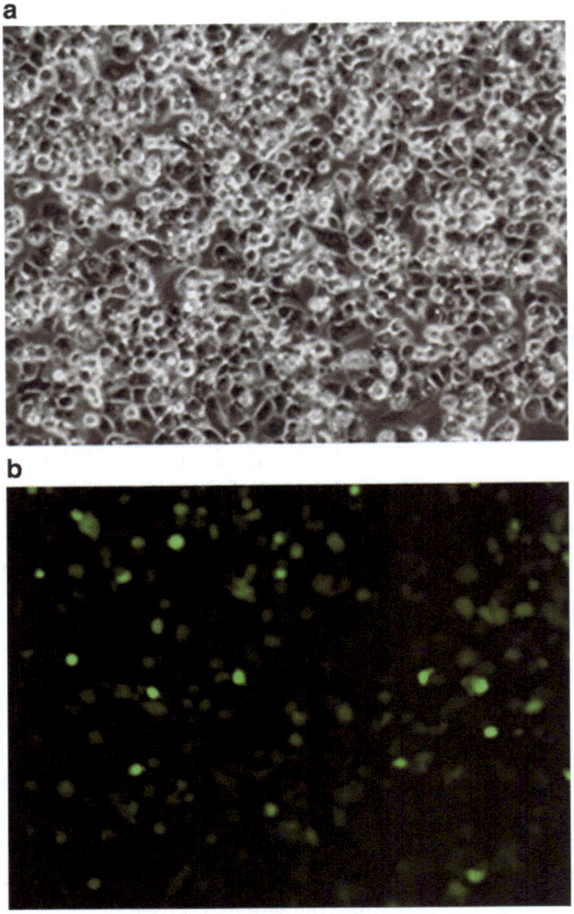

Fig. 2 Phase contrast (**a**) and fluorescent (**b**) images showing transfection efficiency of vaccinia-T7 infected cells. BHK cells were infected with Vaccinia-T7 at an MOI of 5 and then transfected with 4 μg of pTM1-GFP using PEI transfection reagent. Images were taken 20 h post-transfection at 10× magnification

3.7 Observing the Transfection Control

The transfection control should be checked at 24 h post-transfection for fluorescence. At least 50% of the cells transfected with pTM1-GFP should show fluorescence, however 70–90% is better. Figure 2b shows an example of cells transfected with pTM1-GFP (*see* **Note 10**). Moreover, nearly 100% of the cells (in all wells) should show vaccinia CPE indicated by cell rounding.

3.8 Amplification of rVSV

3.8.1 Clarifying Transfection Supernatants

1. At 48 h post-transfection, transfer the supernatant from each transfected well into individual 15 ml polystyrene conical tubes.
2. Pellet cell debris by spinning the conical tubes at 5000 × *g* for 5 min.
3. Transfer each clarified supernatant into a sterile collection tube.

4. If VV-T7 was not used (e.g., BSR-T7/5 cells) or Ara-C was added during the VV-T7 infection and transfection steps, then the supernatants do not need to be filtered after they have been clarified. Proceed to Subheading 3.8.3 to add the supernatants to new cells for rVSV amplification.
5. If VV-T7 was used then proceed to Subheading 3.8.2 to remove vaccinia from the supernatants by filtration.

3.8.2 Removal of Vaccinia by Filtration

Vaccinia virions are large enough that filtering the transfection supernatant through a 0.22 μm syringe-filter should remove most or all of them, while allowing the smaller VSV virions to flow though.

1. Remove the plunger from a sterile 5 ml Luer-lock syringe.
2. Attach a 0.22 μm Millex-GS syringe filter to the syringe tip.
3. Carefully pour or pipette the clarified transfection supernatant into the 5 ml syringe. Use a new syringe for each sample.
4. Position the filter-syringe directly over a sterile collection tube.
5. Carefully place the plunger back into the syringe and push down slowly and evenly to expel the supernatant through the filter. If the filter feels like it is becoming clogged, replace with a new filter. Do not push down on the plunger with heavy force or the membrane may tear (*see* **Note 11**).

3.8.3 Adding Transfection Supernatants to New Cells for Amplification of rVSV

1. Remove the media from each well of the amplification cells that were seeded in Subheading 3.6 (*see* **Note 12**).
2. Add 0.5 ml of each transfection supernatant to the amplification cells in correlating wells. If larger plates were seeded, larger volumes of the transfection supernatants can be added (*see* **Note 13**).
3. Shake plates in an X–Y motion for 5 min and then intermittently every 5–10 min during the virus absorption period (1 h).
4. Allow virus absorption to proceed for 1 h at 37 °C.
5. After the virus absorption period, add 2–3 ml of fresh prewarmed DMEM on top of the supernatant for each well. Add an adequate amount of DMEM if larger plates are used for the amplification (e.g., 10 ml for 10 cm dishes).
6. Do not add Ara-C during the amplification step. If Ara-C was used during the transfection step, *see* **Note 14**.
7. Incubate the plates at 37 °C during the amplification step.
8. Freeze the remaining unused transfection supernatants at −80 °C (*see* **Note 15**).
9. Check for VSV-induced CPE at 24 h post-amplification (*see* Fig. 3b).

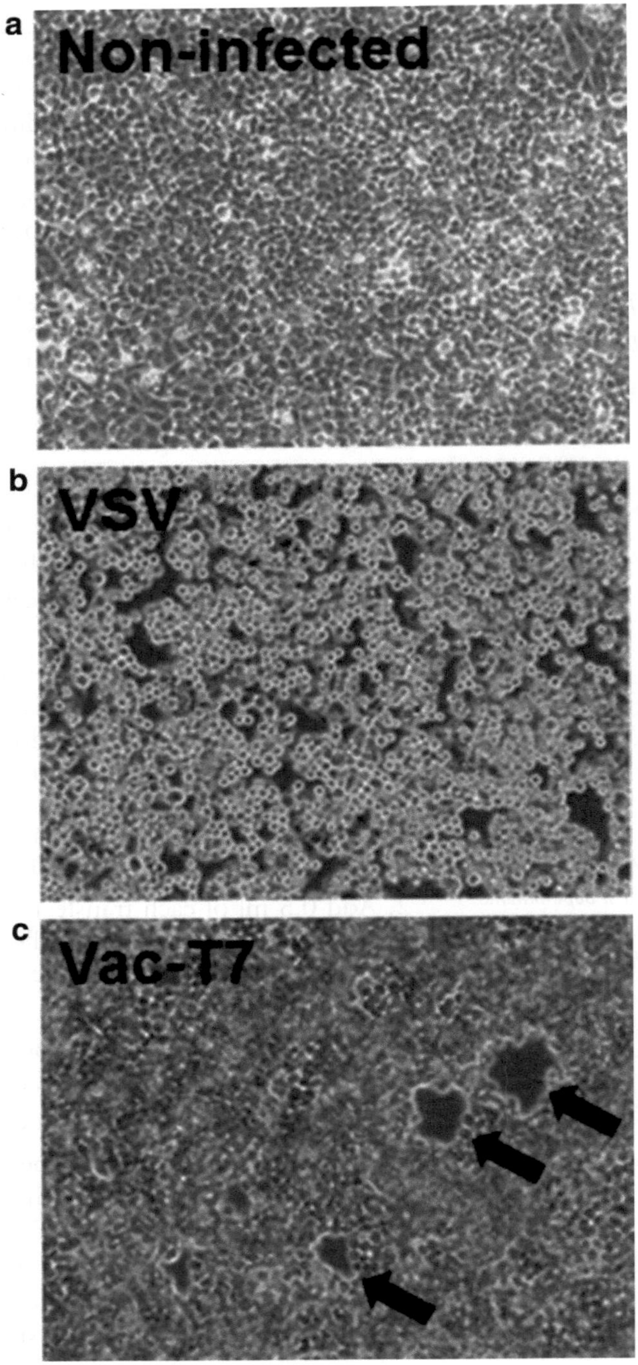

Fig. 3 Cytopathic effect caused by VSV and vaccinia. (**a**) Non-infected BHK cells. BHK cells were infected with VSV (**b**) or vaccinia-T7 (**c**) at an MOI of 0.1. Phase-contrast images were taken 20 h post-infection at 10× magnification. *Arrows* point to foci of vaccinia infected cells

3.9 Visual Confirmation of rVSV Recovery

Successful generation of rVSV can be confirmed by searching for CPE, or fluorescence if applicable, in the amplification plates. It is important to note that some vaccinia particles could manage to pass though the filter. This should be kept in mind when searching for CPE in the amplification step. VSV-infection typically spreads rapidly and is widespread across a monolayer even at low MOI. Vaccinia infections on the other hand do not spread as quickly at low MOI and are first evident by the presence of foci or syncytia (compare Fig. 3b and c). Note that pseudotyped VSV growing in certain cell lines may produce CPE that appears different than that of wild-type VSV growing in BHK cells. While a trained eye may be able to differentiate between vaccinia and VSV CPE in a coinfected monolayer, significant vaccinia contamination can still make it difficult to determine if successful recovery of the rVSV has been achieved. The "No L" control will serve as a useful control in this aspect as filtrate from this sample will not have rVSV and should be free of vaccinia if the filtration process worked effectively. Thus, cells treated with the "No L" supernatant should not show any CPE. Fluorescent protein genes encoded in the rVSV genome can also be very useful for confirming generation of rVSV, although fluorescent proteins may not be desired in recombinant viruses intended for human use. Successful generation of the rVSV can also be confirmed by immunofluorescence staining of the amplified cells using a VSV-specific antibody. Make sure to save the amplified supernatant before staining the cells.

VSV-induced CPE should be visible within 24–48 h post-amplification, although mutants with slower growth kinetics may require more time to produce visible CPE. In general, if VSV-induced CPE is not visible after 72 h then rVSV is not present in the amplification, indicating that generation of the rVSV was not successful.

3.9.1 Storing rVSV from the Amplification Supernatant

1. Once successful generation of the rVSV is confirmed, the amplification supernatant(s) should be transferred to a sterile 15-ml conical tube.
2. If multiple wells produce rVSV, keep the supernatants separate and treat as separate clones (*see* **Note 16**).
3. Remove cell debris by spinning the conical tube(s) at 5000 × *g* for 5 min.
4. Dispense the clarified supernatants in 0.1–0.5 ml aliquots.
5. Freeze at −80 °C (*see* **Note 17**).

3.10 Growing rVSV Stocks

To ensure homogeneity of the virus population in a working stock, it is best to generate stocks from single plaque isolates grown from the transfection supernatant. A standard plaque assay is done with the transfection supernatant and individual plaque colonies are captured by aspirating with a Pasteur pipette. As in the case for the amplification, the cells used in the plaque assay should be a permissive cell line for the target agent that the heterologous glycoprotein originates from. The plaque colonies are then frozen in culture media and used to infect cell monolayers to generate new working stocks.

3.10.1 Plaque Assay to Collect Plaque Purified Isolates

1. Seed the same cell line used in the amplification step into two 6-well plates so that they will be confluent the next day.
2. The following day confirm that each well is greater than 90% confluent.
3. Thaw an aliquot from a transfection supernatant sample that was confirmed to have rVSV present in the amplification step.
4. Make a 10^{-1} dilution by taking 0.5 ml of the transfection supernatant and mixing with 4.5 ml of DMEM in 15 ml conical tubes or similar-sized culture tubes.
5. Mix well by vortex.
6. Make additional tenfold serial dilutions as described in **steps 4** and **5** until a 10^{-6} dilution has been made.
7. Aspirate the media off each well and add 0.2 ml of each dilution into duplicate wells. Make sure to pre-label the wells with the dilution number.
8. Shake both plates constantly in an X–Y direction for 5 min.
9. Incubate at 37 °C in 5% CO_2 for 1 h while shaking the plates intermittently every 5–10 min to spread the viral inoculum and prevent the cells from drying.

3.10.2 Preparing Agarose Overlay

1. During the virus absorption period make a 2% agarose solution in PBS or saline (150 mM sodium chloride) by adding 2 g of agarose for every 100 ml of solution.
2. Before heating, record the weight of the vessel containing the agarose solution. Water evaporated during heating will be replenished back to this original weight.
3. Heat the solution in the microwave until the agarose is fully dissolved (typically 1–2 min). Be sure to use a large enough vessel so the solution will not overflow during heating.
4. Carefully remove the heated agarose solution from the microwave with the open end facing away from any personnel. Wear autoclave gloves as the vessel will be very hot to touch.
5. Add sterile water to the solution to bring the vessel back to its original weight.
6. Keep the melted agarose solution heated by submersing in a water bath at 55 °C until it is ready for use.
7. Pre-warm 31 ml of DMEM at 37 °C.
8. Five minutes prior to the end of the virus absorption period, add 9 ml of the agarose solution to the DMEM to make a

0.45% agarose solution in DMEM. Mix well but avoid the accumulation of air bubbles (*see* **Note 18**).

9. Keep the agarose–DMEM mix heated between 37 and 42 °C until it is used.

3.10.3 Overlaying Agarose Plug on Cells

1. Remove the virus inoculum from the wells.
2. Wash each well with 3 ml of warm PBS.
3. Quickly add 3 ml of the agarose–DMEM solution to each well. Pipette the solution along the side of the wells to avoid knocking cells off of the surface.
4. Allow the agarose plugs to solidify. To avoid excessive condensation avoid covering the plates during this time.
5. After the agarose plugs are solidified (about 5–10 min) cover the plates and incubate overnight at 37 °C, CO_2.
6. Avoid tilting the plates during incubation so that newly budded virus does not slide under the plug to infect other regions of the monolayer.

3.10.4 Picking Primary Plaque-Isolates

1. At approximately 30 h post-infection, plaques will be visible by lifting the plate up to a light source and looking from the bottom up through the monolayer (*see* **Note 19**). Tilt the plate at various angles to view the plaques. Plaques will appear as hazy circular patches in the monolayer and should be about 1–5 mm in diameter. *See* Fig. 4a.
2. *Do not* fix or stain the cells before picking plaques.
3. Choose a dilution where the plaques are easily and discretely visible (*see* **Note 20**).
4. Use a fine-point marker to trace the edges of 5–10 well defined plaques.
5. Add 0.5 ml of DMEM to individual microcentrifuge tubes to collect the plaques. Label these tubes accordingly and with the description “primary plaques”.
6. Fix a rubber bulb to a sterile Pasteur pipette and carefully puncture through the agarose plug directly over the top of a plaque.
7. With the tip of the pipette in contact with the well surface, gently suck up the plaque. A very small volume of liquid (~10–30 μl) will be sucked into the pipette.
8. Transfer the liquid to one of the microcentrifuge tubes containing DMEM and rinse the pipette tip several times to wash the virus particles into the media.
9. Repeat for each plaque using a new pipette and tube each time.
10. Freeze each of the plaque isolates at −80 °C.

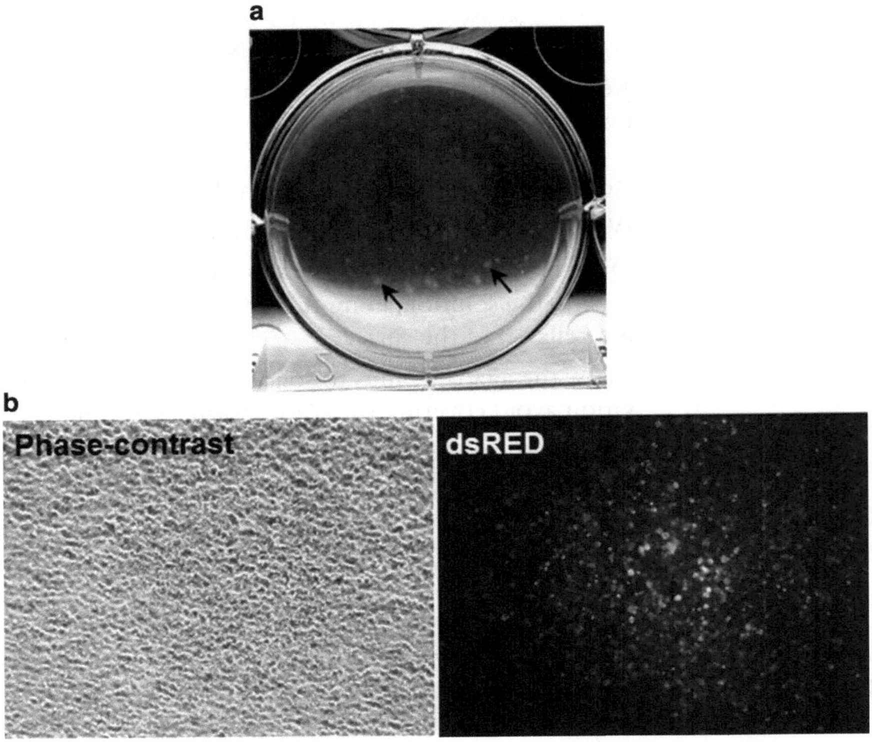

Fig. 4 Visualizing pre-stained plaques to pick plaque isolate clones. A plaque assay was done on BHK cells infected with serially diluted VSV-dsRed. A 0.45% agarose overlay with DMEM was added on top of cells and incubated for 24 h. (**a**) Plaques appear as hazy circular patterns at the bottom of the well as indicated by *arrows*. (**b**) An isolate plaque colony viewed with phase-contrast and fluorescence microscopy at 10× magnification

3.10.5 Growing rVSV Stocks

1. Seed a T-75 or T-150 flask with cells that are permissive for the target agent that the heterologous protein is derived from. The flasks should be nearly confluent by the next day.
2. When the flasks are nearly confluent thaw a tube containing a plaque isolate.
3. Add 100 μl of the plaque isolate to a volume of DMEM that is just enough to cover the cells. Generally, 3 and 5 ml is sufficient for T-75 and T-150 flasks, respectively.
4. Remove the growth media from the flask and add the virus inoculate onto the cells.
5. Allow the virus absorption to occur for 1–1.5 h while shaking intermittently to prevent the monolayers from drying.
6. After the virus absorption period, add additional DMEM for overnight incubation of the cells. Avoid adding large volumes of media. Generally, 10 and 15 ml is enough media for T-75 and T-150 flasks, respectively.

3.10.6 Harvesting rVSV Stocks

Typically, maximum titers are achieved for VSV at approximately 30 h post-infection for a low MOI-infection as described above. However, some mutant rVSV viruses may require a longer incubation time to reach maximum titer levels. Growth kinetics for each rVSV should be characterized to ascertain the time point that produces the greatest yield of virus. If an optimal collection time has not predetermined for a given rVSV it is advised to harvest the virus stock at 40–45 h post-infection. Note that prolonged incubation of wild-type VSV at 37 °C for greater than 48 h has been shown to reduce the peak titers [16].

1. Observe the cells for CPE when maximum titers are expected.
2. Nearly 100% of the cells should be rounded and a substantial portion of cells should be detached from the surface.
3. If significant areas of the monolayer still appear healthy then the infection requires a longer incubation time to reach completion.
4. Transfer the supernatant to a 50 ml conical tube.
5. Clarify the supernatant of cell debris by centrifugation at 5000 × *g* for 5 min.
6. Aliquot the supernatant into sterile tubes for single-use aliquots ranging between 0.1 and 0.5 ml per tube.
7. Note on the tube labels that the stock is a primary amplification from a primary plaque isolate.
8. Freeze aliquots at −80 °C for long-term storage.

4 Notes

1. A plasmid encoding a fluorescent protein gene expressed by T7 RNA polymerase can serve as a transfection control for a T7-driven expression system. In particular, a pTM1 plasmid is useful because it contains an internal ribozyme entry site (IRES), which is needed for expression of T7 transcripts in BSR-T7 cells. Such plasmids may not be available commercially but may be available through various research laboratories. This chapter will refer to a pTM1-GFP plasmid as a transfection control.
2. The type of membrane material used is crucial as it has been observed that certain membrane types may reduce VSV concentration in the flow-thru. Millex-GS syringe filters are recommended for this step as per Whitt [9].
3. BHK-21 cells from the ATCC can be used. However, a commercial source of BHK cells specifically shown to support VSV generation, are available through Kerafast.

4. Some researchers report using the DNA synthesis inhibitor Cytosine D-arabinofuranoside (Ara-C) during the infection and transfection step to inhibit late-stage expression of VV-T7 genes, hence inhibiting VV-T7 production in the transfected cells. Since the T7 RNAP gene is expressed during the early-stage of VV-T7 expression, T7 synthesis is not affected by the addition of Ara-C. Using Ara-C can be advantageous by limiting the synthesis of unwanted VV-T7 and eliminating the need to filter the transfection supernatant before the amplification step. However, Ara-C is cytotoxic at high concentrations and it could complicate the search for VSV-specific CPE. *See* **Note 14** for additional information. If Ara-C is used, it should be added to the master mix and the volume of DMEM adjusted accordingly. Ruedas and Perrault report using Aca-C at a concentration of 40 μg/ml during the VV-T7 infection [16].
5. Various transfection reagents such as TransfectACE, Lipofectamine, and polyethyleneimine (PEI) have been used successfully to generate rVSV. This chapter describes a method that utilizes an affordable and easy to make PEI transfection reagent [17].
6. High-quality plasmids should be used for optimal results. Maxi-preps done by column purification or cesium chloride gradient are recommended.
7. A master mix of all four plasmids can be made and then individually dispensed into each microcentrifuge tube.
8. Plasmid amounts used here are reported by Ruedas and Perrault [17] and can be adjusted for troubleshooting purposes. Note that plasmid amounts reported for rVSV recovery vary considerably throughout the literature.
9. Larger plates such as 6- or 10-cm dishes can be used. This will allow for larger volumes of the supernatants to be added and increase the chance of virus amplification, particularly if the virus concentration is very low in the transfection supernatant.
10. The fluorescent control pTM1-GFP is an indicator of both the transfection efficiency and the efficiency of T7-driven expression in VV-T7 infected cells or BSR-T7 cells. If the fluorescence appears to be suboptimal, these two processes can be separately tested by using a second fluorescent control where a pol-II driven promoter (i.e., CMV or Chicken Actin) is used to drive GFP. The pol-II driven plasmid will serve as a transfection control since it is independent of T7 expression and the pTM1-GFP control will then be an indicator of T7-driven expression.
11. Failure to clarify the supernatants before filtering could result in the filter becoming clogged.

12. If cells are not ready for amplification, the clarified supernatants can be chilled on ice for 24 h or frozen at −80 °C for longer periods.
13. Add a volume that is just enough to cover the monolayer. Adding larger volumes will decrease the chance of interaction between virus particles and the cell monolayer.
14. Cytotoxicity caused by residual Ara-C from the transfection supernatant may result in cell rounding during the amplification step, making it difficult to identify CPE induced by VSV. If Ara-C was used in the transfection step, remove the transfection supernatant after virus absorption on the amplification cells and wash the cells twice with 3 ml of PBS before replenishing with fresh DMEM.
15. Virus present in the transfection supernatant is unpassaged and therefore less likely to contain mutations that may accumulate during passaging of VSV stocks.
16. VSV is noted for having a high mutation rate [13]. It is possible that viruses generated in different wells could conceivably have unique mutations. Therefore, each successful recovery per well should be treated as a unique clone until its genomic sequence is verified.
17. Viruses present in the amplified supernatant are a first-passaged stock. While this stock can be used for growing second-passaged stocks if necessary, it is recommended to use plaque purified isolates from the transfection supernatant to generate working stocks. *See* Subheading 3.10 for making plaque isolates.
18. Before adding to cells, a small drop of the agarose–DMEM mix can be placed on a smooth surface to test its hardness. Upon solidifying the drop should be hard enough to be pushed along the surface without breaking apart. Generally, agarose concentrations between 0.45% and 0.5% are adequate for VSV plaques to form. If needed, more agarose can be added to reach the desired rigidity.
19. The specific rVSV and cell type used may require a longer period before plaques are visible. In most cases, plaques should be evident by 48 h.
20. Plaques may also be viewed under a microscope at low power.

Acknowledgements

The authors acknowledge funding through NIH R21 AI121933 and NIH RO1 to JHC. We also acknowledge support through the National Institute of Allergy and Infectious Diseases of the National Institutes of Health under award UC6AI058618.

References

1. Marzi A, Feldmann F, Geisbert TW, Feldmann H, Safronetz D (2015) Vesicular stomatitis virus-based vaccines against Lassa and Ebola viruses. Emerg Infect Dis 21(2):305–307
2. Lichty BD, Power AT, Stojdl DF, Bell JC (2004) Vesicular stomatitis virus: re-inventing the bullet. Trends Mol Med 10(5):210–216
3. Geisbert TW, Feldmann H (2011) Recombinant vesicular stomatitis virus-based vaccines against Ebola and Marburg virus infections. J Infect Dis 204(Suppl):S1075–S1081
4. Fuchs JD, Frank I, Elizaga ML, Allen M, Frahm N, Kochar N, Li S, Edupuganti S, Kalams SA, Tomaras GD, Sheets R, Pensiero M, Tremblay MA, Higgins TJ, Latham T, Egan MA, Clarke DK, Eldridge JH, Mulligan M, Rouphael N, Estep S, Rybczyk K, Dunbar D, Buchbinder S, Wagner T, Isbell R, Chinnell V, Bae J, Escamilla G, Tseng J, Fair R, Ramirez S, Broder G, Briesemeister L, Ferrara A (2015) First-in-human evaluation of the safety and immunogenicity of a recombinant vesicular stomatitis virus human immunodeficiency virus-1 gag vaccine (HVTN 090). Open Forum Infect Dis 2(3):ofv082
5. Henao-Restrepo AM, Longini IM, Egger M, Dean NE, Edmunds WJ, Camacho A, Carroll MW, Doumbia M, Draguez B, Duraffour S, Enwere G, Grais R, Gunther S, Hossmann S, Kondé MK, Kone S, Kuisma E, Levine MM, Mandal S, Norheim G, Riveros X, Soumah A, Trelle S, Vicari AS, Watson CH, Kéïta S, Kieny MP, Røttingen J-A (2015) Efficacy and effectiveness of an rVSV-vectored vaccine expressing Ebola surface glycoprotein: interim results from the Guinea ring vaccination cluster-randomised trial. Lancet 386(9996):857–866
6. Huttner A, Dayer J-A, Yerly S, Combescure C, Auderset F, Desmeules J, Eickmann M, Finckh A, Goncalves AR, Hooper JW, Kaya G, Krähling V, Kwilas S, Lemaître B, Matthey A, Silvera P, Becker S, Fast PE, Moorthy V, Kieny MP, Kaiser L, Siegrist C-A (2015) The effect of dose on the safety and immunogenicity of the VSV Ebola candidate vaccine: a randomised double-blind, placebo-controlled phase 1/2 trial. Lancet Infect Dis 15(10):1156–1166
7. Mire CE, Geisbert JB, Versteeg KM, Mamaeva N, Agans KN, Geisbert TW, Connor JH (2015) A single-vector, single-injection trivalent filovirus vaccine: proof of concept study in outbred guinea pigs. J Infect Dis 212(Suppl): S384–S388
8. Lawson ND, Stillman EA, Whitt MA, Rose JK (1995) Recombinant vesicular stomatitis viruses from DNA. Proc Natl Acad Sci U S A 92:4477–4481
9. Whitt MA (2010) Generation of VSV pseudotypes using recombinant ΔG-VSV for studies on virus entry, identification of entry inhibitors, and immune responses to vaccines. J Virol Methods 169(2):365–374
10. Fuerst TR, Niles EG, Studier FW, Moss B (1986) Eukaryotic transient-expression system based on recombinant vaccinia virus that synthesizes bacteriophage T7 RNA polymerase. Proc Natl Acad Sci U S A 83(21): 8122–8126
11. Buchholz UJ, Finke S, Conzelmann K-K (1999) Generation of Bovine Respiratory Syncytial Virus (BRSV) from cDNA: BRSV NS2 is not essential for virus replication in tissue culture, and the human RSV leader region acts as a functional BRSV genome promoter. J Virol 73(1):251–259
12. Harty RN, Brown ME, Hayes FP, Wright NT, Schnell MJ (2001) Vaccinia virus-free recovery of vesicular stomatitis virus. J Mol Microbiol Biotechnol 3(4):513–517
13. Knipe DM, Howley PM (2007) Fields virology, 5th edn. Lippincott Williams & Wilkins, Philadelphia
14. Barr JN, Whelan SPJ, Wertz GW (2002) Transcriptional control of the RNA-dependent RNA polymerase of vesicular stomatitis virus. Biochim Biophys Acta 1577:337–353
15. Isaacs SN (ed) (2004) Vaccinia virus and poxvirology: methods in molecular biology, vol 269. Hamana Press, Totowa
16. Ruedas JB, Perrault J (2009) Insertion of enhanced green fluorescent protein in a hinge region of vesicular stomatitis virus L polymerase protein creates a temperature-sensitive virus that displays no virion-associated polymerase activity in vitro. J Virol 83(23): 12241–12252
17. Ruedas JB, Perrault J (2014) Putative domain-domain interactions in the vesicular stomatitis virus L polymerase protein appendage region. J Virol 88(24):14458–14466

Part III

Positive Sense Single-Stranded RNA Viruses

Chapter 13

Alphavirus-Based Vaccines

Kenneth Lundstrom

Abstract

Alphavirus-based vectors have been engineered from Semliki Forest virus, Sindbis virus, and Venezuelan equine encephalitis virus and applied for vaccine development. Immunization in preclinical animal models has been conducted with naked RNA replicons, recombinant viral particles and layered DNA–RNA vectors. Most commonly, the targets for the immunization have been viral surface proteins and tumor antigens, which have elicited strong immune responses and even provided protection against challenges with lethal doses of virus and tumor cells, respectively. As alphaviruses also cause epidemics, vaccines have been developed against Chikungunya virus. Despite the success in several animal smodels only a few clinical trials have been conducted in humans, so far.

Key words Alphaviruses, Immunization, Viral vaccines, Cancer vaccines, Neutralizing antibodies, Protection

1 Introduction

Since the introduction of genetic engineering immunization with expressed recombinant antigens has become an important part of vaccine development. Typically, targets have consisted of viral surface and core proteins [1] and tumor antigens [2]. Among the numerous expression systems applied, alphavirus vectors have proven efficient for eliciting immune responses and protection against challenges with lethal doses of viral pathogens and cancer cells in various animal models [3]. Semliki Forest virus (SFV) [4], Sindbis virus (SIN) [5], and Venezuelan equine encephalitis virus (VEE) [6] are the most frequently used alphaviruses applied for immunization.

Three types of expression systems have been commonly engineered for alphaviruses (Fig. 1).

I. Replication-deficient recombinant particles are generated by in vitro transcription of RNA from expression and helper vectors followed by electroporation of mammalian host cells. The produced recombinant particles are capable of one round of infection of a broad host range of mammalian and nonmammalian cells, but

Maureen C. Ferran and Gary R. Skuse (eds.), *Recombinant Virus Vaccines: Methods and Protocols*, Methods in Molecular Biology, vol. 1581, DOI 10.1007/978-1-4939-6869-5_13, © Springer Science+Business Media LLC 2017

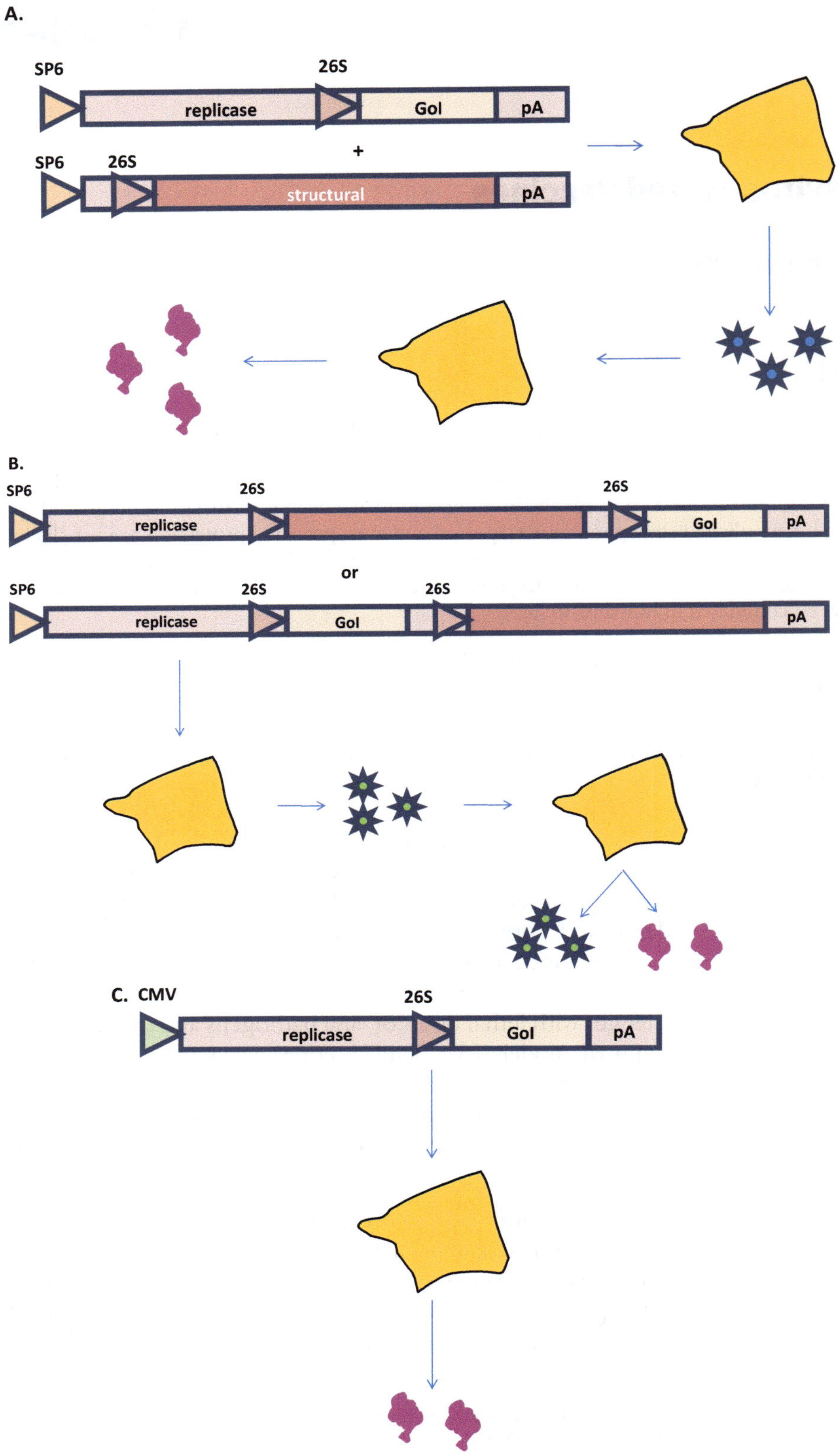
A.
SP6
26S
replicase
GoI
pA
+
SP6
26S
structural
pA
B.
SP6
26S
26S
replicase
GoI
pA
or
SP6
26S
26S
replicase
GoI
pA
C. CMV
26S
replicase
GoI
pA

because no RNA coding for the viral structural genes is present in the particles, no new virus progeny will be generated, but high level recombinant protein expression is obtained. **II. Replication-proficient recombinant particles** are produced from the full-length alphavirus RNA genome into which the gene of interest has been introduced either downstream of a second sub-genomic promoter or fused to one of the structural genes. Application of these vectors provides simultaneously transgene expression and production of virus progeny. **III. Layered DNA–RNA vectors** comprise plasmid DNA where the SP6 RNA polymerase promoter has been replaced by a CMV promoter which allows their direct use as transfectable plasmids. Additionally, DNA-based helper and full-length vectors have been engineered to allow for production of virus progeny.

Dependent on which target (i.e., cell lines, tissue) the best type of vector can be chosen. Moreover, in the context of immunization it is possible to choose between gene delivery by naked RNA replicons, recombinant particles or DNA plasmids for vaccine development (Fig. 2) [3]. For instance, influenza virus HA (hemagglutinin) [7] and NA (neuraminidase) [8], HIV envelope (Env) [9] and glycoprotein 41 (gp41) [10], and Ebola virus nucleoprotein (NP) [11] and glycoprotein (GP) [12] have been expressed from alphavirus vectors and subjected to immunization studies in a variety of animal models. Moreover, when primates were vaccinated with VEE particles protection from intramuscular and aerosol challenges with Ebola virus was obtained [13].

Recombinant alphavirus-based vaccines have applications beyond their use to immunize against pathogenic viruses. In relation to cancer vaccines, a number of cancer antigens have been subjected to immunization studies, resulting in therapeutic efficacy and protection against challenges with tumor cells in animal models [14]. When mice were immunized with VEE particles expressing the neu (neuroectodermal) gene, tumor regression was observed [15]. Likewise, protection of mice challenged with neu overexpressing cancer cells was achieved after immunization with SIN-HER2 (human epidermal growth factor receptor)/neu carrying DNA plasmids [16]. Moreover, complete tumor protection was obtained in mice after a single injection with SFV-LacZ (structural gene of the lac operon coding for β-galactosidase) RNA. Vaccination 2 days after tumor cell administration extended animal survival for 10–20 days [17].

Fig. 1 Alphavirus vector systems. Replication-deficient expression system (**a**). In vitro-transcribed RNA from expression and helper vectors is electroporated into mammalian host cells resulting in replication-deficient particles enabling transduction of a broad range of host cell for recombinant protein expression. However, no virus progeny is generated. Replication-proficient expression system (**b**). Transduction of full-length SFV RNA including insert of gene of interest (GoI) generates replication-proficient particles for both recombinant protein production and generation of new virus progeny. Layered DNA–RNA transfection system (**c**). Plasmid DNA vectors can be used for transfection of host cells for recombinant protein expression

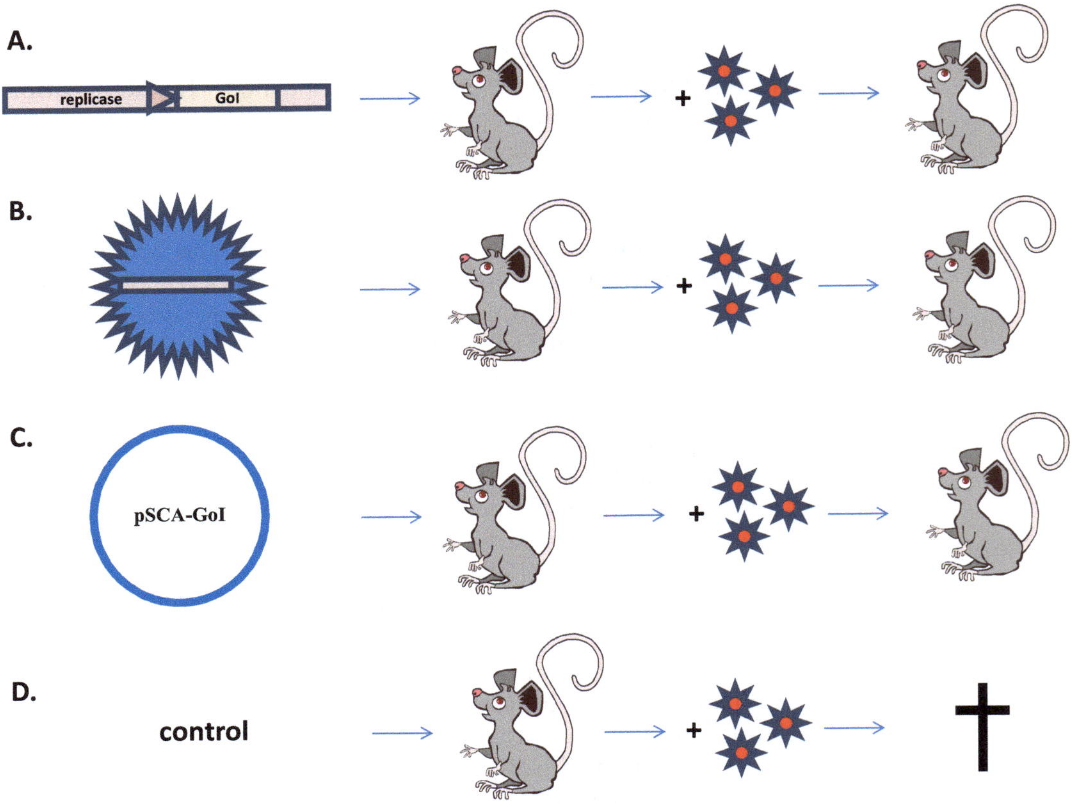

Fig. 2 Alphavirus immunization strategies. Immunization with RNA replicon (**a**), recombinant SFV particles (**b**), and layered DNA–RNA vector (**c**); control (**d**). Challenge with lethal dose of virus. *GoI* gene of interest

Alphaviruses have been identified as the cause of several recent epidemics [18], which has accelerated the development of vaccines. In this context, the live attenuated VEE V3526 vaccine provided protection against VEE challenges [19]. Moreover, a synthetic DNA vaccine has been engineered based on Chikungunya (CHIK) virus isolated from an acutely infected human patient [20].

Only a limited number of clinical vaccine trials have been conducted so far. Safety and immunogenicity was studied in volunteers subjected to subcutaneous injection of a serially passaged, plaque-purified live CHIK vaccine in a human phase II, randomized, double-blind, placebo-controlled study [21]. After vaccination, neutralizing antibodies were detected in 98% of the individuals and 85% of those remained seropositive a year later. In another study, VEE replicons expressing cytomegalovirus (CMV) gB or pp65/IE1 (immediate early protein 1) fusion proteins were subjected to a phase I randomized, double-blind clinical trial [22]. After intramuscular or subcutaneous administration, induced neutralizing antibodies and multifunctional T-cell responses were detected in CMV seronegative adult volunteers. Furthermore, patients with metastatic cancers were immunized with VEE replicons expressing the prostate-specific membrane antigen (PSMA) in another phase I clinical trial [23]. Disappointingly, the vaccination elicited only a weak PSMA-specific signal with no clinical benefits.

2 Materials

2.1 Reagents and Equipment

1. Restriction endonucleases *Nru*I, *Sap*I, *Spe*I.
2. 0.8% agarose gel.
3. Gel electrophoresis apparatus.
4. Phenol–chloroform–isoamyl alcohol 25:24:1 (v/v/v).
5. 3 M sodium acetate, pH 4.8.
6. 95% and 70% (v/v) ethanol.
7. 10× SP6 Buffer: 400 mM HEPES, pH 7.4, 60 mM magnesium acetate, 20 mM spermidine.
8. 10 mM m7G(5′) ppp (5′) G sodium salt (Roche Molecular Biochemicals).
9. 50 mM dithiothreitol (DTT).
10. rNTP Mix: 10 mM rATP, 10 mM rCTP, 10 mM rUTP, 5 mM rGTP.
11. 10–50 U/μl RNase inhibitor.
12. 10–20 U/μl SP6 RNA polymerase (Amersham Pharmacia Biotech).
13. RNase-free water (DEPC treated).
14. Phosphate buffered saline (PBS).
15. Trypsin–ethylenediamine tetraacetic acid (EDTA): 0.25% trypsin, 1 mM EDTA × 4 Na.
16. Sterile electroporation cuvettes, 0.2 and 0.4 cm (Bio-Rad or BTX).
17. Electroporator (Bio-Rad Gene Pulser).
18. Tissue culture flasks (T25, T75, and T175).
19. Microwell plates (6-, 12-, and 24-well plates).
20. Falcon tubes (15 and 50 ml).
21. Plastic syringes (1, 10, and 50 ml).
22. Sterile 0.22 μm filters.
23. MicroSpin™ S-200 HR Columns (Amersham).
24. Dulbecco's modified F-12 medium.
25. Iscove's modified Dulbecco's medium.
26. Opti-MEM I reduced-serum medium.
27. X-gal stock solution: 50 mM K ferricyanide, 50 mM K ferrocyanide, 1 M MgCl, 2% X-gal in DMF or DMSO.

28. X-gal staining solution: 1× PBS, 5 mM K ferricyanide, 5 mM K ferrocyanide, 2 mM MgCl, 1 mg/ml X-gal.
29. Moviol 4-88 containing 2.5% DABCO (1,4-diazobicyclo-[2.2.2]-octane).
30. Lysis buffer: 50 mM Tris–HCl pH 7.6, 150 mM NaCl, 2 mM EDTA, 1% (v/v) Nonidet P-40 (NP40).
31. Hybond ECL nitrocellulose filter.
32. TBST: Tris-buffered saline with 0.1% Tween 20.
33. ECL Chemiluminescence kit (Amersham).
34. Starvation medium: methionine-free MEM, 2 mM glutamine, 20 mM HEPES.
35. Chase medium: E-MEM, 2 mM glutamine, 20 mM HEPES, 150 μg/ml unlabelled methionine.

2.2 Cell Lines

The following cell lines are commonly used for alphavirus production and studies on expression of recombinant proteins:

1. BHK-21 cells (ATCC CCL-10) (Baby hamster kidney).
2. CHO-K1 cells (ATCC CCL-61) (Chinese hamster ovary).
3. COS7 cells (ATCC CRL-1651) (African green monkey kidney).
4. HEK293 cells (ATCC CRL-1573) (Human embryonic kidney).

2.3 Cell Culture Media

1. BHK-21, CHO-K1, and HEK293 cells are cultured in a 1:1 mixture of Dulbecco's modified F-12 medium (Gibco BRL) and Iscove's modified Dulbecco's medium (Gibco BRL) supplemented with 4 mM glutamine and 10% fetal calf serum (FCS).
2. COS7 cells are cultured in DMEM (Dulbecco's Modified Eagles Medium) supplemented with 5% fetal calf serum, 5 mM glutamine, and 0.1% penicillin/streptomycin.

2.4 Alphavirus Plasmid Vectors

As SFV-, SIN-, and VEE-based expression and helper vectors share common features the focus will be on SFV only here. The following vectors are applied for generation of replicon RNA and recombinant viral particles:

1. pSFV1 (basic vector, minimal cloning sites: *Bam*HI, *Sma*I) [4].
2. pSFV2gen (multilinker cloning sites: *Apa*I, *Bam*HI, *Xho*I, *Spe*I, *Sma*I) [24].
3. pSFV-Helper2 (second generation helper vector) [25].
4. pSFV4 (full-length vector) [26].
5. VA7(74) (full-length vector from avirulent strain) [27].
6. pSCA1 (layered DNA–RNA vector with CMV promoter) [28].
7. pSCA-Helper (layered DNA–RNA helper vector with CMV promoter) [29].
8. pCMV-SFV4 (full length layered DNA–RNA vector) [30].

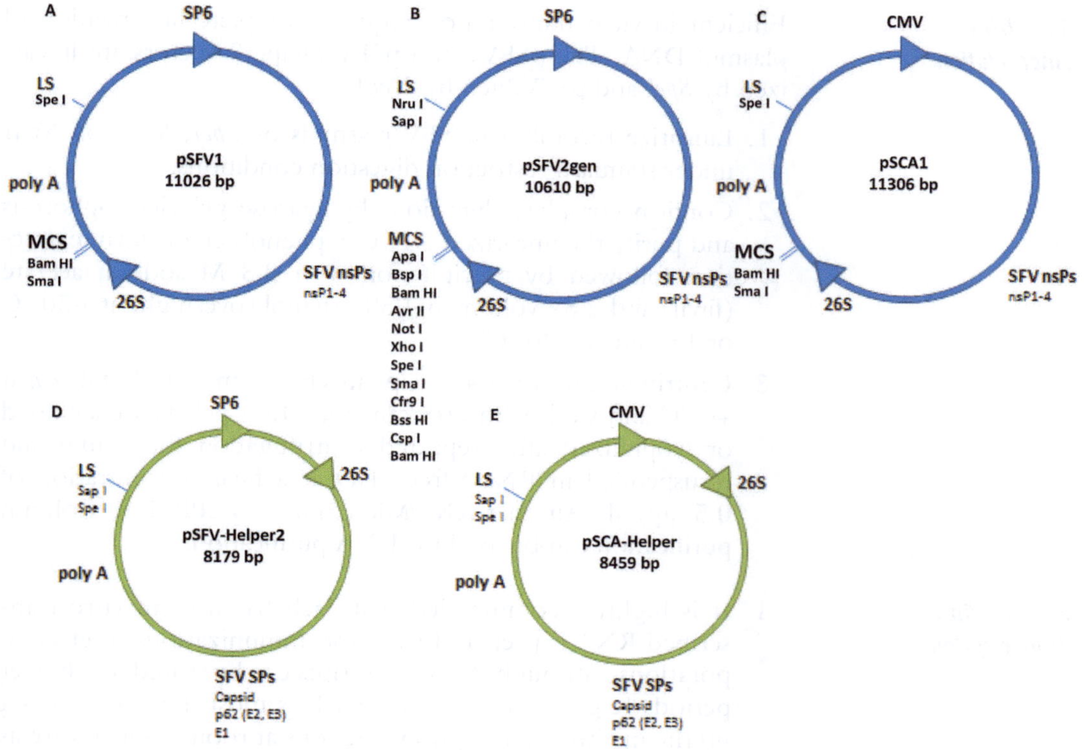

Fig. 3 SFV plasmid vector maps. Replication-deficient expression vectors pSFV1 (**a**) and pSFV2gen (**b**) and layered DNA–RNA vector pSCA1 (**c**). Helper vectors pSFV-Helper2 (**d**) and pSCA-Helper (**e**). *LS* linearization sites, *MCS* multiple cloning sites, *poly A* polyadenylation signal, *SFVnsPs* SFV nonstructural proteins, *SFVsPs* SFV structural proteins

Replication-deficient recombinant particles are generated from expression vectors pSFV1 or pSFV2gen (also called pSFV4.2) together with the pSFV-Helper2 vector, whereas pSFV4 or VA7(74) vectors are applied for the production of full-length replication-proficient particles (Fig. 3). Layered DNA–RNA vectors can be used directly for transfection of host cells for recombinant proteins or alternatively together with the layered DNA–RNA helper vector or as a full-length layered DNA–RNA vector for production of replication-proficient and deficient particles, respectively.

3 Methods

3.1 Subcloning into SFV Vectors

Genes of interest are introduced into the cloning sites of the chosen SFV expression vector and restriction endonuclease digestions and nucleotide sequencing are used for verification of inserts. Preparation of high purity DNA (Midiprep or Maxiprep DNA) is highly recommended to provide the best possible quality and yields of in vitro-transcribed RNA for immunization and/or recombinant viral particle production (*see* **Note 1**).

3.2 DNA Linearization

Efficient in vitro transcription requires complete linearization of plasmid DNA. The pSFV1 and pSFV-Helper2 vectors are linearized by *Spe*I and pSFV2gen by *Nru*I.

1. Linearize recombinant SFV plasmids by *Spe*I, *Sap*I, or *Nru*I under standard restriction digestion conditions.
2. Confirm complete digestions by agarose gel electrophoresis and purify the linearized DNA by phenol/chloroform extraction followed by precipitation with 0.3 M sodium acetate (final) and 2.5× volume of 95% ethanol (overnight at −20 °C or 15 min at −80 °C).
3. Centrifuge the ethanol precipitates for 15 min at 18,000 × *g* at +4 °C and wash with 70% ethanol. DNA pellets are air-dried or lyophilized after repeated centrifugation for 5 min and resuspended in RNase-free H_2O at a final concentration of 0.5 μg/μl. Alternatively, MicroSpin™ S-200 HR Column purification can be used for DNA purification.

3.3 In Vitro Transcription

1. It is highly recommended that each batch of in vitro-transcribed RNA is prepared fresh for immunizations or electroporations, although RNA transcripts can be stored for shorter periods (e.g., weeks) at −80 °C. It is most important to set up the in vitro transcription reactions at room temperature as the spermidine in the SP6 buffer might precipitate at lower temperatures. It is recommended that the optimized SP6 RNA polymerase buffer be used instead of available commercial in vitro transcription buffers (*see* **Note 2**). Add enzyme components last because they are the least stable reactants in the reaction.
2. In vitro transcription reaction

   5 μl (2.5 μg) linearized plasmid DNA.

   5 μl 10× SP6 buffer.

   5 μl 10 mM $m^7G(5')ppp(5')G$.

   5 μl 50 mM DTT.

   5 μl rNTP mix.

   x μl RNase-free H_2O to reach a final volume of 50 μl.

   1.5 μl (50 U/μl) RNase inhibitor.

   3.5 μl (20 U/μl) SP6 RNA polymerase.

1. Mix all reaction components and incubate for 1 h at 37 °C (*see* **Note 3**).
2. Assess the quality of in vitro-transcribed RNA by loading 1–4 μl aliquots on 0.8% agarose gels. High-quality RNA is visible as thick bands without smearing along the axis of migration with an approximate mobility of 8 kb (compared to DNA markers) from the expression vector and a slightly faster mobility of

helper RNA. Each in vitro transcription reaction is anticipated to generate 20–50 μg of RNA.

3. Apply in vitro-transcribed RNA directly to electroporation or lipid-mediated transfection. In case RNA transcripts are stored at −80 °C, the quality of RNA should be reevaluated by agarose gel electrophoresis before use.

3.4 Electroporation of RNA

Generally, the use of BHK-21 cells is preferred for alphavirus production as they are known to produce high-titer virus stocks. Alternative host cells can be considered, however, the process needs to be optimized for any other cell type employed. The following conditions have been found optimal for obtaining high-titer SFV stocks (e.g., 1×10^9 infectious particles/ml) in BHK-21 cells.

1. Culture cells with a low passage number in T175 flasks to no more than 80% confluency, wash once with PBS, and trypsinize with 6 ml trypsin–EDTA per T175 flask for 5 min at 37 °C.
2. Resuspend cells in 25 ml cell culture medium, centrifuge for 5 min at 800 × *g* and resuspend cell pellets in a small volume (<5 ml) of PBS.
3. Increase the volume to 25 ml with PBS and recentrifuge for 5 min at 800 × *g*.
4. Resuspend cells in approximately 2.5 ml PBS per T175 flask, equivalent to $1–2 \times 10^7$ cells per ml. Use cells immediately for electroporation although short term storage (<1 h) on ice is acceptable.
5. Transfer 0.4 ml BHK-21 cell suspension to 0.2 cm cuvettes (0.8 ml to 0.4 cm cuvettes). Add in vitro-transcribed recombinant RNA (20–45 μl) and helper RNA (20 μl) to the cell suspension and apply two consecutive pulses with the following settings for the Bio-Rad Gene Pulser:

	0.2 cm cuvette	0.4 cm cuvette
Capacitance extender	960 μF	960 μF
Voltage	1500 V	850 V
Capacitor	25 μF	25 μF
Resistance (pulse controller)	∝ Ω	Disconnected
Expected time constant (TC)	0.8 s	0.4 s

The Bio-Rad Gene Pulser II requires the following modifications:

- Set the pulse controller to "high range" and "∝."
- Set the capacitance rotary switch to "high capacitance."
- Apply the following settings: 360 V and 75 μF.
- The resistance for 0.2 cm cuvettes should be 10 Ω and the time constant 0.7–0.8 s.

6. Immediately dilute cells 25-fold in cell culture medium and transfer to T25 flasks or 100 mm culture plates for overnight incubation at 37 °C in an incubator with 5% CO_2.

3.5 Lipid-Mediated Transfection of RNA

Alternatively to electroporation, DMRIE-C and other transfection reagents can be used to transfect BHK-21, COS7, or CHO-K1 cells.

1. Culture BHK-21 cells ($1.5–3 \times 10^5$) in 35 mm petri dishes or on six-well plates to approximately 80% confluency.
2. Wash cells with Opti-MEM I reduced-serum medium.
3. To prepare the cationic lipid–RNA complexes:
   (a) For each transfection sample, add 0, 3, 6, 9, 12, or 15 μl of DMRIE-C to a 1.5 ml microcentrifuge tube containing 1 ml Opti-MEM I reduced-serum medium at room temperature.
   (b) Mix 10 μl (~5 μg) in vitro-transcribed recombinant RNA and 5 μl (~2.5 μg) helper RNA per sample to be transfected,
   (c) Add the RNA (15 μl total) to each tube containing the DMRIE and vortex briefly.
4. Add the lipid–RNA complex immediately to the cells and incubate at 37 °C for 4 h.
5. Replace the transfection medium with pre-warmed (37 °C) complete BHK medium and incubate the BHK-21 cells at 37 °C overnight in an incubator with 5% CO_2.

3.6 Harvest of Recombinant SFV Particles

Production of recombinant SFV particles occurs within the first 24 h resulting in titers of approximately 10^9 infectious particles/ml. The titers can be modestly increased by extending the incubation time by another 24 h.

1. Harvest virus particles by carefully removing the medium from the BHK-21 cells.
2. Sterilize and purify the virus stock by forcing the harvested medium through a 0.22 μm filter to remove cell debris and possible contaminants.
3. Aliquot virus stocks before storage at −20 °C (for weeks) or at −80 °C (for years) as repeated cycles of freezing and thawing can reduce the titers significantly.

3.7 Activation of Recombinant SFV Particles

Although the conventional pSFV-helper vector has been used it is recommended to utilize the second generation vector pSFV-Helper2 [25]. In contrast to SFV particles generated with the pSFV-helper vector, the particles produced with pSFV-Helper2 are conditionally infectious and thereby prevent accumulation of replication-proficient particles through recombination. Instead, particles generated with pSFV-Helper2 need to be activated as described below.

1. Activate particles by addition of α-chymotrypsin at a final concentration of 500 μg/ml for 20 min at room temperature.
2. Terminate the reaction by adding aprotinin (trypsin inhibitor) at a final concentration of 250 μg/ml

3.8 Verification of Virus Titers

The titers of replication-proficient virus can be verified by standard plaque assay methods [31]. In contrast, replication-deficient particles that do not generate plaques place restrictions on titer determination. Instead, indirect titer estimations are possible by determining of the number of infected cells visualized by reporter gene expression.

1. Culture BHK-21 (or other) cells to a defined confluency on 6- or 12-well plates or on sterile coverslips before infection with serial dilutions (e.g., fivefold dilutions in the range expected to give 20–50 positive cells per microscope field) of virus stocks expressing green fluorescent protein (GFP) or β-galactosidase.
2. Count cells expressing the reporter gene (fluorescent or stained cells, *see* below) after 24 h incubation at 37 °C. Certain SFV mutant vectors may provide a weak signal at 24 h post-infection and should be incubated for 48 h to reach optimal expression levels (*see* **Note 4**).

3.8.1 GFP Detection

1. Count the number of GFP positive cells applying fluorescence microscopy.
2. Estimate the approximate titers as infectious particles/ml based on the number of GFP.
   - Positive cells per well, taking into account the virus dilution.

3.8.2 X-Gal Staining

1. Wash SFV-infected cells with PBS, fix in cold methanol (99.8%) at −20 °C for 5 min and wash again three times with PBS.
2. Stain cells for at least 2 h in X-gal staining solution at 37 °C or at room temperature.
3. Count the number of β-galactosidase (blue) positive cells applying light microscopy.
4. Estimate the approximate titers as described for GFP detection above.

3.8.3 Immunofluorescence

If antibodies are available against the recombinant protein itself, or against tags engineered in the vector construct, immunofluorescence methods can be applied for titer determination.

1. Culture SFV-infected cells on sterile coverslips, rinse twice with PBS and fix for 6 min at −20 °C in methanol.

2. Wash coverslips three times in PBS and incubate for 30 min at room temperature in PBS containing 0.5% gelatin and 0.25% BSA to prevent nonspecific binding.
3. Replace the blocking buffer with a primary antibody in the same buffer for 30 min at room temperature.
4. Wash three times with PBS and incubate with a secondary antibody for 30 min at room temperature.
5. Wash coverslips again three times with PBS, once more with H_2O, and air-dry.
6. Mount the coverslips on glass slides using 10 μl Moviol 4-88 containing 2.5% DABCO (1,4-diazobicyclo-[2.2.2]-octane), count the number of positive cells and estimate the titers as described for GFP detection above.

As alphavirus infections cause changes to the cell morphology (i.e., they round up) microscopic examination can also be applied to provide an approximate estimate of titers. Similar to fluorescence and staining (described above) the titers can be estimated by counting the number of rounded cells.

3.8.4 RT-PCR-Based Titer Determination

Another alternative for titer determination is to apply RT-PCR [32].

1. Extract RNA from SFV stocks using the RNeasy Kit (Qiagen).
2. Apply qRT-PCR for sequence amplification within the nsP1 gene of SFV.
3. Make a serial dilution of pSFV plasmid DNA to obtain a standard curve for SFV-RNA.
4. Apply mean Cts to a standard curve equation to determine the cDNA copy number in each sample.
5. Calculate the total SFV RNA copy number present in the original SFV sample by multiplying the cDNA copy number by the conversion factor specific to each sample considering all dilutions made and the yield of RNA extraction.

3.9 Evaluation of Gene Expression

Initial confirmation of recombinant protein expression is recommended before proceeding to immunization studies. It enables verification of expression levels and the size of gene products. Expression evaluation can be performed by Western blotting if antibodies are available against the target protein or the tag fusions engineered. Alternatively, expression can be evaluated by metabolic labeling of SFV-infected cells with ^{35}S-methionine.

3.9.1 Western Blotting

1. Infect host cells (BHK-21, CHO-K1, HEK293) cultured on 6-, 12-, or 24-well plates with serial dilutions of virus stocks and incubate for 1–2 days at 37 °C.
2. Lyse cells with 250, 125, and 62.5 μl of lysis buffer per 6-, 12-, and 24-well plate, respectively. Incubate for 10 min on ice

and load samples on to 10–12% SDS-PAGE s. PAGE = polyacrylamide gel electrophoresis

3. Transfer electrophoresed protein material to Hybond ECL nitrocellulose filters for 30 min.
4. Treat filters with 5% nonfat dry milk in TBST at +4 °C for 30 min followed by primary and secondary antibody treatment, each for 30 min at room temperature.
5. Visualize specific bands with the ECL Chemiluminescence kit.

3.9.2 Metabolic Labeling

1. Infect host cells (BHK-21, CHO-K1, or HEK293) cultured on 6-, 12-, or 24-well plates with serial dilutions of virus stocks and incubate for 1–2 days at 37 °C.
2. Remove the medium, wash cells once with PBS, and add Starvation medium. Incubate for 30 min at 37 °C.
3. Replace the medium with Starvation medium containing 50–100 μCi/ml of ^{35}S methionine. Incubate for 20 min at 37 °C.
4. Remove the medium, wash cells twice with PBS, and add Chase medium for appropriate time (e.g., 15 min to 3 h).
5. Remove the Chase medium, wash cells once with PBS, add 250 μl lysis buffer per six-well plate, and incubate for 10 min on ice.
6. Load samples on 10–12% SDS-PAGE under standard conditions, fix in 10% acetic acid, 30% methanol for 30 min at room temperature and replace with Amplify® for 30 min at room temperature.
7. Dry the gel and expose on Hyperfilm-MP for 2–24 h (depending on signal) at room temperature or at −80 °C applying radioactivity-intensifying screens for visualization (*see* **Note 5**).

3.10 Virus Stock Purification

Although alphavirus particles are ready to use for expression in cell lines after a single filter-sterilization procedure, in vivo applications for immunization in animal models gain from additional purification steps. Moreover, rigid purification procedures are mandatory for application of alphavirus particles for clinical trials. For this purpose, various methods based on ultracentrifugation and affinity chromatography can be employed as described below.

3.10.1 Ultracentrifugation of Virus Stocks

1. Prepare a step gradient in ultracentrifuge tubes by addition of 1 ml of 50% sucrose solution (bottom) and 3 ml of 20% sucrose solution (top).
2. Add virus stock solution (9 ml for SW 40 Ti or 8 ml for SW 41 Ti) onto the sucrose gradient.
3. Centrifuge at 160,000 x *g* (30,000 rpm in SW 40 Ti or SW41 Ti rotor) for 90 min at +4 °C.

4. Collect the virus settled near the interface between the 20% and 50% sucrose layers by discarding the medium fraction and the bottom 0.8 ml consisting of 50% sucrose.

3.10.2 Centriprep Concentration

1. Load virus stocks onto the sample container of the Centriprep concentrator as described by the manufacturer.
2. Centrifuge the assembled concentrator at an appropriate *g*-force (according to the manufacturer's recommendations), until the fluid levels inside and outside the filtrate collector equilibrate.
3. Remove the device, snap off the airtight seal cap, decant the filtrate, replace the cap, and centrifuge the concentrator a second time.
4. Decant the filtrate, loosen the twist-lock cap, and remove the filtrate collector.
5. Collect the concentrated virus sample with a 1 ml disposable plastic pipette. If further concentration of virus is desired, centrifuge again after decanting the filtrate.

3.10.3 Affinity Chromatography Concentration

Matrex® Cellufine™ Sulfate columns allows for efficient removal of endotoxins and other contaminants and provide a convenient procedure for concentrating virus stocks. The manufacturer's recommendations should be followed as described below.

1. Equilibrate the affinity matrix column with adsorption buffer (0.01 M phosphate, 0.1 M NaCl, pH 7.5) and load samples at pH 7.5.
2. Wash the column with several bed volumes of adsorption buffer to remove nonbinding contaminants and elute the concentrated virus with elution buffer (1–2 M NaCl or KCl).

3.11 Immunizations

In the context of vaccine development, a large number of immunization studies have been conducted with alphaviruses [3]. The type of vector used will obviously dictate the immunization procedure; as the requirements for delivery varies between RNA replicons, recombinant viral particles and layered DNA–RNA vectors. Therefore, the various immunization methods used to immunize different hosts are described below.

3.11.1 Immunization of Mice with RNA

In the case of applying RNA replicons for immunization experiments in mice, in vitro-transcribed RNA can be directly used for administration as follows [17].

1. Administer 100 μg of in vitro-transcribed SFV-LacZ RNA intramuscularly into BALB/c mice.
2. Evaluate the immune response by monitoring the presence of IgG antibodies against recombinant β-galactosidase protein by ELISA 21 days post-injection.

3. Isolate splenocytes 21 days after immunization and restimulate in vitro for 6 days in the presence of Ld-restricted peptide β-gal 876–884 (1 μg/ml) for monitoring of β-galactosidase-specific $CD8^+$ T cell recognition.

Evaluation of tumor protection of mice immunized with in vitro-transcribed RNA can be performed as follows.

1. Administer mice intravenously with 5×10^5 CT26.CL25 tumor cells (from mouse colon) and evaluate tumor protection 21 days post-immunization.
2. Count the number of pulmonary metastases after 12 days.
3. In case of preestablished tumors, inject BALB/c mice intravenously with 1×10^5 CT26.CL25 cells and grow tumors for 2 days before immunization with 100 μg SFV-LacZ RNA.
4. Assess the animals for survival.

3.11.2 Immunization of Mice with Recombinant VEE Particles

1. Dilute 10^6 VEE particles in PBS and inject subcutaneously into the plantar surface of each footpad of C57BL/6 mice three times at 2 weeks intervals [33].
2. Challenge vaccinated mice with 7.5×10^4 B16F10 tumor cells (from mouse melanoma) intradermally 2 weeks after immunization for tumor protection evaluation.
3. Address therapeutic efficacy by an initial inoculation of 7.5×10^4 B16F10 tumor cells (either intradermally or intravenously) followed by 3 weekly vaccinations with VEE particles.

3.11.3 Immunization of Macaques with Recombinant VEE Particles

1. Inoculate intramuscularly 10^{10} VEE-EBOV GP focus forming units (FFUs) in the quadriceps muscle of naïve cynomolgus macaques for vaccine development against Ebola virus [13].
2. Challenge vaccinated animals intramuscularly and intranasally with approximately 1000 PFU of Ebola virus and monitor closely for at least 28 days.

3.11.4 DNA Immunization of C57BL/6 mice with DNA

1. Immunize C57BL/6 mice with 3 μg layered DNA–RNA plasmid vectors by five weekly intramuscular injections, which can be enhanced by plasmid-coated gold particles applying gene gun technology [34].
2. Inoculate mice with 1×10^5 B16F10 tumor cells 1 week after the last immunization and monitor tumor growth for at least 3 weeks.

3.11.5 DNA Immunization of BALB/c Mice with Recombinant VEE Particles

1. Dilute SFV plasmid DNA vectors expressing membrane proteins PrM and E of Murray Valley encephalitis virus (MVE) in saline to a concentration of 1 mg/ml and 100–125 mg DNA doses and inject intramuscularly into BALB/c mice [35].

2. Challenge immunized mice intraperitoneally with 1.3×10^8 PFU of MVE and observe signs of encephalitis for 21 days. Alternatively, immunize intramuscularly SPF mice with 100 mg DNA into multiple sites in the hind leg muscles and boost after 21 days.
3. Challenge mice intracranially with 1000 TCID50 of MVE 2 weeks after the final immunization and monitor for signs of encephalitis for 21 days.

3.12 Conclusions

Alphavirus vectors have been engineered as RNA replicons, recombinant viral particles, and layered DNA–RNA plasmids for efficient expression of recombinant proteins. Moreover, alphaviruses have been subjected to expression of antigens to elicit immune responses in various animal models. In this context, overexpression of viral and tumor antigens from alphavirus RNA replicons, recombinant particles, and layered DNA–RNA vectors has generated strong immune responses in rodents and primates. Furthermore, immunization has provided protection against challenges with lethal doses of viruses and tumor cells in vaccinated animals. The rapid RNA and virus production, high transgene expression, and strong immune responses make alphaviruses attractive vectors for vaccine development.

4 Notes

1. High purity plasmid DNA preparations are essential for the production of both high quality and quantity of in vitro-transcribed RNA.
2. In vitro transcription yields can be optimized by titration of the CAP analogue $m^7G(5')ppp(5')G$ concentration and the use of appropriate transcription buffer. Although commercially available buffers might generate superior RNA yields, the quality is not always compatible with high titer virus production.
3. Special attention should be paid to the size of genes introduced into the expression vector as it might affect the RNA yields. Inserts exceeding 4 kb generally reduces the RNA yields. This can to some extent be compensated for by extension of the incubation time for in vitro transcription reactions.
4. Alphaviruses cause cytopathic effects on host cells, which may reduce the time of host cell survival and reduce transgene expression levels. A number of mutant SFV [36] and SIN [37] vectors have been engineered to address these problems, which might also be used for enhanced efficacy in immunization studies. Additionally, vectors with translation enhancement signals have been developed for increased expression levels [38].

5. Radioactive signals of ^{35}S methionine from SDS-PAGE can efficiently be enhanced by application of X-ray intensifying screens [39]. Cassettes for film exposure are equipped with double-sided screens, which enhance the radioactive signal.

References

1. Deng MP, Hu ZH, Wang HL, Deng F (2012) Developments of subunit and VLP vaccines against influenza A virus. Virol Sin 27:145–153
2. Butterfield LH (2015) Cancer vaccines. Br Med J 350:h988
3. Lundstrom K (2014) Alphavirus-based vaccines. Viruses 6:2392–2415
4. Liljestrom P, Garoff H (1991) A new generation of animal cell expression vectors based on the Semliki Forest virus replicon. Bio/Technology 9:1356–1361
5. Xiong C, Levis R, Shen P, Schlesinger S, Rice CM, Huang HV (1989) Sindbis virus: an efficient, broad host range vector for gene expression in animal cells. Science 243:1188–1191
6. Davies NL, Brown KW, Johnston RE (1989) In vitro synthesis of infectious Venezuelan equine encephalitis virus RNA from a cDNA clone: analysis of a viable deletion mutant. Virology 171:189–204
7. Schultz-Cherry S, Dybing JK, Davis NL, Williamson C, Suarez DL, Johnston R, Perdue ML (2000) Influenza virus (A/HK/156/97) hemagglutinin expressed by an alphavirus replicon system protects against lethal infection with Hong Kong-origin H5N1 viruses. Virology 278:55–59
8. Zhou X, Berglund P, Rhodes G, Parker SE, Jondal M, Liljestrom P (1994) Self-replicating Semliki Forest virus RNA as recombinant vaccine. Vaccine 12:1510–1514
9. Brand D, Lemiale F, Turbica I, Buzelay L, Brunet S, Barin F (2000) Comparative analysis of humoral immune responses to HIV type 1 envelope glycoproteins in mice immunized with a DNA vaccine, recombinant Semliki Forest virus RNA, or recombinant Semliki Forest virus particles. AIDS Res Hum Retroviruses 14:1369–1377
10. Giraud A, Ataman-Onal Y, Battail N, Piga N, Brand D, Mandrand B, Verrier B (1999) Generation of monoclonal antibodies to native human immunodeficiency virus type 1 envelope glycoprotein by immunization of mice with naked RNA. J Virol Methods 79:75–84
11. Wilson JA, Hart MK (2001) Protection from Ebola virus mediated by cytotoxic T-lymphocytes specific for the viral nucleoprotein. J Virol 75:2660–2664
12. Pushko P, Bray M, Ludwig GV, Parker M, Schmaljohn A, Sanchez A, Jahrling PB, Smith JF (2000) Recombinant RNA replicons derived from attenuated Venezuelan equine encephalitis virus protect guinea pigs and mice from Ebola hemorrhagic fever virus. Vaccine 19:142–153
13. Herbert AS, Kuehne AI, Barth JF, Ortiz RA, Nichols DK, Zak SE, Stonier SW, Muhammad MA, Bakken RR, Prugar LI, Olinger GG, Groebner JL, Lee JS, Pratt WD, Custer M, Kamrud KI, Smith JF, Hart MK, Dye JM (2013) Venezuelan equine encephalitis virus replicon particle vaccine protects nonhuman primates from intramuscular and aerosol challenge with Ebolavirus. J Virol 87:4952–4964
14. Lundstrom K (2015) Alphaviruses in gene therapy. Viruses 7:2321–2333
15. Moran TP, Burgents JE, Long B, Ferrer I, Jaffee EM, Tisch RM, Johnston R, Serody JS (2007) Alphaviral vector-transduced dendritic cells are successful therapeutic vaccines against neu-overexpressing tumors in wild-type mice. Vaccine 25:6604–6612
16. Lachman LB, Rao XM, Kremer RH, Ozpolat B, Kiriakova G, Price JE (2001) DNA vaccination against neu reduces breast cancer incidence and metastasis in mice. Cancer Gene Ther 8:259–268
17. Ying H, Zaks TZ, Wang RF, Irvine KR, Kammula US, Marincola FM, Leitner WW, Restifo NP (1999) Cancer therapy using a self-replicating RNA vaccine. Nat Med 5:823–827
18. Jansen KA (2013) The 2005–2007 Chikungunya epidemic in Reunion: ambiguous etiologies, memories, and meaning-making. Med Anthropol 32:174–189
19. Hart MK, Caswell-Stephan K, Bakken R, Tammariello R, Pratt W, Davis N, Johnston RE, Smith J, Steele K (2000) Improved mucosal protection against Venezuelan equine encephalitis virus is induced by the molecularly defined, live-attenuated V3526 vaccine candidate. Vaccine 18:3067–3075
20. Mallilankaraman K, Shedlock DJ, Bao H, Kawalekar OU, Fagone P, Ramanathan AA, Ferraro B, Stabenow J, Vijayachari P, Sundaram SG, Muruganandam N, Sarangan G, Srikanth P, Khan AS, Lewis MG, Kim JJ, Sardesai NY,

Muthumani K, Weiner DB (2011) A DNA vaccine against chikungunya virus is protective in mice and induces neutralizing antibodies in mice and nonhuman primates. PLoS Negl Trop Dis 5:e928

21. Edelman R, Tacket CO, Wasserman SS, Bodison SA, Perry JG, Mangiafico JA (2000) Phase II safety and immunogenicity study of live chikungunya virus vaccine TSI-GSD-218. Am J Trop Med Hyg 62:681–685
22. Bernstein DI, Reap EA, Katen K, Watson A, Smith K, Norberg P, Olmsted RA, Hoeper A, Morris J, Negri S, Maughan MF, Chulay JD (2009) Randomized, double-blind, Phase 1 trial of an alphavirus replicon vaccine for cytomegalovirus in CMV seronegative adult volunteers. Vaccine 28:484–493
23. Slovin SF, Kehoe M, Durso R, Fernandez C, Olson W, Gao JP, Israel R, Sher HI, Morris S (2013) A phase I dose escalation trial of vaccine replicon particles (VRP) expressing prostate-specific membrane antigen (PSMA) in subjects with prostate cancer. Vaccine 31:943–949
24. Schweitzer C, Kratzeisen C, Adam G, Lundstrom K, Malherbe P, Ohresser S, Stadler H, Wichmann J, Woltering T, Mutel V (2000) Characterization of [^{3}H] LY-354740 binding of rat $mGlu_2$ and $mGlu_3$ receptors expressed in CHO cells using Semliki Forest virus vectors. Neuropharmacology 39:1700–1706
25. Berglund P, Sjöberg M, Garoff H, Atkins GJ, Sheahan BJ, Liljestrom P (1993) Semliki Forest virus expression system: production of conditionally infectious recombinant particles. Bio/Technology 11:916–920
26. Lijestrom P, Lusa S, Huylebroeck D, Garoff H (1991) In vitro mutagenesis of a full-length cDNA clone of Semliki Forest virus: the small 6,000-molecular weight membrane protein modulates virus release. J Virol 65:4107–4113
27. Vähä-Koskela MJ, Tuittila MT, Nygardas PT, Nyman JK, Ehrengruber MU, Renggli M, Hinkkanen AE (2003) A novel neurotropic expression vector based on the avirulent A7(74) strain of Semliki Forest virus. J Neurovirol 9:1–15
28. DiCiommo DP, Bremner R (1998) Rapid, high-level protein production using DNA-based Semliki Forest virus vectors. J Biol Chem 273:18060–18066
29. DiCiommo DP, Duckett A, Burcescu I, Bremner R, Gallie BR (2004) Retinoblastoma protein purification and transduction of retina and retinoblastoma cells using improved alphavirus vectors. Invest Ophthalmol Vis Sci 45:3320–3329
30. Ulper L, Sarand I, Rausalu K, Merits A (2008) Construction, properties, and potential application of infectious plasmids containing Semliki Forest virus full-length cDNA with a n inserted intron. J Virol Methods 148:265–270
31. Puglia AL, Rezende AG, Jorge SA, Wagner R, Pereira CA, Astray RM (2013) Quantitative RT-PCR for titration of replication-defective recombinant Semliki Forest virus. J Virol Methods 193:647–652
32. Juare D, Long KC, Aguilar P, Kochel TJ, Halsey JS (2013) Assessment of plaque assay methods for alphaviruses. J Virol Methods 187:185–189
33. Avogadri F, Merghoub T, Maughan MF, Hirschhorn-Cymerman D, Morris J, Ritter E, Olmsted R, Houghton AN, Wolchok DJ (2010) Alphavirus replicon particles expressing TRP-2 provide potent therapeutic effect on melanoma through activation of humoral and cellular immunity. PLoS One 5:e12670
34. Leitner WW, Hwang NL, de Veer MJ, Zhou A, Silverman RH, Williams BR, Dubensky TW, Ying H, Restifo NP (2003) Alphavirus-based DNA vaccine breaks immunological tolerance by activating innate antiviral pathways. Nat Med 5:33–39
35. Colombage G, Hall R, Pavy M, Lobigs M (1998) DNA-based and alphavirus-vectored immunization with PrM and E proteins elicits long-lived and protective immunity against the flavivirus, Murray Valley encephalitis virus. Virology 250:151–163
36. Lundstrom K, Abenavoli A, Malgaroli A, Ehrengruber MU (2003) Novel Semliki Forest virus vectors with reduced toxicity and temperature-sensitivity for long-term enhancement of transgene expression. Mol Ther 7:202–209
37. Agapov EV, Frolov I, Lindenbach BD, Pragal PM, Schlesinger S, Rice CM (1998) Noncythopathic Sindbis virus RNA vectors for heterologous gene expression. Proc Natl Acad Sci U S A 95:12989–12994
38. Sjöberg EM, Suomalainen M, Garoff H (1994) A significantly improved Semliki Forest virus expression system based on translation enhancer segments from the viral capsid gene. Bio/Technology 12:1127–1131
39. Voytas, D, and Ke, N, (2001) Detection and quantitation of radiolabeled proteins and DNA in gels and blot. Curr Protoc Mol Biol, Appendix 3, 3A

Part IV

Bacteriophage

Chapter 14

Display of HIV-1 Envelope Protein on Lambda Phage Scaffold as a Vaccine Platform

Jonelle L. Mattiacio, Matt Brewer, and Stephen Dewhurst

Abstract

The generation of a strong antibody response to target antigens is a major goal for vaccine development. Here we describe the display of the human immunodeficiency virus (HIV) envelope spike protein (Env) on a virus-like scaffold provided by the lambda phage capsid. Phage vectors, in general, have advantages over mammalian virus vectors due to their genetic tractability, inexpensive production, suitability for scale-up, as well as their physical stability, making them an attractive vaccine platform.

Key words Bacteriophage lambda, Virus-like particle, Envelope protein

1 Introduction

The generation of a robust, neutralizing antibody response to virus infection is a major goal of vaccine research. Low spike immunogenicity, like that for HIV, complicates the generation of broadly neutralizing antibodies [1–3]. The repetitive, high density display of viral surface proteins can result in greatly increased immune responses and has been exemplified by the success of virus-like particles (VLPs) or nanoparticles both for hepatitis B virus [4] and human papillomavirus (HPV) [5–7] and more recently with the obligate intracellular parasite *Toxoplasma gondii* [8]. Bacteriophage vectors are being explored as VLP-like scaffolds for vaccine applications and have been experimentally administered to animals and safely used in humans for several decades, for the treatment of bacterial infections [9] and the assessment of immune responses in immunocompromised individuals [10]. Phage capsids have the flexibility to be used to display not only short peptides but also intact proteins. Systems have been developed for lambda phage that permit the display of foreign proteins by fusing them to the gpD major coat protein [11–14]. gpD is a trimeric, 109 amino acid protein that is required for the packaging of full-length genomes. Lambda gpD is unusual, however, among phage display

Maureen C. Ferran and Gary R. Skuse (eds.), *Recombinant Virus Vaccines: Methods and Protocols*, Methods in Molecular Biology, vol. 1581, DOI 10.1007/978-1-4939-6869-5_14, © Springer Science+Business Media LLC 2017

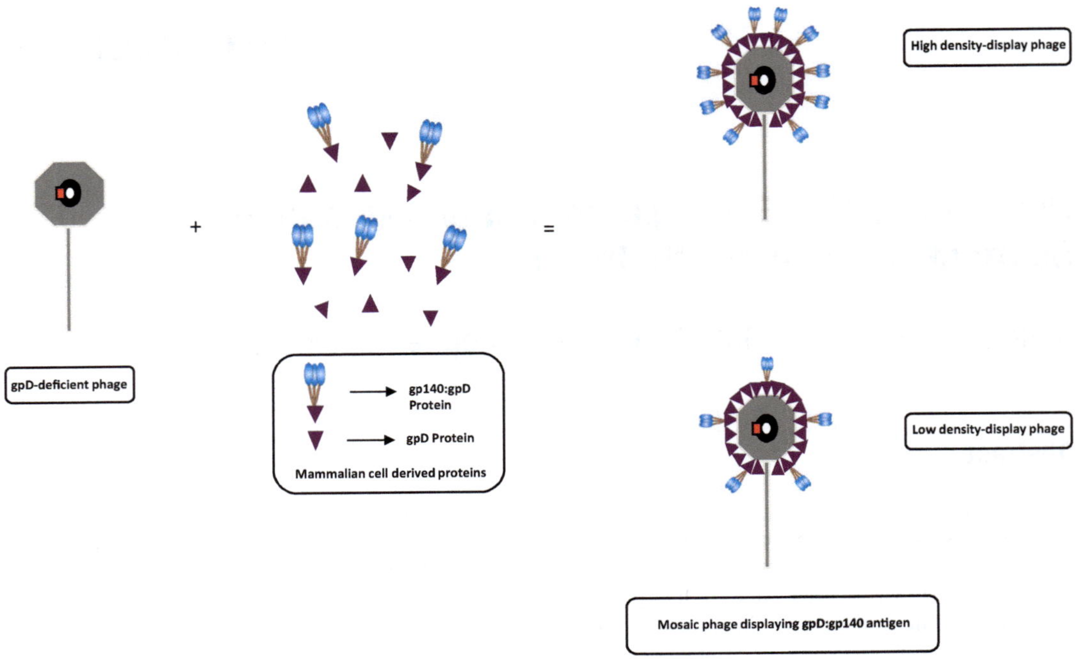

Fig. 1 Schematic diagram of the in vitro decoration of gpD deficient lambda phage particles with recombinant gpD and gp140:gpD fusion proteins. gpD-deficient phage are decorated with mammalian derived gpD and gp140:gpD fusion protein at different ratios to produce phage particles displaying gp140:gpD at either high (10:1) or low density (1:1), relative to wildtype gpD

systems in being tolerant of large peptides or fusion proteins, which can then be displayed at high copy number and density. gpD-deficient lambda phage capsids can also be decorated in vitro with exogenously supplied gpD, which allows for considerable flexibility with respect to the display of antigens such as the highly glycosylated envelope spike protein of HIV-1 or the hemagglutinin (HA) of influenza A virus. Here, we describe a simple in vitro complementation system to decorate lambda phage capsids with mammalian cell-derived HIV-1 envelope spike protein (Fig. 1). Very similar methods can also be used to derive phage capsids bearing mammalian cell-derived influenza A virus hemagglutinin (HA) or other proteins of interest, not only for vaccination purposes, but also for detection of antigen-specific serologic responses (e.g., detection of hemagglutination-inhibition antibodies) [14].

2 Materials

Prepare all solutions using ultrapure water and analytical grade reagents. Store all reagents at room temperature, unless otherwise indicated.

2.1 Envgp140, Envgp140:gpD, and gpD Protein Expression and Purification

1. A human codon-optimized derivative of the clade B HIV-1 isolate YU2 envelope gene, and the wild type λ gpD gene (synthesized by GeneArt, Regensburg, Germany). *See* Subheading 3.1 for more details on these constructs.
2. pcDNA3 mammalian expression vector (Invitrogen).
3. Freestyle™ 293 Expression System (Invitrogen): HEK293-F cells (293F), Freestyle 293 Expression Medium, Freestyle Max reagent.
4. Ni-NTA resin (Qiagen).
5. Ni-NTA wash buffer (4×): 50 ml of 50 mM sodium phosphate buffer pH 8.0, 17.53 g NaCl, 1.36 g imidazole. Add water to a volume of 250 ml and filter-sterilize or autoclave. Dilute 125 ml 4× wash buffer into 375 ml double distilled water and filter-sterilize for 1× wash buffer (20 mM imidazole). Prepare a stock of 3 M imidazole and filter-sterilize or autoclave. For 1× wash buffer (40 mM imidazole), dilute 125 ml of 4× wash buffer and 3.2 ml of 3 M imidazole into 371.8 ml double distilled water and filter-sterilize. For 1× elution buffer (250 mM imidazole) dilute 125 ml of 4× wash buffer and 41.7 ml of 3 M imidazole into 333.3 ml water and filter-sterilize. Store all 1× buffers at 4 °C.
6. Dialysis buffer: 50 mM Tris–HCl pH 8.0, 10 mM NaCl, 10 mM $MgCl_2$. Prepare 2 L of solution, adjust the pH to 8.0, autoclave and store at 4 °C.
7. Slide-A-Lyzer cassettes 10K/30K MWCO (Thermo Fisher).
8. Amicon Ultra centrifugal filter devices 10K/30K MWCO (Millipore).

2.2 Generation of Decorated Bacteriophage Particles

1. *E. coli* TOP10 competent cells (Invitrogen).
2. NZCYM (Difco): Dissolve 22 g of powder per 1 L of water and autoclave at 121 °C for 15 min.
3. Phage suspension media (SM with gelatin): 50 mM Tris–HCl pH 7.5, 100 mM NaCl, 10 mM $MgSO_4$, 0.01% gelatin. Weigh 5.8 g NaCl and 7.3 g $MgSO_4 \cdot 7H_2O$ and mix with 25 ml of 2 M Tris–HCl (pH 7.5) and 5 ml 2% w/v gelatin. Bring to 1 L with water and autoclave.
4. DNase I (Code DPRF, catalog number LS006333, Worthington Biochemical Corporation, Lakewood, NJ): Dissolve entire 10,000 unit vial in 5 ml of buffer (2 M Tris–HCl pH 8, 1 mM $MgCl_2$, 50 mM NaCl, 80% glycerol) for 1 mg/ml final concentration solution.
5. CsCl solution (in SM with gelatin): Weigh 178.57 g of molecular grade CsCl and add 250 ml SM with gelatin. Filter-sterilize using a 0.45 μm filter. It is best to prepare a 50 ml batch fresh each time and not use after 1 week old.

6. Quick-Seal®, polypropylene, 13.5 ml 16 × 76 mm ultracentrifuge tubes (Beckman Coulter catalog number 342413).
7. Phage dialysis buffer: 50 mM Tris–HCl pH 8.0, 10 mM NaCl, 10 mM $MgCl_2$. Mix 6 ml of 5 M NaCl, 75 ml of 2 M Tris–HCl (pH 8.0) and 30 ml of 1 M $MgCl_2$. Bring the volume up to 3 L with water, autoclave and store at 4 °C.
8. LB phage plates: Weigh 20 g of LB Broth and 15 g of Bacto agar in a flask. Bring volume to 1 L with water and autoclave. Pour 7 ml into each plate (normally makes 6–7 sleeves of plates) and store at 4 °C.
9. Top agar: Weigh 20 g of LB Broth, 1 g $MgCl_2$ and 7 g of Bacto agar in a flask. Bring the volume to 1 L with water and autoclave. Pour slightly cooled agar into 4 × 250 ml bottles and store at room temperature. Before use, microwave in 1 min intervals to melt the agar completely and place in a 55 °C water bath until ready to use.
10. LE392 (*supE*, *supF*) *E. coli* host cells (Stratagene).
11. Tris–MgCl buffer (TM): 10 mM Tris, pH 7.5, 10 mM $MgCl_2$. Tris buffer with EDTA (TE): 10 mM Tris, pH 7.5, 100 mM EDTA.
12. EndoTrap red® Endotoxin Removal kit (Hyglos GmbH, Germany).

3 Methods

3.1 Cloning Envelope Glycoprotein into −/+ gpD Expression Plasmids

To generate mammalian expression constructs, HIV-Envgp140, Envgp140:gpD fusion and gpD were all cloned into the multiple cloning site of pcDNA3 vector. *See* Mattiacio et al. [15] for further details on these constructs.

1. To generate a mammalian expression construct that encodes a cleavage deficient, trimeric HIV-Envgp140, fuse human codon-optimized Env in frame to the human tissue plasminogen activator (TPA) leader sequence (*see* **Note 1**).
2. Position the trimeric motif derived from T4 bacteriophage fibritin (FT) after lysine 683 of HIV-Envgp140 (YU2) followed by a 6× His tag and stop codon.
3. To produce gp140:gpD fusion protein, add a short flexible linker peptide $[Gly_4Ser]_2$ following the FT domain and then fuse gpD to the C-terminus along with the 6× His tag and stop codon.
4. Clone both gp140 and gp140:gpD fusion constructs into pcDNA3 vector for expression in mammalian cells.

5. For a construct that expresses gpD alone, use a human codon-optimized derivative of wild type λ gpD gene with a short flexible linker peptide [Gly_4Ser]$_1$ followed by a 6× His tag and stop codon.

3.2 Expression and Purification of Envgp140gpD and gpD Proteins

All proteins were expressed in serum-free medium by transient transfection of suspension-adapted FreeStyle HEK 293-F cells and purified by metal affinity chromatography using Ni-NTA resin.

1. Seed 293-F cells at a density of 7.0×10^5 cells per ml the day before transfection. After overnight incubation at 37 °C with 8% CO_2, 125 rpm, adjust cell density to 1.0×10^6 cells/ml by the addition of fresh medium, just prior to transfection.
2. Use FreeStyle MAX reagent as directed by the manufacturer for transfection of the various DNA constructs (*see* **Note 2**).
3. Five to 6 days post-transfection, depending on cell viability, collect the cell culture supernatant and centrifuge at 3500 × *g* to remove cell debris. Do not allow the cell viability to reach below 70%.
4. Secreted proteins in the supernatant are purified by metal affinity chromatography using Ni-NTA resin by gravity flow. Perform all steps at room temperature but keep buffers and cell culture supernatant on ice.
5. Equilibrate 2 ml of Ni-NTA resin with 1× wash buffer (20 mM imidazole) per 250 ml of cell culture supernatant and then add the clarified cell supernatant to the column resin bed.
6. After binding the protein to the resin bed, wash the column with 30 ml of Ni-NTA wash buffer containing 20 mM imidazole and then 30 ml of buffer containing 40 mM imidazole followed by elution in the presence of 250 mM imidazole (*see* **Note 3**).
7. Analyze elution fractions for yield and purity by performing SDS-PAGE and Coomassie blue staining.
8. Pool fractions containing purified protein and dialyze, using a 30K Slide-A-Lyzer cassette for Envgp140:gpD and 10K for gpD, against 1 L of dialysis buffer overnight at 4 °C. Change buffer and dialyze an additional 1 h.
9. Following dialysis, concentrate purified protein with Amicon Ultra centrifugal filter devices to concentrations of ~1 mg/ml (*see* **Note 4**). Store protein aliquots at −80 °C.

3.3 Generation of Mosaic Env Decorated Phage: gpD-Deficient Phage Preparation

1. Grow lysogens of TOP10 cells containing λ D1180 [16], which is deficient in gpD, overnight at 32 °C (*see* **Note 5**). The resulting culture is then used to inoculate 4 × 1 L flasks of fresh NZCYM medium the next day (at a dilution of 1:100). Grow the cultures at 32 °C with vigorous shaking (300 rpm) until an OD_{600} of between 0.5 and 0.6 is reached.

2. Induce the lysogen by transferring the bacteria to a water bath set between 51 and 53 °C, followed by gentle shaking for 15 min. After thermal induction, vigorously shake (300 rpm) the cultures for an additional 3 h at 38 °C.
3. Pellet the bacteria at 5000 rpm (4400 × *g*) for 10 min at 4 °C (Beckman JA-10 rotor) and resuspend in phage suspension media (SM). Lyse with the addition of chloroform (12% of resuspended pellet volume). Following chloroform treatment, digest bacterial DNA with DNase I to a final concentration of 10 μg/ml and mix gently at room temperature for 30 min.
4. Clear the lysate of cellular debris by low speed centrifugation (10,000 rpm or 17,600 × *g* for 10 min at 4 °C). Transfer the supernatant to ultra clear centrifuge tubes (for Beckman SW28 rotor).
5. Add 15 ml of fresh SM to the pellet in **step 4**, vortex, and then spin again as above. Combine the supernatant with the supernatant from **step 4** and add additional SM until the tube is full to the top. Centrifuge at 25,000 rpm (110,000 × *g*) for 1 h at 4 °C. Pour off the supernatant and add 2 ml of SM to the phage pellet.

3.4 Generation of Mosaic Env Decorated Phage: In Vitro Phage Decoration

1. For phage decoration, add 2 ml of SM to the phage pellet along with recombinant proteins (WT gpD, gp140:gpD) and allow decoration to occur overnight at 4 °C with gentle shaking (*see* **Note 6**).
2. Purify decorated phage by cesium chloride equilibrium density gradient ultracentrifugation (*see* **Note 7**) at 38,000 rpm (148,000 × *g*) for 24 h at 4 °C with no brake (Beckman Ti70.1 rotor).
3. Remove the phage band with a 5 ml syringe and 18-gauge needle, transfer the extracted band to a 10K Slide-A-Lyzer cassette and dialyze against 1 L of phage dialysis buffer at 4 °C with at least three buffer changes, one being overnight. Store phage at 4 °C.
4. Titer serial dilutions of the decorated phage on LE392 *E.coli* bacteria to determine the plaque forming units (PFU) (*see* **Note 8**).
5. For any subsequent in vivo studies, remove endotoxins (ET) using an EndoTrap red® Endotoxin Removal kit according to the product manual; measure the final ET content using the limulus amebocyte lectin (LAL) assays (Associates of Cape Cod).

3.5 Determining Stability of Env Decorated Phage Particles: EDTA Treatment

Test the effectiveness of the decoration reaction by measuring the titers of the resulting phage preparations before and after exposure to a high concentration (100 mM) of EDTA, which inactivates gpD-deficient capsids. In order to confirm that gpD and gp140:gpD fusion proteins are incorporated and stable on the phage capsid,

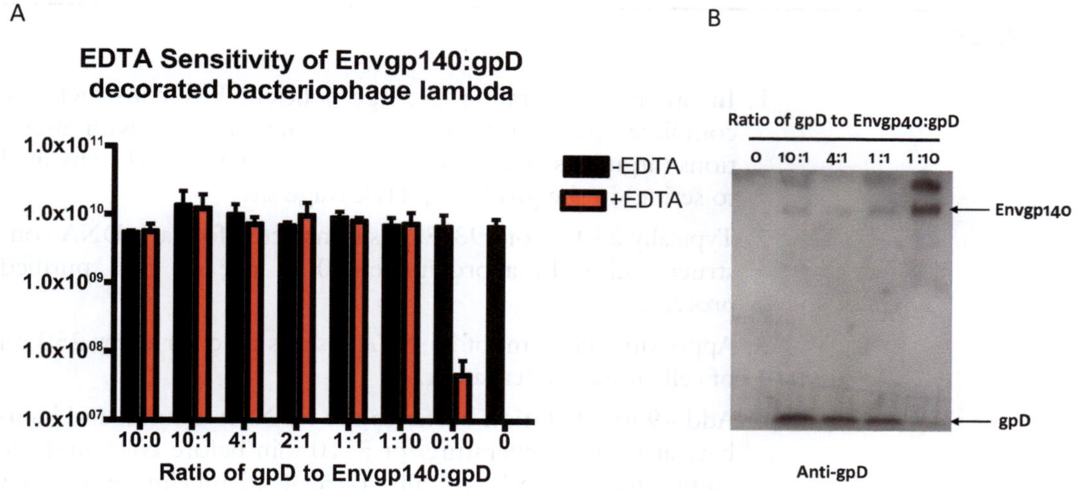

Fig. 2 Stability of Envgp140:gpD decorated phage. (**a**) Phage decorated with various ratios of gpD to Envgp140:gpD were incubated in the presence or absence of EDTA and titered on LE392 *E. coli* host cells to determine PFU per ml. (**b**) Phage titered on LE392 *E. coli* host cells loaded on a 12.5% SDS-PAGE gel (1–2 × 10^9 PFU/lane). Phage protein is analyzed by immunoblot analysis, using antiserum directed against gpD. Incorporation of both wild-type gpD and gp140:gpD fusion protein in the phage preparations decorated with the different molar ratios of protein is indicated by the *arrows*

subject equal amounts of CsCl-gradient purified (*see* **Note** 7) decorated phage particles to SDS-PAGE and immunoblot analysis using gpD-specific antiserum (Fig. 2).

1. Take 1 × 10^9 PFU of gpD-deficient bacteriophage lambda and decorate with varying molar ratios of WT gpD protein and gp140:gpD fusion protein.
2. Perform decorations by incubating the desired molar ratios of proteins with gpD-deficient phage at 30 °C for 20 min.
3. Test decorated phage samples using EDTA by diluting the phage samples in either the absence (TM buffer) or presence of EDTA (TE) and incubate for 30 min at 37 °C.
4. Use equal amounts (PFU) of undecorated gpD-deficient phage as a control group (EDTA sensitive).
5. Titer serial dilutions (10^{-1}, 10^{-2}, 10^{-3}, 10^{-4}, 10^{-5}, 10^{-6}, 10^{-7}) of the treated phage on LE392 *E.coli* host cells to determine PFU per ml.

3.6 Determining Stability of Env Decorated Phage Particles: SDS-PAGE Analysis

1. Take 1–2 × 10^9 PFU of phage decorated with either WT gpD alone or ratios of gpD and gp140:gpD fusion protein and denature by separation on a 12.5% SDS-PAGE.
2. Use rabbit antiserum for gpD to detect the phage gpD and gp140:gpD fusion protein by western blotting [17].

4 Notes

1. In order to generate a cleavage deficient Env construct, the complete gp120 and gp41 ectodomain was used with alterations (arginines at amino acid positions 508 and 511 changed to serine) in the gp120/gp41cleavage site.
2. Typically 250 ml of 293-F cells transfected for each DNA construct will yield approximately 0.25 mg of each purified protein.
3. Approximately 2 ml of Ni-NTA resin is used for every 250 ml of cell culture supernatant.
4. Add ~9 ml of elution buffer to the Ni-NTA column and incubate at room temperature for 5–10 min before collecting the elution fractions. We typically collect 4 × 2 ml elution fractions that are pooled, dialyzed and concentrated to ~0.25 ml yielding a protein concentration of ~ 1 mg/ml.
5. For wildtype phage preparations, lysogen λ D1180 is transformed with a gpD expression plasmid [18].
6. For high density-display phage, gpD and Env:gpD fusion proteins were mixed at a 1:1 molar ratio. For low density-display phage, gpD and Env:gpD were mixed at a 10:1 molar ratio.
7. Purify the phage by cesium chloride equilibrium density gradient centrifugation as described [19]. Briefly, bring volume of phage up to 2.5 ml with SM, and then add 10 ml of CsCl solution. Transfer to quick seal ultracentrifuge tube using 5 ml syringe and 18G needle. Seal the top of the tube using a flat top metal sealer and centrifuge for 24 h at 38,000 rpm (Ti70.1 rotor) at 4 °C with no brake. Remove the blue phage band with a 5 ml syringe and 18-gauge needle after centrifugation. Use a small 23-gauge needle to vent the top of the tube while doing this.
8. To perform the plaque assay, make serial tenfold dilutions of the phage from 10^{-2} to 10^{-10} in SM buffer in a total 200 μl volume. Mix 100 μl of each phage dilution with 100 μl of LE392 *E. coli*. Add 3 ml of cooled top agar to each dilution tube, pour onto labeled LB plates and swirl the plate to distribute the soft agar over the entire surface. Allow the top agar to harden before inverting and incubating at 37 °C overnight. After the overnight incubation, count the number of plaques on each plate. Choose plates that have between 20–200 plaques and determine the number of phage particles by multiplying the plaque number by the dilution factor on the plate and by 10 to get the plaque forming units (PFU) per ml (plaque # × plate dilution × 10). Typical titers for CsCl-banded WT phage are 1×10^{12} PFU/ml, while Env decorated phage titers are normally 5×10^{11} PFU/ml.

Acknowledgment

This work was supported by NIH grant R21A1074351 (S.D.), T32DE007202 (J.M.) and T32AI049815 (M.B.).

References

1. Burton DR (2006) Structural biology: images from the surface of HIV. Nature 441(7095): 817–818
2. Pantophlet R, Burton DR (2006) GP120: target for neutralizing HIV-1 antibodies. Annu Rev Immunol 24:739–769
3. Zolla-Pazner S (2004) Identifying epitopes of HIV-1 that induce protective antibodies. Nat Rev Immunol 4(3):199–210
4. McAleer WJ, Buynak EB, Maigetter RZ, Wampler DE, Miller WJ, Hilleman MR (1984) Human hepatitis B vaccine from recombinant yeast. Nature 307(5947):178–180
5. Evans TG, Bonnez W, Rose RC, Koenig S, Demeter L, Suzich JA et al (2001) A Phase 1 study of a recombinant virus like particle vaccine against human papillomavirus type 11 in healthy adult volunteers. J Infect Dis 183(10):1485–1493
6. Harper DM, Franco EL, Wheeler C, Ferris DG, Jenkins D, Schuind A et al (2004) Efficacy of a bivalent L1 virus-like particle vaccine in prevention of infection with human papillomavirus types 16 and 18 in young women: a randomised controlled trial. Lancet 364(9447): 1757–1765
7. Villa LL, Costa RL, Petta CA, Andrade RP, Ault KA, Giuliano AR et al (2005) Prophylactic quadrivalent human papillomavirus (types 6, 11, 16, and 18) L1 virus-like particle vaccine in young women: a randomised double-blind placebo-controlled multicentre phase II efficacy trial. Lancet Oncol 6(5):271–278
8. Lee DH, Lee SH, Kim AR, Quan FS (2016) Virus-like nanparticle vaccine confers protection against *Toxoplasma gondii*. PLoS One. 11(8). doi:10.1371/journal.pone.0161231
9. Merril CR, Scholl D, Adhya SL (2003) The prospect for bacteriophage therapy in Western medicine. Nat Rev Drug Discov 2(6):489–497
10. Fogelman I, Davey V, Ochs HD, Elashoff M, Feinberg MB, Mican J et al (2000) Evaluation of CD4+ T cell function In vivo in HIV-infected patients as measured by bacteriophage phiX174 immunization. J Infect Dis 182(2):435–441
11. Piersanti S, Cherubini G, Martina Y, Salone B, Avitabile D, Grosso F et al (2004) Mammalian cell transduction and internalization properties of lambda phages displaying the full-length adenoviral penton base or its central domain. J Mol Med 82(7):467–476
12. Yang F, Forrer P, Dauter Z, Conway JF, Cheng N, Cerritelli ME et al (2000) Novel fold and capsid- binding properties of the lambda-phage display platform protein gpD. Nat Struct Biol 7(3):230–237
13. Sternberg N, Hoess RH (1995) Display of peptides and proteins on the surface of bacteriophage lambda. Proc Natl Acad Sci 92(5): 1609–1613
14. Domm W, Brewer M, Baker SF, Feng C, Martinez-Sobrido L, Treanor J, Dewhurst S (2014) Use of bacteriophage particles displaying influenza virus hemagglutnin for the detection of hemagglutination-inhibition antibodies. J Virol Methods 197:47–50 Vaccine 29(14):2637–2647
15. Mattiacio J, Walter S, Brewer M, Domm W, Friedman AE, Dewhurst S (2011) Dense display of HIV-1 envelope spikes on the lambda phage scaffold does not result in the generation of improved antibody respones to HIV-1 Env. Vaccine 29(14):2637–2647
16. Eguchi A, Akuta T, Okuyama H, Senda T, Yokoi H, Inokuchi H et al (2001) Protein transduction domain of HIV-1 Tat protein promotes efficient delivery of DNA into mammalian cells. J Biol Chem 276(28):26204–26210
17. Zanghi CN, Lankes HA, Bradel-Tretheway B, Wegman J, Dewhurst S (2005) A simple method for displaying recalcitrant proteins on the surface of bacteriophage lambda. Nucleic Acids Res 33(18):e160. doi:10.1093/nar/gni 158
18. Zanghi CN, Sapinoro R, Bradel-Tretheway B, Dewhurst S (2007) A tractable method for simultaneous modifications to the head and tail of bacteriophage lambda and its application to enhancing phage-mediated gene delivery. Nucleic Acids Res 35(8):e59. doi:10.1093/nar/gkm146
19. Sambrook J, Russell DW (2006) Purification of bacteriophage λ particles by isopycnic centrifucation through CsCl gradients. Cold Spring Harb Protoc. doi:10.1101/pdb.prot3968

Chapter 15

Bacteriophage T4 as a Nanoparticle Platform to Display and Deliver Pathogen Antigens: Construction of an Effective Anthrax Vaccine

Pan Tao, Qin Li, Sathish B. Shivachandra, and Venigalla B. Rao

Abstract

Protein-based subunit vaccines represent a safer alternative to the whole pathogen in vaccine development. However, limitations of physiological instability and low immunogenicity of such vaccines demand an efficient delivery system to stimulate robust immune responses. The bacteriophage T4 capsid-based antigen delivery system can robustly elicit both humoral and cellular immune responses without any adjuvant. Therefore, it offers a strong promise as a novel antigen delivery system. Currently *Bacillus anthracis*, the causative agent of anthrax, is a serious biothreat agent and no FDA-approved anthrax vaccine is available for mass vaccination. Here, we describe a potential anthrax vaccine using a T4 capsid platform to display and deliver the 83 kDa protective antigen, PA, a key component of the anthrax toxin. This T4 vaccine platform might serve as a universal antigen delivery system that can be adapted to develop vaccines against any infectious disease.

Key words Bacteriophage T4, Virus decoration proteins, Nanoparticle vaccine platform, PA, Anthrax vaccine

1 Introduction

Vaccines represent one of the most important contributions to the prevention of infectious disease in humans. Currently, there are mainly three types of licensed vaccines: (1) inactivated whole-pathogen vaccines, (2) live-attenuated whole-pathogen vaccines, and (3) protein-based subunit vaccines [1]. The majority of vaccines fall into the first two categories and are therefore considered whole-pathogen vaccines. Unfortunately, these whole pathogen vaccines pose significant safety concerns including reversion to a pathogenic form, reactions in immunocompromised hosts, and other adverse effects such as allergic and autoimmune reactions. Only a few protein-based subunit vaccines such as virus-like particles (VLPs), detoxified toxoids/toxins, and polysaccharide–protein

Maureen C. Ferran and Gary R. Skuse (eds.), *Recombinant Virus Vaccines: Methods and Protocols*, Methods in Molecular Biology, vol. 1581, DOI 10.1007/978-1-4939-6869-5_15,

conjugates have been approved for administration to humans. Generally these subunit vaccines have low immunogenicity and stability, thus requiring an efficient delivery system and/or an adjuvant to overcome these limitations. If delivered efficiently, these protein-based subunit vaccines should be safer than the more traditional whole pathogen vaccines.

Recently, we have developed a novel antigen delivery system using the bacteriophage T4 capsid [2–4]. Antigens were displayed on the T4 capsid at a high density, and, upon immunization, they elicited robust humoral and cellular immune responses without any adjuvant, making T4 a robust antigen display and delivery system [2, 3, 5, 6]. The T4 capsid (head) is composed of three essential capsid proteins: gp23*, gp24*, and gp20 ("*" refers to the cleaved and matured form). There are 930 copies of the major capsid protein, gp23*, 55 copies of the vertex protein, gp24*, and 12 copies of the portal protein, gp20. In addition, the capsid also contains two nonessential proteins: *h*ighly antigenic *o*uter *c*apsid protein (Hoc) and *s*mall *o*uter *c*apsid protein (Soc). There are 870 copies of Soc (10 kDa), and 155 copies of Hoc (39 kDa) [7, 8]. Both Hoc and Soc are dispensable. Mutant phage in which both these genes are defective (amber or deletion) do not show a significant loss of infectivity or replicative capacity under laboratory conditions [9]. Furthermore, purified recombinant Soc and Hoc proteins can be assembled on $Hoc^{-}Soc^{-}$ capsids in vitro with high specificity and nanomolar affinity [10]. The phage T4 capsid nanoparticle, thus, provides an ideal platform to display foreign antigens as Soc or Hoc fusion proteins [2, 11, 12]. Large full-length proteins as well as multi-protein complexes can be displayed without compromising the ability of Soc and Hoc to bind to the capsid [6, 12]. All 1025 copies of Soc and Hoc can be replaced either with a single antigen or with multiple antigens [2, 10–12].

Bacillus anthracis is the etiological agent of anthrax, a highly lethal infection and also a serious biothreat as evident from the 2001 anthrax attacks in the USA [13, 14]. An alum-adsorbed anthrax vaccine (AVA) was approved in the 1970s for military use, and a reformulated version has recently been approved for civilian adults. This vaccine is based on crude bacterial culture supernatant containing secreted protective antigen (PA). PA is one of the components of the anthrax toxin that consists, in addition, of lethal factor (LF) and edema factor (EF) [15, 16]. Previous studies demonstrated that PA alone is sufficient to provide complete protection against anthrax [16–18]. AVA requires a long immunization regimen and causes significant side reactions in vaccinated individuals [19]. Therefore, recent efforts have been directed to developing a safer next generation subunit vaccine using recombinant PA (rPA) (*see* reviews [15, 16, 19–21]).

Results from our laboratory and others have demonstrated that soluble rPA adjuvanted with alum, as well as bacteriophage

T4-displayed rPA can protect macaques against aerosol challenge with Ames *Bacillus anthracis* spores [5, 17, 18, 21–24]. In this chapter, we describe the methods to generate T4 nanoparticle rPA conjugate that might serve as a candidate for the next generation anthrax vaccine.

2 Materials

2.1 Construction of Plasmids

1. Vector, gene DNA, and cells: *E. coli* expression vector pET28b (Novagen, MA), bacteriophage RB69 Soc gene DNA and *Bacillus anthracis* PA gene DNA (prepared in our lab), competent *E. coli* DH5α cells (New England Biolabs, MA).
2. Growth media: SOC medium (Quality Biologicals, MD) and Luria–Bertani (LB) medium (Quality Biological, MD).
3. 1000× kanamycin (50 mg/mL): Add 0.5 g kanamycin (Gold Biotechnology, MD) to 10 mL Milli-Q water.
4. Kanamycin LB plates: Add 2 g LB powder (Affymetrix, OH) and 1.5 g agar to 100 mL Milli-Q water, autoclave for 15 min at 121 °C. When cooled to about 50 °C, add 0.1 mL 1000× kanamycin. Mix and pour into sterile petri plates (Akro-Mils, OH).
5. Enzymes: 2× Phusion High-Fidelity PCR Master Mix (Thermo Scientific), FastDigest *Nhe*I (Thermo Scientific), FastDigest *Hind*III (Thermo Scientific), FastDigest *Xho*I (Thermo Scientific), FastAP Thermosensitive Alkaline Phosphatase (Thermo Scientific), and T4 DNA Ligase (Thermo Scientific).
6. Agarose gel running buffer: add 100 mL 10× AccuGENE™ Tris–borate–EDTA (TBE) agarose gel running buffer (Lonza Chemicals Company, Switzerland) to 900 mL Milli-Q water to make 1× agarose gel running buffer.
7. Kits: GeneJET Gel Extraction Kit (Thermo Scientific) and GeneJET Plasmid Miniprep Kit (Thermo Scientific).

2.2 Protein Purification

1. Expression cell: Competent *E. coli* BL21-CodonPlus (DE3)-RIPL cells (Agilent Technologies, CA).
2. Growth media: SOC medium (Quality Biologicals, MD) and Moore's medium (1 L medium contains 20 g tryptone, 15 g yeast extract, 8 g NaCl, 2 g dextrose, 2 g Na_2HPO_4 and 1 g KH_2PO_4; add 1 mL 1000× (50 mg/mL) kanamycin and 1 mL 1000× (50 mg/mL) chloramphenicol before use. The final concentration of each antibiotic is 50 μg/mL.
3. Antibiotics: 1000× kanamycin (50 mg/mL): Add 0.5 g kanamycin (Gold Biotechnology, MD) to 10 mL Milli-Q water;

1000× chloramphenicol (50 mg/mL): Add 0.5 g chloramphenicol (Amresco) to 10 mL ethanol.

4. Kanamycin–chloramphenicol LB plates: Add 2 g LB powder (Affymetrix, OH) and 1.5 g agar to 100 mL Milli-Q water, autoclave for 15 min at 121 °C. When cooled to about 50 °C, add 0.1 mL 1000× kanamycin and 0.1 mL 1000× chloramphenicol. Mix and pour into sterile petri plates (Akro-Mils, OH).
5. Chemical reagents: 1 M isopropyl β-D-1-thiogalactopyranoside (IPTG) (add 238 mg IPTG [Gold Biotechnology, MO] to 1 mL Milli-Q water), Coomassie blue R-250 staining solution (Teknova, CA), complete proteinase inhibitor cocktail (Roche), and acetylated bovine serum albumin (BSA) standard (Affymetrix, OH).
6. Buffers (*see* **Note 1**): HisTrap binding buffer (50 mM Tris–HCl pH 8.0, 300 mM NaCl, and 20 mM imidazole); HisTrap washing buffer (50 mM Tris–HCl pH 8.0, 300 mM NaCl, and 50 mM imidazole); HisTrap elution buffer (50 mM Tris–HCl pH 8.0, 300 mM NaCl, and 400 mM imidazole); Gel filtration buffer (20 mM Tris–HCl, pH 8.0 and 100 mM NaCl); SDS-loading buffer (20 mM Tris–HCl pH 6.8, 100 mM dithiothreitol, 2.5% β-mercaptoethanol, 1% SDS (w/v), 0.1% bromophenol blue, and 10% glycerol); Tris–glycine running buffer (add 100 mL 10× Tris–glycine running buffer (Bio-Rad) to 900 mL Milli-Q water to make 1× Tris–glycine running buffer).
7. Destaining solution: Add 100 mL methanol and 100 mL acetic acid to 800 mL Milli-Q water.
8. Columns: 1 mL HisTrap HP Nickel affinity chromatography column (GE Healthcare) and Hi-load 16/60 Superdex 200 gel filtration chromatography column (GE Healthcare).
9. Amicon Ultra-4 centrifugal filter units (Millipore, MA).
10. 4–20% (w/v) polyacrylamide gel (Life Technologies).

2.3 T4 Phage Purification

1. Phage and *E. coli*: Hoc$^-$Soc$^-$ phage T4 mutant (constructed in our laboratory) and *E. coli* P301.
2. Growth media: LB medium (Quality Biological, MD) and M9CA medium (to 800 mL Milli-Q water, add 12.5 g M9CA medium powder [Amresco, OH], adjust to 1 L with Milli-Q water, and autoclave for 15 min at 121 °C).
3. LB plates: Add 2 g LB powder (Affymetrix, OH) and 1.5 g agar to 100 mL Milli-Q water, and autoclave for 15 min at 121 °C. Mix and pour into sterile petri plates.
4. Top-Agar: Add 2 g LB powder (Affymetrix, OH) and 0.75 g agar to 100 mL Milli-Q water, sterilize, and keep it at 42 °C.

5. Chemical reagents: Deoxyribonuclease I (DNase I) (Sigma-Aldrich) and HPLC-grade chloroform (Thermo Fisher Scientific).
6. Buffers: Pi-Mg buffer (26 mM Na_2HPO_4, 22 mM KH_2PO_4, 70 mM NaCl, and 1 mM $MgSO_4$); Dialysis buffer I (10 mM Tris–HCl pH 7.5, 200 mM NaCl, and 5 mM $MgCl_2$); Dialysis buffer II (10 mM Tris–HCl pH 7.5, 50 mM NaCl, and 5 mM $MgCl_2$).
7. Cesium chloride (CsCl) stock solution: 8 M CsCl, 100 mM Tris–HCl, pH 7.5, 85 mM NaCl, and 20 mM NH_4Cl.
8. Slide-A-lyzer dialysis cassette with molecular weight cut-off (MWCO) of 10 K (3–12 mL capacity; Thermo Scientific™ Pierce™ Protein Biology, IL).

2.4 Antigen Preparation

1. 1× PBS pH 7.4: Add 100 mL 10× PBS pH 7.4 (Quality Biological, MD) to 900 mL Milli-Q water to make 1× PBS buffer.
2. 5 M NaCl (Quality Biological, MD).
3. Protein LoBind Eppendorf tube 1.5 mL (Hamburg, Germany).

3 Methods

Both Hoc and Soc can be used to display antigens. Here we use Soc to display PA, because it has 5.6 times more binding sites (870 per capsid) compared with Hoc (155 per capsid). Thus, through Soc, antigens can be displayed on T4 capsid at a higher density.

3.1 Construction of pET-Soc-PA

A universal vector, pET-Soc-N, is first constructed such that it contains a multiple cloning site (MCS) at the COOH-terminus of Soc by inserting Soc (*see* **Note 2**) into pET28b expression vector with *Nhe*I/*Hind*III. PA or any other antigen genes can be amplified by PCR and cloned into pET-Soc-N to generate an in-frame fusion with the C-terminal end of Soc (*see* **Note 3**).

1. Use Thermo 2X Phusion High-Fidelity PCR Master Mix to amplify RB69 Soc gene DNA from RB69 phage genome DNA, using the following primers, where the underlined sequences correspond to the recognition sequences for the respective restriction enzymes:

   Soc *Nhe*I Forward:

   5′-GCATCC<u>GCTAGC</u>GGTGGTTATGTAAACATCAAA-3′.

   Soc *Hind*III Reverse:

   5′-GCAG<u>AAGCTT</u>CACCACTTACTGGTGTAGGGGTAAAC-3′.

2. Add 10 μl 10× DNA loading buffer to 90 μl PCR product, load onto 2% agarose gel, and separate by agarose gel electrophoresis.
3. Cut out the expected DNA band and extract DNA using Thermo gel extraction kit according to the manufacturer's instructions.
4. Cut 1 μg purified PCR product with *Nhe*I and *Hind*III at 37 °C for 2 h. At the same time, cut 1 μg pET28b vector plasmid DNA using the same restriction enzymes at 37 °C for 2 h.
5. Directly add 1 μl FastAP thermosensitive alkaline phosphatase into *Nhe*I- and *Hind*III-digested pET28b vector without changing the restriction enzyme buffer and incubate at 37 °C for 30 min.
6. Load the digested insert and vector onto 2% and 1% agarose gel respectively and separate by agarose gel electrophoresis.
7. Cut out the expected DNA bands and extract DNA using Thermo gel extraction kit according to the manufacturer's instructions.
8. Ligate insert and vector at a molar ratio of 3:1 using T4 DNA ligase for 1 h at 22 °C.
9. Transform *E. coli* DH5α with the ligation product according to the manufacturer's instructions. Incubate the LB-kanamycin plate overnight at 37 °C.
10. Pick a single colony and inoculate into a 125 mL flask containing 10 mL LB medium containing 50 μg/mL of kanamycin. Incubate the flask in a shaking incubator overnight at 220 rpm and 37 °C.
11. Isolate the plasmid DNA using Thermo GeneJET plasmid miniprep kit according to the manufacturer's instructions. The thus generated plasmid was named pET-Soc-N, which contained a hexa-histidine tag at the NH2-terminus and a MCS at the COOH-terminus of Soc.
12. Use Thermo 2× Phusion High-Fidelity PCR Master Mix to amplify the PA DNA from the template (pET-F1mutV-PA) using the following primers, where the underlined sequences correspond to the recognition sequences for the respective enzymes:

    *Hind*III Forward:5′-ACCC<u>AAGCTT</u> CTGCTGAAGTTAA ACAGGAGAACCGGTTATT-3′.

    *Xho*I Reverse: 5′-GCC<u>CTCGAG</u>TTATCCTATCTCATAGCC TTTTTTAG-3′.
13. Repeat **steps 2–3**.
14. Digest 1 μg purified PCR product with *Hind*III and *Xho*I at 37 °C for 2 h. At the same time, digest 1 μg pET-Soc-N plasmid DNA using the same restriction enzymes at 37 °C for 2 h.

15. Directly add 1 μl FastAP Thermosensitive Alkaline Phosphatase into *Hind*III- and *Xho*I-digested pET-Soc-N without changing the restriction enzyme buffer and incubate at 37 °C for 30 min.
16. Repeat **steps 6–10**.
17. Isolate the plasmid DNA using Thermo GeneJET plasmid miniprep kit according to the manufacturer's instructions. The resulting clone, pET-Soc-PA, contains PA fused in-frame to the COOH-terminus of RB69 Soc.

3.2 Purification of Recombinant Soc-PA from E. coli BL21-CodonPlus (DE3)-RIPL

1. Transform 10 ng of pET-Soc-PA into 25 μl BL21-CodonPlus (DE3)-RIPL competent cells according to the manufacturer's instructions. Incubate on LB-kanamycin/ chloramphenicol plates overnight at 37 °C.
2. Pick a single colony and inoculate into 30 mL Moore's medium with 50 μg/mL kanamycin and 50 μg/mL chloramphenicol. Incubate the flask overnight in a shaking incubator at 220 rpm and 37 °C.
3. Inoculate 20 mL of overnight cultures into a 2 L flask containing 1 L of Moore's medium supplemented with 50 μg/mL kanamycin and 50 μg/mL chloramphenicol. Incubate the flask in a shaking incubator at 220 rpm and 37 °C until the cell density reaches 1.5–2.0×10^8 cells/mL.
4. Change the temperature of the shaking incubator to 28 °C and keep shaking for 30 min at 220 rpm before adding IPTG (*see* **Note 4**).
5. Add 1 mL IPTG (isopropyl β-D-1 thiogalactopyranoside) (1 M) to the culture and induce protein expression for 2 h at 28 °C.
6. Distribute the culture into 500 mL centrifuge bottles and collect the cells by centrifugation at 7000 rpm (8288 × *g*) for 10 min at 4 °C with GS3 rotor in Sorvall RC-5C plus centrifuge or equivalent.
7. Discard the supernatant and resuspend the pellet with 40 mL HisTrap binding buffer supplemented with one pill of complete proteinase inhibitor cocktail (*see* **Note 5**).
8. Set up French press (Thermo Scientific) and lyse the cells at 12,000 psi twice.
9. Distribute the cell lysate into 30 mL centrifuge tubes and centrifuge at 17000 rpm (34,572 × *g*) for 22 min at 4 °C with SS34 rotor in Sorvall RC-5C plus centrifuge or equivalent.
10. Collect the supernatant which contains soluble Soc-PA protein, and filter it through 0.22 μm filters before loading onto the HisTrap column (*see* **Note 6**).
11. Set up 1 mL HisTrap HP column on AKTA-prime system. First, wash the column with 20 mL of water, and then equilibrate the column with 20 mL of HisTrap binding buffer.

12. Load the supernatant collected in **step 10** onto the HisTrap HP column at a loading speed of 1 mL/min.
13. Wash the column with 20 mL HisTrap washing buffer (*see* **Note 7**).
14. Elute the protein with 20–400 mM linear imidazole gradient with the HisTrap binding buffer as buffer A and the HisTrap elution buffer as buffer B. AKTA-prime was set as follows:

    Concentration (% Buffer B): 0; Gradient Length: 40; Target (% Buffer B): 100; Flow Rate: 1 mL/min; Fraction Base: mL; Fraction Size: 1; Pressure Limit: 0.3.
15. Collect and pool the peak fractions (*see* **Note 8**).
16. Wash the Hi-load 16/60 Superdex 200 column with 150 mL Gel filtration buffer. Load the HisTrap peak fractions onto the Hi-load 16/60 Superdex 200 column with a flow rate of 1.0 mL/min.
17. Collect and pool the peak fractions from gel filtration elution, and concentrate using Amicon Ultra-4 centrifugal filtration (10 kDa cut-off).
18. Quantify concentration of the Soc-PA protein using Nanodrop (Thermo Scientific) (*see* **Note 9**).
19. Aliquot the concentrated Soc-PA protein and store at −80 °C for future use.

3.3 Purification of Hoc⁻Soc⁻ Phage T4

1. Use sterilized plain wood applicator (Fisher Scientific) to streak the glycerol stock of *E. coli* P301 cells on an LB plate. Incubate the plate at 37 °C overnight (*see* **Note 10**).
2. Pick a single colony, inoculate into 20 mL LB medium, and incubate the flask in a shaking incubator at 220 rpm and 37 °C for 8 h. Store the culture at 4 °C cold room for use the following day.
3. Inoculate 10 mL of cultures into a 2 L flask containing 500 mL of LB and M9CA medium (250 mL LB + 250 mL M9CA). Incubate the flask in a shaking incubator at 220 rpm and 37 °C until the cell density reaches 2.0×10^8 cells/mL.
4. Infect *E. coli* P301 with Hoc^-Soc^- phage T4 at multiplicity of infection (MOI) of 0.2 by adding 2×10^{10} plaque forming units (PFU) of Hoc^-Soc^- phage T4 (*see* **Note 11**), and keep the flask shaking in a 37 °C incubator at 200 rpm for 2–3 h.
5. Observe phage growth (*see* **Note 12**) during incubation. After confirmation of phage growth, add 20 mL chloroform into the flask, and keep it shaking at 200 rpm for 10 min at 37 °C.
6. Collect the phages by centrifuging the culture for 45 min at 12,000 rpm (23,440 × *g*) at 4 °C with GSA rotor in Sorvall RC-5C plus centrifuge or equivalent.

7. Resuspend the pellet in 30 mL Pi-Mg buffer, add 500 μl chloroform and 43 μl of 7 mg/mL DNase I (final concentration of 10 μg/mL), and keep shaking at 220 rpm in 37 °C for 30 min.
8. Transfer the phage suspension to a 30 mL centrifuge tube, and centrifuge at 6000 rpm (4300 × *g*) for 10 min at 4 °C with SS34 rotor in Sorvall RC-5C plus centrifuge or equivalent to remove any cell debris.
9. Transfer the supernatant containing the phages to a new 30 mL centrifuge tube, and centrifuge at 16,000 rpm (30,624 × *g*) for 45 min at 4 °C with SS34 rotor in Sorvall RC-5C plus centrifuge or equivalent to pellet the phages.
10. Discard the supernatant and resuspend the phage pellet in 2 mL Pi-Mg buffer.
11. Prepare CsCl gradient for phage purification. First, prepare layer buffer according to the table below (Table 1). Then, from the bottom to the top, sequentially add 750 μl of layer buffer No.6, No.5, No.4, No.3, No.2, and No.1 to a 5 mL Beckman centrifuge tube.
12. For each Beckman centrifuge tube, load 0.5 mL resuspended phage sample from **step 10** onto the top of the CsCl gradient solution, centrifuge at 35,000 rpm (148,596 ×*g*) for 1 h at 4 °C using SW55 Ti rotor in Beckman L-60 Ultracentrifuge or equivalent.
13. Fasten the Beckman centrifuge tube to a vertical holder after centrifugation. Pierce the wall of centrifuge tube at the bottom of the turbid phage band using a 5 mL syringe needle. Aspirate the phage band into the syringe.
14. Transfer the phage sample into a 3–12 mL Slide-A-lyzer dialysis cassette and dialyze first against dialysis buffer I for 5 h at 4 °C and then against dialysis buffer II overnight at 4 °C.
15. Collect the phage sample, quantify the concentration of phages, and store at 4 °C for future use. The following steps

Table 1
Prepare CsCl gradient layers for phage purification

Layer No.	Stock CsCl (mL)	H_2O (mL)	Total volume (mL)
1	1	4	5
2	1.5	3.5	5
3	2	3	5
4	2.5	2.5	5
5	3	2	5
6	3.5	1.5	5

(**steps 16–21**) will determine the concentration of the phage by SDS-PAGE with BSA (1 mg/mL) as a standard.

16. Mix equal volume of Hoc⁻Soc⁻ T4 phage or BSA with 2× SDS loading buffer and boil for 5 min.
17. Load 1, 2, 3, and 4 μl of Hoc⁻Soc⁻ phage, as well as 1, 2, 4, and 8 μg of BSA to different wells of an SDS-PAGE gel (4–20% Tris-Gly gel), and electrophorese according to the manufacturer's instructions.
18. Disassemble the gel and transfer it into a clean tray. Add Coomassie blue R-250 staining solution to the tray after rinsing with water, microwave for 1 min, and keep shaking gently at room temperature for 15 min.
19. Discard the Coomassie blue R-250 staining solution, add destain solution to the tray, microwave for 1 min, and keep shaking gently at room temperature until the background becomes clean.
20. Scan the gel with laser densitometry (PDSI, GE Healthcare) and quantify the protein bands with ImageQuant 5.2 software (GE Healthcare) according to the manufacturer's instructions.
21. Generate a BSA standard curve using Microsoft Excel with the numbers calculated in **step 20** and calculate the concentration of Hoc⁻Soc⁻ T4 phage based on the BSA standard curve (*see* **Note 13**).

3.4 Preparation of Antigen for Immunizations

The exact amount of Hoc⁻Soc⁻ T4 phages and protein depends on how many animals will be used. The dose we mention here is for one animal (10 μg antigen/animal).

1. Take about 6.0×10^{11} phage particles and centrifuge at 15,000 rpm (21,130 ×*g*) in 1.5 mL LoBind Eppendorf tubes for 45 min at 4 °C using AM 2.18 rotor in Jouan MR-23i centrifuge or equivalent (*see* **Note 14**).
2. Discard the supernatant and wash the pellet by adding 1.0 mL PBS and one more round of centrifugation as in **step 1**.
3. Discard the supernatant, add 200 μl PBS to the tube, and leave it at 4 °C overnight to completely resuspend the phage pellet.
4. Add 1.16 mg Soc-PA to the resuspended phage, adjust the volume to 800 μl with PBS, gently vortex to mix, and incubate at 4 °C for 45 min.
5. Sediment the phage particles with Soc-PA bound at 15,000 rpm (21,130 × *g*) for 45 min at 4 °C using AM 2.18 rotor in Jouan MR-23i centrifuge or equivalent.
6. Wash the phage pellet containing the bound Soc-PA twice as in **step 1**.

7. Add 50 μl PBS to the pellet, leave it at 4 °C overnight to completely resuspend the phage pellet, and analyze it by SDS-PAGE as described in procedures from **steps 16** to **21** under Subheading 3.3. Determine the copy number of PA per capsid.
8. Immunize the animals by intramuscular injection with 10 μg T4-displayed PA. The immunization regimens, analyses of PA antibody and lethal toxin neutralizing antibody titers, and anthrax challenge models have been described previously [17, 18, 22].

4 Notes

1. All buffers used for protein purification have to pass through 0.22 μm filter in order to avoid clogging the column.
2. We used RB69 Soc instead of T4 Soc to construct Soc fusion. RB69 phage is a relative of T4 and previous studies found that recombinant RB69 Soc is more soluble than T4 Soc and binds to T4 capsid at nearly the same affinity as recombinant T4 Soc [10].
3. We had also constructed a universal vector, pET-Soc-C, which contains a multiple cloning site (MCS) at NH2-terminus of Soc [4]. Any other antigen gene can be amplified by PCR and cloned into pET-Soc-C to generate an in-frame fusion with the NH2-terminal end of Soc.
4. The purpose of this step was to cool down the *E. coli* to 28 °C before IPTG induction. Higher induction temperature may increase the chance of partitioning the overexpressed Soc-PA into the inclusion bodies, thus reducing the yield of soluble protein.
5. Add proteinase inhibitor cocktail to binding buffer right before use. Proteinase inhibitors are necessary during purification to prevent protein degradation.
6. All samples to be loaded onto HisTrap column or Hi-load 16/60 Superdex 200 column have to go through 0.22 μm filter to prevent clogging the columns.
7. After washing with 20 mL HisTrap washing buffer, the A280 reading of the HisTrap HP column flow through should be stable with minute variations. If not, keep washing with HisTrap washing buffer until the A280 reading becomes stable.
8. The maximum loading volume of Hi-load 16/60 Superdex 200 column is 5 mL. If the volume of the pooled peak fractions is more than 5 mL, concentrate them to 5 mL so that the pooled peak fractions can be loaded onto the Hi-load 16/60 Superdex 200 column.

9. Each protein has its own molar extinction coefficient, which is 91,680 M^{-1} cm^{-1} in the case of Soc-PA. The default extinction coefficient of NanoDrop is based on BSA. Remember to change the extinction coefficient and molecular weight when using NanoDrop.
10. $Hoc^{-}Soc^{-}$ phage T4 is an amber mutant, not a gene deletion mutant. In order to produce $Hoc^{-}Soc^{-}$ capsid, only non-suppressor *E. coli*, such as P301, can be used as the host cell to propagate $Hoc^{-}Soc^{-}$ phage T4.
11. Mix it immediately after adding the phage so as to distribute the phage uniformly.
12. The growth of phage can be assessed by (1) looking for turbidity and floating cell debris in the culture flask, (2) chloroform treatment, or (3) observing under light microscope.

    Chloroform treatment: Take 1 mL of culture in a test tube and add four drops of chloroform. If the cells are infected well, they lyse instantly, clearing the cell suspension, and cellular debris can be seen floating in the sample.

    Observation under light microscope: Put a drop of culture on the chamber of the cell counter and cover it with a cover slip. Focus at individual *E. coli* cells by fine adjustment. The appearance of clear center and black/dark spots at the poles (ends) of the cells indicate good phage infection.
13. Each T4 capsid has 930 molecules of major protein gp23 *("*" refers to the cleaved and matured form), whose molecular weight is 48 kDa; thus, 0.78 μg gp23* equal to 1×10^{10} phages.
14. Proteins may nonspecifically bind to a regular Eppendorf tube. Thus, it is highly recommended to use low-binding tubes such as Protein LoBind Eppendorf tube.

Acknowledgments

This work was supported by grants from the National Institutes of Health (NIAID U01-AI082086 and R01-AI111538). The authors thank Dr. Ayca Akal-Strader for assistance with the preparation of this article.

References

1. Andrew R, Michael JH, Martin PC (eds) (2003) Vaccine protocols, vol 87, 2nd edn. Humana Press Inc., Totowa, NJ
2. Sathaliyawala T et al (2006) Assembly of human immunodeficiency virus (HIV) antigens on bacteriophage T4: a novel in vitro approach to construct multicomponent HIV vaccines. J Virol 80(15):7688–7698
3. Tao P et al (2013) Mutated and bacteriophage T4 nanoparticle arrayed F1-V immunogens from Yersinia pestis as next generation plague vaccines. PLoS Pathog 9(7):e1003495
4. Tao P, Mahalingam M, Rao VB (2016) Highly effective soluble and bacteriophage T4 nanoparticle plague vaccines against Yersinia pestis. Methods Mol Biol 1403:499–518

5. Shivachandra SB et al (2006) In vitro binding of anthrax protective antigen on bacteriophage T4 capsid surface through Hoc-capsid interactions: a strategy for efficient display of large full-length proteins. Virology 345(1):190–198
6. Tao P et al (2013) In vitro and in vivo delivery of genes and proteins using the bacteriophage T4 DNA packaging machine. Proc Natl Acad Sci U S A 110(15):5846–5851
7. Black LW, Rao VB (2012) Structure, assembly, and DNA packaging of the bacteriophage T4 head. Adv Virus Res 82:119–153
8. Fokine A et al (2004) Molecular architecture of the prolate head of bacteriophage T4. Proc Natl Acad Sci U S A 101(16):6003–6008
9. Ishii T, Yanagida M (1977) The two dispensable structural proteins (soc and hoc) of the T4 phage capsid; their purification and properties, isolation and characterization of the defective mutants, and their binding with the defective heads in vitro. J Mol Biol 109(4):487–514
10. Qin L, Fokine A, O'Donnell E, Rao VB, Rossmann MG (2010) Structure of the small outer capsid protein, Soc: a clamp for stabilizing capsids of T4-like phages. J Mol Biol 395(4):728–741
11. Li Q, Shivachandra SB, Leppla SH, Rao VB (2006) Bacteriophage T4 capsid: a unique platform for efficient surface assembly of macromolecular complexes. J Mol Biol 363(2): 577–588
12. Li Q, Shivachandra SB, Zhang Z, Rao VB (2007) Assembly of the small outer capsid protein, Soc, on bacteriophage T4: a novel system for high density display of multiple large anthrax toxins and foreign proteins on phage capsid. J Mol Biol 370(5):1006–1019
13. Hsu VP et al (2002) Opening a bacillus anthracis-containing envelope, Capitol Hill, Washington, D.C.: the public health response. Emerg Infect Dis 8(10):1039–1043
14. Doolan DL et al (2007) The US capitol bioterrorism anthrax exposures: clinical epidemiological and immunological characteristics. J Infect Dis 195(2):174–184
15. Moayeri M, Leppla SH, Vrentas C, Pomerantsev AP, Liu S (2015) Anthrax pathogenesis. Annu Rev Microbiol 69:185–208
16. Williamson ED, Dyson EH (2015) Anthrax prophylaxis: recent advances and future directions. Front Microbiol 6:1009
17. Rao M et al (2011) Highly effective generic adjuvant systems for orphan or poverty-related vaccines. Vaccine 29(5):873–877
18. Peachman KK et al (2012) Anthrax vaccine antigen-adjuvant formulations completely protect New Zealand white rabbits against challenge with Bacillus anthracis Ames strain spores. Clin Vaccine Immunol 19(1):11–16
19. Scorpio A, Blank TE, Day WA, Chabot DJ (2006) Anthrax vaccines: pasteur to the present. Cell Mol Life Sci 63(19–20):2237–2248
20. Kaur M, Singh S, Bhatnagar R (2013) Anthrax vaccines: present status and future prospects. Expert Rev Vaccines 12(8):955–970
21. Grabenstein JD (2008) Vaccines: countering anthrax: vaccines and immunoglobulins. Clin Infect Dis 46(1):129–136
22. Shivachandra SB et al (2007) Multicomponent anthrax toxin display and delivery using bacteriophage T4. Vaccine 25(7):1225–1235
23. Bellanti JA et al (2012) Phase 1 study of a recombinant mutant protective antigen of Bacillus anthracis. Clin Vaccine Immunol 19(2):140–145
24. Peachman KK et al (2006) Correlation between lethal toxin-neutralizing antibody titers and protection from intranasal challenge with Bacillus anthracis Ames strain spores in mice after transcutaneous immunization with recombinant anthrax protective antigen. Infect Immun 74(1):794–797

Index

Maureen C. Ferran and Gary R. Skuse (eds.), *Recombinant Virus Vaccines: Methods and Protocols*, Methods in Molecular Biology, vol. 1581, DOI 10.1007/978-1-4939-6869-5,

MIX
Papier aus verantwortungsvollen Quellen
Paper from responsible sources
FSC® C105338

FSC
www.fsc.org

If you have any concerns about our products,
you can contact us on
ProductSafety@springernature.com

In case Publisher is established outside the EU,
the EU authorized representative is:
Springer Nature Customer Service Center GmbH
Europaplatz 3, 69115 Heidelberg, Germany

Printed by Libri Plureos GmbH
in Hamburg, Germany